Acute and Chronic Pancreatitis

Edited by Luis Rodrigo

Published in London, United Kingdom

Acute and Chronic Pancreatitis
http://dx.doi.org/10.5772/intechopen.1005706
Edited by Luis Rodrigo

Contributors
Afag Jabbarova, Ahmet Ziya Bayhan, Alexey Severtsev, Alicia Goya Pacheco, Alim Huseynov, Armando Di Dato, Atanas S. Yonkov, Betsabé Reyes Correa, Chih-Yang Wang, Chung-Che Tsai, Demet Kacaroglu, Dimitar I. Bulanov, Elena Arabadjieva, Elena Ramírez-Maldonado, Evgeni E. Zhivkov, Farajee Soheyla, Gulcin Ercan, Hung-Yun Lin, Irakly Kitiashvili, Jaqueline Whang-Peng, Javier Padilla Quintana, Ju-Ku Mo, Juan Francisco Merino-Torres, Karl Heinz Leonhardt Rowika, Kuan Wang, Maria Argente-Pla, Naren S. Nallapeta, Nazir Najeeb Kapadia, Radoslav S. Todorov, Riccardo Bellino, Rosa Jorba, Sanal Byurchiev, Sandica Bucurica, Sandra López Gordo, Shukhrat Dzhurakulov, Srushti Sahukar, Sándor Márton, Valery Vechorko, Vania Myralda Giamour Marbun, Viktor Anosov, Wen-Long Wang, Ya-Jung Shih, Yi-Hua Wu, Zi-Lin Li

First published in London, United Kingdom, 2025 by IntechOpen
IntechOpen is the global imprint of INTECHOPEN LIMITED, registered in England and Wales, registration number: 11086078, 167-169 Great Portland Street, London, W1W 5PF, United Kingdom

For EU product safety concerns: IN TECH d.o.o., Prolaz Marije Krucifikse Kozulić 3, 51000 Rijeka, Croatia, info@intechopen.com or visit our website at intechopen.com.

British Library Cataloguing-in-Publication Data
A catalogue record for this book is available from the British Library

Acute and Chronic Pancreatitis
Edited by Luis Rodrigo
p. cm.
Print ISBN 978-0-85466-650-8
Online ISBN 978-0-85466-649-2
eBook (PDF) ISBN 978-0-85466-651-5

Meet the editor

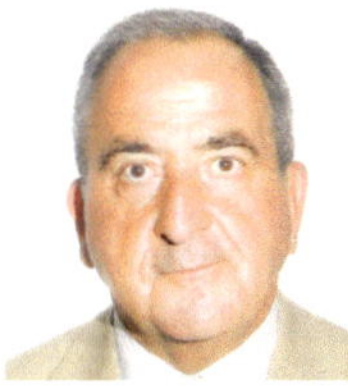

Dr. Luis Rodrigo, MD, is an Emeritus Professor of Medicine at the School of Medicine of the University of Oviedo (Spain). He has been the Chief of Gastroenterology at the HUCA, University Hospital in Oviedo, for over 40 years. He obtained his Ph.D. in 1975 and has developed a long teaching and research career over nearly four decades. Dr. Rodrigo has published a total of 600 scientific papers, 420 written in English and the rest in Spanish. He has participated as the main investigator in a total of 45 clinical trials and has directed a total of 40 Doctoral theses. He has contributed actively to the formation of around 100 specialists in Gastroenterology. He has authored 35 chapters in various books on his speciality and related diseases, and has served as the Main Editor of 25 books in his speciality. His areas of interest are mainly related to Celiac Disease and Autoimmune Diseases.

Contents

Preface

Acute Pancreatitis is a common inflammatory disease of the pancreatic gland. Although it is a benign process, it can be associated with some complications and mortality. This event is usually preceded by multi-organ failure, so prevention, early diagnosis and aggressive treatment are essential.

The incidence of BP varies depending on the geographical areas studied, ranging from 13 to 45 cases per 100,000 inhabitants per year.

Areas studied ranged from 13 to 45 cases per 100,000 inhabitants per year. An increase in incidence has been observed in recent years, which could be due to improved diagnoses, together with a greater increase in the consumption of alcoholic beverages, among other factors.

There is a relationship between aetiology, sex and age. Thus, the most frequent variant is alcoholic BP in male patients aged between 45 and 55 years, with biliary BP being more frequent in women over this age.

Enzymatic activation of pancreatic acini contributes to some of the early glandular damage (acinar cell death). Still, the local inflammation (late glandular damage) and systemic inflammation that occur in AP progress independently of this phenomenon. Nuclear factor-kappa beta (NF-kappa beta) is a protein complex that controls DNA transcription and is involved in the cellular stress response, playing a key role in the regulation of the immune response.

In Western countries, the most frequent causes of BP are biliary (50-60%), followed at some distance by alcoholic aetiology (15-20%) and idiopathic forms or those of unknown aetiology. Other causes of BP include those related to hypertriglyceridaemia, drugs, tumours, and iatrogenic (post-ERCP). In recent years, smoking has been identified as an independent cause of BP. Other rarer causes are anecdotal.

Diagnosis is based on the presence of at least two of the following three criteria: 1) Elevation of serum lipase and/or lipase at least 3 times the upper limit of normal (ULN). 2) Presence of abdominal pain radiating to the back) Imaging is compatible with AP (abdominal ultrasound, CT scan, MRI), with the last two being more reliable.

The spectrum of severity of the disease is very broad, as it can range from mild forms, manifested by pain of varying intensity and lasting a few hours, to dramatic conditions associated with hospital admissions that can last for several weeks.

Predicting severity consists of identifying predictors (clinical, analytical, radiological, etc.) associated with an increased risk of an unfavourable course. This is because the circumstances that define severity (necrosis, organ failure) often take time to appear before they can be detected.

Certain situations define a worse evolution, for example, a patient with infected necrosis with persistent organ failure requires a more extended hospital stay and has a higher mortality risk than other patients without these complications.

The severity classifications are based on published studies, the natural history of the disease, and expert consensus.

Abdominal pain is the patient's primary symptom in the early phase, yet there are not many studies on which firm recommendations can be based. NSAIDs are more effective than a placebo and opioids. Morphine is not currently discouraged in BP. In refractory cases, after a good differential diagnosis and ruling out serious local complications, epidural analgesia may be used.

There are generally two schools of thought on managing fluid therapy in AP: The classical one is based on the hypothesis that aggressive fluid therapy initiated early improves the prognosis by increasing perfusion of pancreatic necrosis and thus preventing its development and systemic complications.

Apart from this debate, it is essential to actively administer fluids continuously to improve irrigation of inflamed areas. In patients admitted to the ICU, it is recommended to calculate the systolic volume variation or intrathoracic blood volume determination.

Mild AP does not generally require special nutritional support, as oral or nasogastric tube nutrition can be resumed for the first few days, continuing with a liquid or soft diet as soon as the abdominal pain disappears.

In AP with associated severity criteria, it is generally recommended that adequate nutritional support be provided by administering enteral nutrition.

Generally, most patients will soon tolerate the oral route, unless local complications affecting the passage of food through the pylorus or duodenum develop. In patients with persistent organ failure, early enteral nutrition is prudent.

In all patients with AP, prophylaxis for deep vein thrombosis and possible pulmonary thromboembolism should be considered unless their general condition does not preclude their mobility.

Prophylactic antibiotics are not necessary, as they do not prevent pancreatic infection nor improve the course of the disease.

Endoscopic retrograde cholangiography (ERCP) is only indicated in cases of acute cholangitis associated with AP to improve drainage of the main bile duct.

Luis Rodrigo
Professor,
University of Oviedo,
Oviedo, Spain

Chapter 1

Postoperative Pancreatitis

Radoslav S. Todorov, Evgeni E. Zhivkov, Elena Arabadjieva, Dimitar I. Bulanov and Atanas S. Yonkov

Abstract

At the beginning of the twentieth century, a lot of authors were reporting cases of occurrence of postoperative inflammation of the pancreas after different abdominal operations, which in the early postoperative period evolves into acute pancreatitis and sometimes leads to lethal complications—failures of various organs and even whole systems. In this way, the term postoperative pancreatitis has been introduced in the medical society. With the progress of modern medical art and science, a lot of authors are reporting clinical cases of postoperative transitory hyperamylasemia, which devolves as a condition without any complications. These observations lead to the introduction of the term—"postoperative transitory hyperamylasemia." Nowadays, it is still difficult to distinguish whether there is pancreatitis developing in the early postoperative period or just a transitory hyperamylasemia occurring after the operative intervention.

Keywords: postoperative pancreatitis, hyperamylasemia, interleukin 6, interleukin 10, postoperative hyperenzymemia

1. Introduction

Since the beginning of the twentieth century, many authors have reported on various surgical interventions, which in the postoperative period became complicated by inflammation of the pancreas and associated severe and lethal complications on the part of various organs and systems. Thus, the term "acute postoperative pancreatitis" or "postoperative pancreatitis" gradually took shape in the literature. At the turn of the century, the diagnosis was most often made at the patient's autopsy. Subsequently, as a result of the use of modern laboratory and instrumental diagnostic methods, the disease began to be diagnosed more frequently in the early postoperative period before it became severe and, in most cases, fatal complications occurred. There is some disagreement in scientific circles, with half of the authors believing that only postoperative hyperamylasemia exists and the other half maintaining the theory of the existence of postoperative pancreatitis (POP). In the last 10 years, numerous immunological and biochemical methods have been introduced in the diagnostics of the disease, allowing the demonstration of incipient pancreatitis in the first 6 to 12 hours after surgery, long before the associated complications to occur. Thanks to these methods, it is even possible to answer the question of whether pancreatitis will develop or everything will be limited to postoperative benign hyperamylasemia.

1.1 Definition

Postoperative pancreatitis is a severe complication in the postoperative period. It progresses and develops with a mechanism similar to acute pancreatitis; the differences are only in its etiology [1–6].

In 1949, Millbourn conducted the first study of postoperative pancreatitis after gastrectomies and gastric resections. He reported that the disease occurred in about 90% of cases, and its severity was directly related to elevated serum amylase levels [7–18].

2. Incidence of disease

Cases of postoperative inflammation of the pancreas represent 10% of all cases of acute pancreatitis. According to literature data, this type of pancreatitis occurs in about 1–3% of all cases of pancreatic surgery, having a higher incidence in interventions associated with exploration of the extrahepatic bile ducts. Postoperative pancreatitis occurs in 8% of biliary tree operations. The reason postoperative pancreatic inflammation is so severe is complex. The mortality rate in this disease ranges between 30 and 40%, and according to some authors, it is over 50% [7–9].

3. Etiology of postoperative pancreatitis (POP)

Postoperative pancreatitis is a frequent complication of various abdominal surgical interventions. Surgical interventions that complicate POP can be classified into several groups. The unifying feature for categorizing them into these groups is the etiological causative agent and mechanism of postoperative pancreatitis.

In 1949, Millbourn, based on his research, created a classification of causes that lead to postoperative pancreatitis, which is still valid today and has not undergone changes: [11–19].

1. Mechanical damage directly on the pancreatic parenchyma and pancreatic ducts.

2. Variations in the blood supply to the gland, leading to ischemia.

3. Postoperative causes leading to spasm or obstruction of the sphincter of Oddi.

4. Stasis and reflux of duodenal contents. Interventions on bile ducts and gallbladder—cholecystectomies, biliary tree revisions, and biliary drain placement, bile duct resections and biliodigestive anastomoses, papillosphincterotomies, and papillosphincteroplasties.

3.1 Gallstones in the bile ducts

In many cases of POP, the main reason for its presence is gallstones not detected preoperatively or during the surgical intervention. Passing through the terminal choledochus and common biliopancreatic duct, they obstruct bile outflow and predispose bile reflux into the pancreatic duct. Bile refluxed into the pancreatic duct leads to the activation of pancreatic enzymes intraparenchymal and self-digestion of the gland [1–9]. In 1901, Opie described a case of an incarcerated biliary stone in the papilla in a patient who died as a result of pancreatitis. Opie proposed the thesis that biliary pancreatitis may occur when a stone, edema, or inflammation resulting from the passage of the stone obstructs the outflow of bile to the papilla and duodenum. Due to the obstruction, bile refluxes into the pancreatic duct and activates glandular enzymes [1–23]. This theory is also known as the "common duct theory" because a common biliopancreatic duct is necessary for the mechanism of biliary reflux to occur [12, 23]. Studies conducted in animal models support the theory for the genesis of POP in common biliopancreatic duct obstruction. In addition, these experimental models demonstrate that even pancreatic duct obstruction alone, without bile reflux, results in POP [22–27]. To illustrate this mechanism, models have been described in dogs where the ductus pancreaticus is ligated, and pancreatitis subsequently develops in these experimental models [13]. Thus, POP has been associated with causes as diverse as pancreatic trauma after excision and duodenal ulcer strictures. In the situation described, there are several pathogenic variants for the occurrence of POP. In the excision and suppuration of the ulcer defect, the ductus pancreaticus may be inadvertently sutured directly, thereby leading to its complete or partial obstruction, or mechanical trauma to the pancreas, ductus pancreaticus, or duodenum papilla may occur as a consequence of the excision. When the papilla is traumatized, it undergoes a sustained spasm that leads to obstruction of the outlet of the pancreatic duct and, subsequently, to POP. Mechanical injury to the pancreas is defined either as a direct disruption of the integrity of the parenchyma of the gland or as a consequence of surgical intervention to cause a disruption in the blood supply to a particular area of the parenchyma of the gland and to cause POP. Pancreatic stones formed due to inducible pancreatitis of the pancreas may cause stenosis postoperatively and obstruct the common pancreatic duct, causing POP.

In papillosphincteroplasty performed transduodenally, the opening of the pancreatic duct may be inadvertently misturated, leading to POP by the mechanism described. Papillosphincterotomy can lead to the development of POP by the mechanism of spasm and edema of the papilla due to iatrogenic trauma in the misrecognition and mistaken incision of the sphincter complex of the pancreatic duct [16].

Dilatation of the papilla Fateri in benign stenosis results in spasms of the pancreatic duct sphincter and development of POP [16].

Drains are often placed in the biliary tree during cholecystectomy and extrahepatic bile duct surgery. These drains are of different types - transcystic, T-tube drainage – such as Kehr drainage, Cattell T-tube drainage, Whelan-Moss T-tube, Deaver T-tube, and transpapillary—passing through the papilla Fateri. These drainages can lead to the occurrence of POP. The mechanism of pancreatitis in transcystic and transpapillary drains is as follows—when a drain passes through the papilla Fateri, it mechanically irritates the sphincter complex and causes spasm of the sphincter at the outlet of the pancreatic duct or directly mechanically obturates the latter and hence—POP.

3.2 Interventions on the stomach and duodenum: Gastrectomy, gastric resection, gastro-enterostomies, excision or suturing of duodenal ulcers or tumors

In this heterogeneous group of operative interventions, concentrated in the stomach, duodenum, and initial part of the small intestine, multiple causes lead to inflammation of the pancreas in the postoperative period. The pathogenetic mechanisms are varied but obey Millbourn's classification.

3.3 Mechanical damage directly on the pancreatic parenchyma and pancreatic ducts

Mechanical damage occurs in cases of severe mobilizations of the head of the pancreas and cases of excision of a penetrating gastric ulcer into the parenchyma of the pancreas. Pancreatitis postoperatively is also observed in carcinomatous infiltrations of the tumor through the wall of the stomach into the pancreatic parenchyma, necessitating pancreatic resection to be performed together with gastric resection or gastrectomy. In the described cases, one of the main prerequisites for postoperative pancreatitis is the variability of the anatomy of the ductal system of the pancreas [18, 20–22].

Millbourn describes four varieties of pancreatic duct systems, and Arey adds one more. In all these variations of the anatomy of the ductal system of the pancreas, the possibility is pointed out that during surgical intervention, on account of a gastric ulcer penetrating the head of the pancreas or a gastric tumor infiltrating the pancreatic parenchyma, damage may be done to the more superficially situated ductus pancreaticus minor—Santorini. In about 40% of cases, this "minor" pancreatic duct is the main drainer of pancreatic secretion. Its accidental traumatization, perforation, or ligation leads to the occurrence of POP [18, 20–30].

3.4 Disorders of the blood supply to the gland that leads to ischemia

The pancreatic gland is supplied with blood by several arteries. Those supplying blood to the body and tail of the gland are branches of the lienal artery—a. pancreatica dorsalis, a. pancreatica inferior, a. pancreatica magna, and a. caudae pancreatis. The arteries supplying blood to the head of the pancreas are branches of gastro-duodenalis artery—aa. pancreaticoduodenales superior, anterior et posterior, and a. pancreaticoduodenalis inferior—a branch of a. mesenterica superior. In many cases, the normal anatomy of these arteries is modified due to varieties of the vascular system. Burton, Eckman, and Haxo described several cases of variations in the blood supply to the pancreas due to modifications in the arteries branching off from the truncus coeliacus and a. mesenterica superior [17, 18, 20–24, 28].

- Absence of a. pancreaticoduodenales superior anterior and separation of a. colica media and a. pancreaticoduodenalis inferior from a. gastro-duodenalis. Lack of knowledge of the surgeon of this anatomic variation may result in improper ligation of the gastro-duodenal artery and schematization of the underlying transverse colon. Ziegler describes two such cases discovered intraoperatively.

- Absence of a. pancreaticoduodenalis inferior or its variations in which it originates from a. mesenterica superior or from a. epiploica dextra. Ziegler described 12 cases in a study, including 24 patients, and according to Anson, these variations were found in 51 patients out of 500 who had been operated on in total.

In all cases of variations in the arterial blood supply to the pancreatic gland and the surgeon's lack of knowledge of these changes, there is an increased risk of pancreatic ischemia when any of the described arteries is ligated during surgical intervention.

3.5 Postoperative causes leading to spasm or obstruction of the sphincter of Oddi

In all Billroth II-type gastric resections and all total gastrectomies, the duodenum has to be resected, and the duodenal pouch closed blindly. There are several surgical techniques. Occasionally, the pathological process necessitating the operative intervention is located low in the pyloric and antral regions of the stomach. This necessitates the duodenum being cut lower than usual. This situation poses several risks. On the one hand, the possibility of insufficiency of the duodenal pouch sutures takes place due to the lack of sufficient tissue for its good closure, and on the other hand, creating conditions for POP. Most often, this is achieved by squeezing, stenting, or ligating the papilla duodenis at the closure of the duodenal pouch. This is particularly common when duodenal closure techniques are used without sufficient tissue due to the development of the pathological process in this area—a penetrating duodenal ulcer or tumor process [24–29].

In case of insecure closure of the duodenal pouch as a safety mechanism, cholecystectomy is performed, and biliary drainage—transcystic or T-shaped/Kerr—drainage/ is placed. The aim is to reduce the pressure in the duodenal pouch by draining the bile out. Placing the biliary drain or manipulating the gallbladder and extrahepatic bile ducts may result in pushing out of concrements or bile sludge-slough, which may obstruct the papilla Fateri and lead to the development of POP. The mere insertion of a biliary drain into the bile duct results in mechanical irritation, which causes reflex spasms of the sphincter of Oddi and leads to the preconditions for the development of POP [20–24, 28].

3.6 Stasis and reflux of duodenal contents

Pfeffer's closed duodenal loop is a model of a closed-blind loop. Normally, pancreatic enzymes are secreted in inactive proenzyme forms activated by enterokinase, which occurs in the duodenum. In Billroth II-type gastric resections and gastrectomies with "omega"-type esophagojejunostomy, restoration of intestinal passage sometimes results in conditions leading to obstruction or obstructed passage in the afferent loop. Stasis of activated pancreatic enzymes mixed with bile and food particles results. The stasis leads to hypertension in the duodenal pouch and stretching of its walls. Under these conditions and in the presence of an accessory duodenal papilla minor, which a priori has an imperfect sphincteric apparatus, the conditions are set for reflux of duodenal contents with activated enzymes back to the pancreatic duct. Reflux of activated enzymes to the ductal system of the gland causes POP [21–27, 29].

3.7 Liver resections: This group includes both typical liver resections – Hemihepatectomies, lobectomies, and segmentectomies, as well as atypical liver resections and metastasectomies

As in bile duct surgery, intrahepatic cholangiolithiasis should be noted as a cause of POP in liver resections. Concrements and slough in the intrahepatic bile ducts lead to their pushing out and descending migration during the surgical intervention. These concrements and slough obstruct the papilla Fateri postoperatively, leading to postoperative pancreatitis [9–16, 19].

The liver is an organ with a double blood supply, and due to the specific structural relationship of the parenchyma to the blood vessels and bile ducts, various mechanical damages may occur in liver resections /typical or atypical/, which may subsequently cause postoperative inflammation of the pancreas. The mechanism of POP in hepatic resections depends on the technique used to dissect the liver parenchyma. Different methods have been described for the disconnection of the latter, such as digitoclasia, kerniclasia, and hepatoclasia with Cavitron, cavitron ultrasonic surgical aspirator (CUSA), etc. The mechanism of POP in liver resections is not fully understood; however, according to the theory of Hashimoto et al., depending on the technique used to dissect the parenchyma, blood enters into the open bile ducts during liver resection and plays a significant role in liver resections. This iatrogenically induced hemobilia results in blood coagulomas of different sizes in the biliary tree. These, migrating towards the papilla Fateri in the direction of normal biliary outflow, cause papilla Fateri obstruction. This obstruction leads to reflux of bile into the pancreatic duct and POP.

In major liver resections, various techniques are used to reduce the cessation of blood flow entering the liver. With various modifications, these techniques are mainly based on Pringle's prima to clamp the hepatoduodenal ligament and remove the hepatomegaly blood flow. This results in less intraoperative bleeding and, consequently, less blood loss during liver resection. However, many authors have opined that Pringle maneuver and its various modifications are major causes of POP in liver resections. Abdalla et al. and Kubota et al. theorized that hyperamylasemia after Pringle application is due to the resultant venous congestion in the splanchnicus and pancreas, respectively, after cessation of the hepatofugal blood supply [30–33].

In their study, Omer Vedat Unalp et al. directly demonstrated both a plasma change—an increase in alpha-amylase levels after Pringle mannose administration, and direct histological damage to the pancreas, resulting in epithelial edema and the appearance of infiltrates of inflammatory polymorphonuclear cells within the gland. According to the authors, these changes are directly related to the duration of clamp time and the severity of venous congestion [34].

Regarding the severity of venous congestion achieved with the Pringle application, Kubota et al. present a randomized study of two groups of patients. In the first, they performed hepatic resection with Pringle maneuver application; in the second, they applied a superior mesenteric artery flap, in addition to Pringle. Consequently, venous congestion in the second group was less due to the reduced arterial blood supply to the pancreas. Respectively, serum amylase levels in the second group were less elevated postoperatively [33].

3.8 Pancreatic resections, pancreato-cysto-gastrostomies, pancreato-cysto-jejunostomies, and pancreato-digestive anastomoses

Postoperative pancreatitis in surgical interventions of this group occurs due to direct surgical trauma inflicted on the pancreas [35–41]. The difference comes from the fact that in the other surgical interventions, the inflammation of the pancreas is a consequence of surgical intervention on a nearby, adjacent, or distant organ. Millbourn's classification again applies here but with some exceptions.

3.9 Mechanical damage directly on the pancreatic parenchyma and pancreatic ducts

Direct damage to the pancreatic parenchyma leads to necrosis of its cells. This provokes processes of enzyme activation and autolysis of pancreatic tissue. Necrosis of the pancreatic parenchyma occurs when using the electron knife and plating the resection surface for hemostasis. Failure to recognize the varieties in the ductal system of the pancreas can lead to ligation of the central pancreatic duct and cause obstructive pancreatitis.

3.10 Disorders of the blood supply to the gland that leads to ischemia

In all surgical interventions on the pancreas, whether resections, pancreato-digestive anastomoses, pancreato-cysto-enterostomies, or gastrostomies, gland ischemia may occur postoperatively. This ischemia may be iatrogenically induced as a consequence of the surgical intervention performed. It may also occur as a consequence of embolism or thrombosis. Regardless of the cause, ischemia eventually leads to necrosis of the pancreas and the development of pancreatitis [40–43].

3.11 Postoperative causes leading to spasm or obstruction of the sphincter of Oddi

In surgical interventions on the pancreas, this mechanism of postoperative inflammation of the gland is rare. It refers to cases of resections of the left half of the pancreas. Most often, this is due to the development of inducible pancreatitis or pseudo- or true cysts. In cases with inductive pancreatitis of the body or tail of the pancreas, there may be concretions formed in the pancreatic duct. When a left resection is performed, these concrements may be accidentally pushed in a proximal/to the papilla Fateri/direction. Moving there, they obstruct the papilla, causing obstructive postoperative pancreatitis. Although extremely rare, parasitic cysts of the body and tail of the pancreas, specifically pancreatic echinococcosis, can cause a similar genesis of POP. In the ideal echinococcectomy, the cyst is resected along with the parenchyma into a healthy tissue. This is not always possible, and in some cases, portions of the germinative membrane of the echinococcal cyst may be pushed proximally along the course of the duct of Viersung. Thus, reaching the papilla Fateri it obstructs the papilla and causes POP [41–45]. Identical is the mechanism of POP in left pancreatic resection due to pseudocysts communicating with the pancreatic duct. In this case, the role of the "agent" inducing papilla Fateri obstruction may be detrital and sphacelate material from the pseudocyst.

3.12 Stasis and reflux of intestinal contents

Through this mechanism, POP occurs in many cases with right pancreatic resections, such as the Whipple procedure and its various modifications [39, 40]. In a lesser proportion, the mechanism causes POP in pancreatico-cysto-gastro- and jejuno-stomies and pancreato-digestive anastomoses [38]. Regardless of the type of surgical technique, pancreatic enzymes secreted in an inactive form from the pancreatic remnant are shed into the small bowel through the pancreatico-viersungo-jejunoanastomosis performed. On contact with the intestinal mucosa, they are activated by enterokinase. The activated enzymes are carried with the distal peristalsis of the jejunum. Still, when stasis enters the outflow loop, the activated pancreatic secretion begins to act in the area of the anastomosis. The activated enzymes induce autodigestion of the pancreatic parenchyma and the pancreatico-jejunoanastomosis. The absence of an anatomical sphincter complex of the pancreatic duct after the resection is a prerequisite for the reflux of activated enzymes and the development of POP [37–41, 46]. Using a prosthesis or stent embedded in the pancreatico-viersungo-jejunoanastomosis distances the pancreatic juice from the anastomosis. This method assists in the drainage of pancreatic secretion, and the activation of proteolytic enzymes occurs away from the anastomosis. In addition, because of the better secretion drainage, reflux conditions for activated enzymes back to the pancreatic duct are reduced [37–43, 46].

3.13 Splenectomies

Removal of the spleen is a standard procedure for diseases of the latter. Sometimes, splenectomy is necessary for some surgical interventions on adjacent organs. Postoperative pancreatitis in splenectomy occurs by two mechanisms:

3.13.1 Direct trauma to the pancreatic parenchyma

Traumatization of the pancreatic parenchyma during splenectomy occurs most often in the tail region of the pancreas. According to Skandalakis et al., in about 50% of cases, the tail of the gland is targeted and adheres to the hilus of the spleen. When ligating the pancreatic artery into the hilus of the spleen, most often, a portion of the pancreatic tail parenchyma is clamped and subsequently falls within the range of the ligatures imposed on the pancreatic artery [44, 45, 47]. According to Michels, two variants of arterial branch formation exist in the splenic hilus. The first is a small hilus with several larger branches of the lienal artery entering the parenchyma of the spleen [44, 45, 47]. In the second type, the lienal artery divides into multiple convoluted branches a few centimeters anterior to the splenic hilus. The hilus itself is broad, as in about 50% of cases, the tail of the pancreas lies centrally among the vessels entering the spleen [44, 45]. In this variant, injury to the tail of the pancreas is achieved in a very high percentage, especially in emergency surgical interventions in the splenic region [47–49].

3.13.2 Ischemia of pancreatic tissue

The body and tail of the pancreas are supplied with blood by arteries originating from the artery of lienalis. These are a. dorsalis pancreatis, a. magna pancreatis, a. transversalis pancreatis, and a. cauda pancreatis. The arteries listed exhibit substantial variability in their site of separation and size. Ignorance of the anatomic variations of these arteries can lead to erroneous ligation of any of these arteries and iatrogenic ischemia of the tail and body of the pancreas [47, 48]. According to Skandalakis et al., there are over four pancreatic artery dorsalis arteriosus separation variants. It may be separated, besides the artery of the spleen, from the truncus coeliacus in 28% of cases, from the common hepatic artery in 17%, from the superior mesenteric artery in 15%, and in rarer cases from the accessory hepatic or even the middle colic artery, or from the gastro-duodenal artery. This artery splices blood to the pancreatic neck and part of the processus uncinatus. Its ligation or thrombosis can lead to necrosis of parts of the body and processus uncinatus of the pancreas. The transversal pancreatic artery branches off from the artery dorsalis pancreaticis. It supplies the body and part of the tail of the pancreas. It may anastomose with branches of the splenic artery in the hilus of the spleen. Its ligation or thrombosis results in infarction and necrosis of sections of the body and tail of the pancreas. In some anatomical variants, the artery may be absent, being replaced by several direct small arterial branches from the lienal artery supplying blood to the body of the pancreas. More proximal ligation of the lienal artery in these cases may result in ischemia and necrosis of the pancreas and POP [45, 47–49].

The a. magna pancreatis supplies blood to the distal parts of the body and the tail of the pancreas. If present, it is the largest arterial branch of the splenic artery, situated on the border of the middle distal third. The a. caudae pancreatis is detached from the distal segment of the splenic artery before breaking off into the hilus of the spleen. One (32%), two (/46%), or three (22%) arteries may represent it. These provide the blood supply to the tail of the pancreas and occasionally to the accessory spleen, if present [45]. Ignorance of the anatomical variations of these arteries may lead to ligation of any of them and cause iatrogenic damage and postoperative ischemia of the pancreas, leading to the onset of POP [47–49].

3.14 Large intestinal and small intestinal resections

This group of operations includes colon resections—left and right hemicolectomy and various types of resections of small bowel segments, as well as all bypass anastomoses involving the small bowel. Although surgical interventions are performed on organs anatomically not directly related to the pancreas and located relatively distantly from it, POP is a frequent finding in the postoperative period. The mechanism of the disease occurs in several ways.

3.14.1 Direct mechanical damage to the pancreatic parenchyma

Colon resections and left and right hemicolectomy are combined with paraaortic and paracaval lymph node dissections. The level of retroperitoneal paraaortic lymph node dissection, starting from the bifurcation of the aorta, can reach the level of the duodenum and pancreas. In doing so, conditions for injury, squeezing, and crushing of pancreatic tissue occur. Given sections of pancreatic parenchyma may be mistaken for bundles of lymph nodes and inadvertently damaged. Occasionally, in advanced colorectal carcinoma, conformations of metastatic retroperitoneal lymph nodes infiltrate pancreatic tissue directly. In such cases, partial resection of pancreatic parenchyma divisions is necessary for lymph node dissection [49].

The pancreas may be subjected to ischemia in colonic and small bowel resections and anastomoses. According to Skandalakis et al., in rare cases, a. dorsalis pancreatis, which supplies blood to a large portion of the pancreatic tissue, may separate from a. colica media. Ligation of this artery when performing a right or left hemicolectomy may result in ischemia of the pancreas [45, 49]. In colonic resections and small bowel anastomoses with the stomach and colon, POP is triggered by a mechanism in which duodenostasis plays a significant role. According to David Spector et al., in gastroenterostomies, retention conditions occur in the small bowel region distal to the duodenum. This, in turn, leads to duodenostasis, increased duodenal pressure, and results in reflux through the papilla Fateri of activated pancreatic enzymes and the onset of POP [48]. According to Chun et al., colonic resections—especially proper semicolon mobilization—compress the duodenum and traumatize the pancreatic head. In postoperative intestinal paresis, conditions are created for small bowel obstruction and retrograde pressure increase in the duodenum, enzyme reflux through the papilla Fateri, and the onset of POP [49].

3.15 Operations on organs and structures located anatomically far from the pancreas: Anterior resections and the anterior abdominal wall hernia repairs

There are cases of POP occurrence in surgical interventions on organs located anatomically very far away from the pancreas. Although rare, POP is observed in anterior rectal resections and anterior abdominal wall hernia repairs. In both types of surgical interventions, the POP occurrence mechanism is nonspecific.

3.15.1 Anterior resection of the rectum

In an anterior rectum resection, the small bowel has to be mechanically repositioned to mobilize the colon, creating pressure on the mesentery, duodenum, and pancreas. This causes increased duodenal pressure, reflux through the papilla Fateri, and the onset of POP [50]. In the case of a shorter left half of the colon, a sizeable intestinal segment has to be resected to remove the tumor in healthy organs. The remaining colon is insufficient to make an anastomosis. This necessitates mobilizing the entire left half of the colon and liberating and flexing the ileum. In the latter manipulation, the ligaments between the spleen and the colon and the diaphragm and the colon are cut. The a. caudae pancreatis may be transected and ligated in some during surgery. This leads to ischemia of the pancreas and POP [50–56].

3.15.2 Plastics of the anterior abdominal wall

The increased intra-abdominal pressure syndrome plays a significant role in the occurrence of postoperative pancreatitis in these surgical interventions. Elevated intra-abdominal pressure is suggested by values above 12 mmHg measured at laparocentesis or indirectly by bladder pressure measurement.

- Pathophysiology of increased intra-abdominal pressure—it directly affects the organs themselves. The hollow abdominal organs collapse as the pressure in the abdominal cavity increases. This mechanism causes the retention of secretions in the lumen and their evacuation to spaces with relatively less pressure. In POP caused by increased intra-abdominal pressure, secretions from the collapsed duodenum are directed through the papilla Fateri into the pancreatic duct, where the pressure is relatively lower. This phenomenon explains that the duct of Viersung is located deep within the parenchyma of the retroperitoneally located pancreas, which protects it from rising levels of intra-abdominal tension [51].

- When the intra-abdominal pressure increases, the veins of the portocaval system collapse. This leads to the appearance of venous stasis in the portal circulation. In the pancreas, this venous stasis leads to the development of POP.

4. Clinical picture of postoperative pancreatitis

The clinical picture of evolving postoperative pancreatitis is not presented due to the masking of typical symptoms by complaints related to the recent surgery.

A typical symptom is severe dagger-like pain, most often presented in the epigastrium. It may also involve the lower abdominal floors or the lower chest. Most patients describe the pain as severe, stabbing, and sharp, radiating straight back to the back. The pain often starts suddenly and gradually increases until it reaches maximum levels. Nausea and vomiting are constant, even on an empty stomach. A nasogastric tube inserted before surgery relieves nausea and reduces the urge to vomit. Pain in patients suffering from POP can be masked by the administration of analgesics in the postoperative period, as well as masked by the pain from the surgical wound.

Patients developing postoperative inflammation of the pancreas appear intoxicated and pale, and psychomotor agitation—expressed in nervousness, irritability, and fear—predominates. Often, the body temperature rises, which is explained by the release of pro-inflammatory cytokines from the injured pancreas. Tachycardia, tachypnea, and hypovolemia are observed. Hypovolemia is manifested by collapsed neck veins, dry skin, mucous membranes, and decreased skin turgor. Pleural effusions, either unilateral or bilateral, are frequently seen. Patients with severe postoperative pancreatitis often develop acute lung injury, which may progress to acute respiratory distress syndrome (ARDS). Occasionally, qualitative changes in consciousness are observed in patients who have developed POP as a result of hypotension, hypoxemia, or the release of toxins into the bloodstream from the inflamed pancreas. In postoperative pancreatitis induced by operative interventions on the bile ducts, jaundice may be observed. It may result from obstruction of the distal choledochal duct by concrements. But jaundice can also occur in POP due to operations that do not affect the bile ducts or pancreas directly. In these cases, jaundice is caused by obstruction of the distal choledochus by the inflammation of the pancreatic head itself or by the severe inflammation itself, which damages the organism overall. With the impetus of POP, there is a decline in intestinal motility. Peristalsis decreases—becomes deaf to absent. The abdomen swells, and a tympanic tone is heard concurrently. The symptom of muscle defense may occur. These changes may be localized as a finding only in the epigastrium but are often scattered throughout the abdomen. A palpable epigastric formation, which is most commonly the inflamed pancreas and surrounding tissues, may be a crucial sign for diagnosing POP [57, 58].

5. Diagnosis of postoperative pancreatitis

5.1 Measurement of plasma levels of pancreatic amylase, C-reactive protein, interleukins 6 and 10

Serum amylase activity is consistently increased in postoperative pancreatitis. Amylase levels usually rise 2 to 12 hours after the onset of symptoms, then fall, so levels are generally normal by 3 to 6 days after the push. Elevated levels of more than 4–5 days suggest either progressive inflammation or the development of complications, such as pseudocyst, abscess, or pancreatic ascites. Urinary amylase levels remain elevated longer than serum levels, and therefore, the measurement of urinary amylase activity may be of diagnostic help in patients with persistent amylasuria. Although amylase can invade the circulation from nonpancreatic sources, including the salivary glands, lung, prostate, and ovary, pancreatic amylase is of primary importance for diagnosing pancreatitis.

The mechanisms responsible for hyperamylasemia are not fully understood. Some authors—Guo-Jun Wang et al. —have suggested that during pancreatitis, amylase and other digestive enzymes may be secreted from the basolateral surfaces of acinar cells, and thus, activated digestive enzymes gain access to the lymphatic and vascular systems. From another point of view, some recent studies have demonstrated that during POP, processes leading to loosening of intercellular contacts and desmosomes occur, allowing enzymes from the intraluminal/ductal/space to reach the periacinar lymphatic and intravascular spaces. In some cases, serum amylase activity may be regular, even during POP's development and progression stages. This may be due to prevalent necrosis of the gland or in instances of superimposition of pancreatitis on advancing chronic pancreatitis, as hyperamylasemia does not develop in the latter cases, as the exocrine function of the pancreas is severely impaired.

Other blood tests that have not become established in practice are a parallel study of circulating lipase levels, which changes values equally with amylase but with a significant delay. Other circulating enzymes, such as trypsinogen, phospholipase, chymotrypsinogen, etc., are elevated during POP but have little diagnostic value when tested in blood. According to some authors, the same activated enzymes examined in urine may provide a clue in assessing the severity of POP [59–61].

Interleukin 6 (IL-6) is a pro-inflammatory cytokine and anti-inflammatory myokine. T lymphocytes and macrophages secrete interleukin during infections, trauma, and tissue injury 6. It is also secreted by striated muscle during and after physical activity. However, interleukin 6 secreted by muscle has different properties—it suppresses the immune system and has anti-inflammatory properties. Sathyanarayan et al. demonstrated in a study on 108 patients the role of IL-6 in developing POP. In addition to its role as a predictor of the development of inflammatory processes in the pancreas and its severity, they linked elevated blood IL-6 levels to the development of organ damage and organ failure. Changes in IL-6 levels have been tracked throughout the development of POP, increasing with the development of the inflammatory process and gradually declining as it resolves. Ohmoto et al. Experimentally, a direct relationship was shown between the increase in plasma IL-6 levels and the severity of developing pancreatitis [62–66].

C-reactive protein (CRP) is a pentameric protein found in blood plasma whose levels rise with inflammation. It is an acute-phase protein secreted by the liver whose secretion increases after IL-6 production by macrophages and T lymphocytes. Its biological role is to bind to lysophosphatidylcholine on the membranes of dead and dying cells, activating the complement system and, subsequently, opsonin-mediated phagocytosis [67–76].

In prospective studies of groups of patients who developed acute and postoperative pancreatitis, the sensitivity of CRP as an early marker of the severity of developing pancreatitis, the development of necrosis in the pancreas, and also the development of complications due to pancreatitis, such as subhepatic collections, collections in the bursa omentalis, pleural effusion, etc., have been demonstrated. In their study on 78 patients, Barauskas et al. showed the significance of CRP as an early prognostic marker for developing pancreatic necrosis in pancreatitis and complications due to pancreatitis. They mark the limit of CRP levels significant for pancreatic necrosis or complication above 110 mg/L. Patients with established CRP values below 110 mg/L do not develop pancreatic necrosis, and the inflammation of the pancreas resolves mildly [75].

Interleukin 10 (IL-10) has been called an anti-inflammatory interleukin in the human body due to its ability to suppress the secretion of cytokines by macrophages and T and B lymphocytes. Interleukin 10 is secreted mainly by monocytes, to a lesser extent by lymphocytes, T helper, and mast cells. Its main functions are immunomodulation and regulation of inflammatory responses. This cytokine is one of the main regulators of inflammatory responses in the digestive tract [67–76].

A significant reduction in the severity of pancreatitis onset was found in experimental models, in which interleukin 10 was administered before or after the onset of pancreatitis [71]. In their study, Van Laethem et al. experimentally demonstrated a reduction in the severity of the course of pancreatitis and a histologic reduction in necrosis and pro-inflammatory damage after interleukin 10 administration in cerulein-induced pancreatitis in experimental animals [73].

In their studies, several authors have shown the role of interleukin 10 as an agent reducing the strength of the immune response in inflammatory reactions such as pancreatitis. Thus, the course of pancreatitis is milder without severe complications. In their study, Pezzilli et al. demonstrated increased serum levels of interleukin 10 in the first days in patients with mild pancreatitis and low interleukin levels in patients with complicated forms of pancreatitis in the study group [72–77].

6. Postoperative pancreatitis or postoperative hyperamylasemia

There is no consensus in scientific circles as to which statement is correct. According to most of the authors, the postoperative increase in amylase, regardless of the values it reaches, is considered to be transient postoperative hyperamylasemia in cases where this phenomenon is not accompanied by the development of complications on the part of the patient—Richard Morrissey et al. [78, 79]. In their study, the authors describe a study of a series of 110 postoperative abdominal surgery patients, 10% of whom developed transient hyperamylasemia without the manifestation of clinical complications. According to them, this phenomenon is transient and does not require active treatment. However, according to other authors, any postoperative hyperamylasemia should be considered and treated as postoperative pancreatitis—because it can develop as such—Luca Frulloni et al. [80–84]

7. Imaging studies

7.1 Radiography

Chest and abdominal radiographs do not indicate pancreatitis diagnosis, although they can diagnose several diseases by masking a picture of POP. In patients with pancreatitis, chest radiographs reveal diaphragmatic relaxations causing decreased respiratory motility. Pleural effusions may be seen predominantly on the left. Abdominal radiographs usually show distended intestinal loops of gas due to the paralytic ileus caused by POP. Occasionally, gas collections may be seen forming retroperitoneally due to inflammatory and inflammatory processes of the pancreas in complicated POP. Pancreatic calcifications are pathognomonic of chronic pancreatitis and are caused by the formation of calcified intraductal protein plugs.

7.2 Abdominal ultrasound

Ultrasound examination may help detect gallstones and sludge in the gallbladder. However, the test has limited diagnostic value due to copious amounts of gas in the small bowel during the development of POP and subsequent intestinal paresis.

7.3 Computed tomography

Computed tomography (CT) has excellent application, especially in contrast enhancement. It can show even small changes in the pancreas in mild pancreatitis, regardless of the gas accumulated in the intestine. CT can show changes in the type of pancreatic edema and changes in the peripancreatic fat layers. In more severe cases of pancreatitis, there are variable levels of pancreatic necrosis and peripancreatic or intrapancreatic fluid collections. Both clinical and experimental studies have demonstrated the close relationship between an ischemic pancreas on a CT scan and pancreatic necrosis on morphological examination. In the later stages of POP, CT may show complications following the POP episode, such as pancreatic pseudocyst, and allow fine-needle aspiration biopsy demonstrating areas of incipient pancreatic infection.

7.4 Magnetic resonance imaging

According to several authors, magnetic resonance imaging (MRI) has a higher sensitivity and specificity regarding POP than CT [85]. Some of its characteristics make it indispensable in demonstrating postoperative changes in the pancreas. The sensitivity of magnetic resonance imaging (MRI) may be equal to that of the spiral scanner. The advantages of the method are its high resolution, the possibility of distinguishing inflamed from normal tissue, and the fact that it is radiation-free [86, 87].

8. Changes in the body occurring due to postoperative pancreatitis

Postoperative pancreatitis is not only a locally developing inflammatory change confined to the confines of the pancreas. In postoperative pancreatitis, changes occur in distantly located organs and systems.

8.1 Changes in the kidneys

In acute pancreatitis, tubular nephrosis, tubular interstitial nephritis, and focal glomerulonephritis develop. Clinically, the patients develop oliguria, albuminuria, hematuria, and sometimes cylinders, and an insignificant amount of leukocytes are observed. All these concepts enter into the generalized syndrome complex of toxic nephritis. On microscopic examination, dystrophic changes in the cells, tissue edema, and focal accumulations of leukocytes in the medullary and cortical layers are observed. All these lesions have the character of toxic changes and are not characteristic only of postoperative pancreatitis.

In postoperative pancreatitis, in some cases of a highly severe disease course, focal necrosis is observed in both layers of the kidney and a pronounced polymorphonuclear infiltration of tissues in areas of cell degeneration. Clinically, pancreatic-renal syndrome develops, manifested by oliguria, changes in the composition of urine, and increased blood urea, creatinine, and potassium ion levels.

8.2 Changes in the gastrointestinal tract

Morphologically, they are manifested by focal hemorrhages, hemorrhages in the greater bulla and mesentery of the colon and small intestine, present effusion into the peritoneal cavity, and hyperemia. Steatonecrotic spots, signs of developing peritonitis, and engorged loops of the small and large intestines are not rare findings. Of the functional disorders in acute pancreatitis, paresis of the gastrointestinal tract (GIT) is observed, manifested by abdominal distention, retention of gas and stool, and a sharp weakening of peristalsis, reaching the appearance of dyskinetic syndrome. Pancreatitis is characterized by the appearance of vomiting, which brings no relief. Sometimes, it appears pretty early in the development of the disease as a symptom and even sometimes precedes the pain. This should be considered not only as a symptom of the condition but also as an essential etiological point for the development of pancreatic reflux and postoperative pancreatitis. During vomiting, the pressure in the upper GIT compartments increases 2–3 times.

8.3 Changes in the spleen

In postoperative pancreatitis, changes in the spleen are manifested by increased organ size. Spots of fat necrosis on the spleen capsule are often observed. Occasionally, focal hemorrhages in the parenchyma and dystrophic mansion are also present. In the later stages of the disease, bleeding may occur from the ruptured vessels or parenchyma of the spleen.

8.4 Changes in the lung and pleura

A serous or hemorrhagic effusion may occur in the pleural cavity in POP as a reaction to the condition. Subsequently, these effusions may become a source of purulent pleurisy.

8.4.1 Pathophysiology of pulmonary complications of postoperative pancreatitis

POP is an inflammatory process in the pancreas with relative involvement of organs close to the pancreas as well as the involvement of distant organs and systems. Pulmonary complications of POP occur in about 75% of cases, ranging from hypoxemia to the development of ARDS. Recent models of POP studies have established that it is a disease that proceeds in three phases.

The initial phase is characterized by intrapancreatic activation of digestive enzymes and acinar cell damage. The second phase is characterized by intrapancreatic inflammatory reaction and varying degrees of acinar cell damage. The third phase—with further progression of POP and appearance of extrapancreatic damage—is systemic inflammatory response syndrome (SIRS) and ARDS.

Changes in the lung are clinically divided into three main stages.

8.4.1.1 Hypoxemia without radiological changes

Tachypnea, moderate alkalosis, and hypoxemia are seen in patients who have no changes on lung X-ray and in whom clinical examination also shows no changes.

8.4.1.2 Hypoxemia with radiological changes

Clinical or radiographic signs of pulmonary complications were present in 33% of patients with POP. These are pulmonary infiltrates and atelectasis in 15%, pleural effusions in 4–17%, and pulmonary edema in 8–50%.

The appearance of pleural effusion is a sign of severe pancreatitis. In general, pleural effusions and pancreatic ascites are rare findings in POP. Pleural effusions in POP are small and, in most cases, are serous or serous-hemorrhagic. They occur with high amylase values/above 30 times the normal serum value/and in total protein below 30 mg/L. Most pleural effusions are left-sided. There are two leading causes of pleural effusions: (1) transdiaphragmatic lymphatic obstruction or (2) pancreatic-pleural fistula secondary to a previous episode of POP with pancreatic duct rupture or ruptured pseudocyst secondary to POP. Most commonly, pleural effusion occurs when the ruptured pancreatic duct or pseudocyst site is posterior to the retroperitoneum. Pancreatic enzymes can be traced to the mediastinum where, after pleural rupture, pathological communication between the pleura and the pancreatic duct can result.

8.4.1.3 Atelectasis

Atelectasis is a frequently observed phenomenon in POP. In experimental animal models of cerulein-induced pancreatitis, associated lung injury and atelectasis were found. This occurs due to a decrease in surfactant production and secretion 31. In cerulean-induced models of pancreatitis, a reduction in the strength and endurance of the diaphragm muscle fibers is also found 32. Thus, a stage of rapid diaphragmatic exhaustion is reached by decreasing pulmonary compliance and increasing respiratory work.

Pro-inflammatory enzymes, such as interleukin 1 (IL-1), IL-6, and tumor necrsosis factor alpha (TNF-ά), have been found experimentally to be the primary cause of skeletal muscle dysfunction in pancreatitis. Diaz PT et al. proved experimentally that TNF-ά in low concentrations (50–400 ng/mL) can cause rapid exhaustion of diaphragm muscle fibers. Matuszczak et al. showed in animal experiments that levels of pro-inflammatory cytokines must be at much higher concentrations to obtain a physiological effect on muscle. According to Norman et al., intrapancreatic concentrations of pro-inflammatory cytokines are many times higher in POP than in systemic circulation. Based on these studies, IL-1, IL-6, and TNFά may be present in high enough doses in the pancreatic juice in POP to cause exhaustion of the diaphragm muscle fibers. Diaphragmatic damage—reduced mobility of the latter—is, in turn, a pathophysiological cause of atelectasis in basally located segments of the lungs through reduced ventilation of these areas.

8.4.1.4 Acute respiratory distress syndrome/ARDS/

The most severe pulmonary complication is ARDS. According to the literature, patients who develop POP in about 15 to 20% of cases also develop ARDS. Their mortality rate is about 56%. ARDS manifests 2 to 7 days after the onset of POP. The clinical picture includes acute dyspnea, extreme hypoxemia, and refractory to high-dose oxygen therapy. Multilobular pulmonary infiltrates occur in patients with previously normal radiographs. Pulmonary parenchyma is characterized in this condition by increased capillary permeability and interstitial edema.

ARDS most commonly develops in the necrotizing form of pancreatitis, but it occurs in 10% of patients with the POP interstitially edematous form. ARDS accounts for 50–90% of mortality in pancreatitis.

8.4.1.4.1 Pathophysiology of ARDS

The pathophysiological mechanisms leading to ARDS in POP are related to the combined effects of pancreatic enzymes and pro-inflammatory factors. The main pathophysiological processes in ARDS occurring in the lung are increased vascular permeability leading to the accumulation of protein-rich transudate in the alveolar space and decreased lung compliance, which are manifested clinically by refractory hypoxemia and radiologically by diffuse infiltrates in the lung [88–90].

8.5 Changes on the part of the cardiovascular system

Disorders on the part of the cardiovascular system (CVS) are expressed in rhythm-conduction disorders, heart weakness, and heart failure.

8.5.1 Rhythm-wire disorders

Myocardial biochemistry is altered due to the efflux of various enzymes into the blood serum in pancreatitis, glucose breakdown, tissue acidosis, and lactate accumulation [91, 92].

In acidosis, the oxygen supply to the myocardium is compromised, reducing its contractility and compliance. Cellular nutrition is hampered due to high blood lactate levels and acidosis. The heart cannot switch from steady-state metabolism—based mainly on the breakdown of medium-chain fatty acids—to metabolism under stress—with glucose and lactate as the primary energy sources. This inability of the myocardium to biochemically switch metabolism is not due to the lack of glucose in the blood but to acidosis. This leads to low energy production in the myocardium and cardiac weakness [91, 93–114].

The high levels of lipase and phospholipase in the blood directly attack the cell membranes of the excitation-conduction system of the heart and myocardium, generating the onset of various rhythm-conduction disturbances—paroxysmal atrial fibrillation (AF), atrioventricular (AV) block, fascicular block, intraventricular block, ventricular tachycardia, and the like—Marcelo G Binker et al. [111–116].

8.5.2 Heart weakness and heart failure

In the setting of acute postoperative pancreatitis, complications, such as cardiac weakness and failure—due to reduced myocardial contractility—often develop. The mechanism of these pathological manifestations is explained by both the hypovolemic moment generated by splanchnic and peripheral vascular paresis and by a decrease in cardiac muscle contractility and ventricular dilatation [117–124]. Myocardial contractility is impaired simultaneously because of the lack of energy metabolites and acidosis and because of impaired homeostasis of essential ions, such as K^+ /hyperkalemia/, Mg^+/hypomagnesemia/, and hypophosphatemia [123, 124].

9. Conclusions

Postoperative pancreatitis (POP) is an inflammatory disease that occurs in the postoperative period. Its pathophysiological mechanisms are similar to and different from those of acute pancreatitis. The changes that occur in it affect not only the pancreas but also the whole organism. There is no uniform worldwide classification of POP. There are no clearly defined criteria for assessing the extent and severity of POP. There is no model for risk stratification of complications due to POP.

Diagnostically, imaging and endoscopic examinations have little or, in most cases, no practical use in making the diagnosis. The patient who develops POP in the first 24 to 48 hours after surgery is oxygen-dependent, non-transportable, and needs constant monitoring of vital signs. In these circumstances, instrumental imaging is not feasible in most cases. Blood tests are one of the primary sources of information about the severity of the patient's condition and the development of subsequent complications. Due to the in vitro ability of blood enzymes—trypsinogen, phospholipase, chymotrypsinogen, and proteases, which mainly cause complications in postoperative pancreatitis, they are rarely studied. Another fact that makes them inapplicable is their late positivity in blood samples—only after the development of postoperative pancreatitis and its complications. Consequently, they cannot predict the condition and its complications.

Because of its early positivity in blood and relatively low cost per test, pancreatic amylase has established itself as a significant predictor of the development of postoperative pancreatitis worldwide. By examining its variations in the early postoperative period, one can predict the complications occurring in postoperative pancreatitis, although amylase is not a direct cause of these complications. From the facts described above, we can conclude that postoperative pancreatitis is a severe complication occurring early, in the first 24 to 48 hours after surgery. The changes that occur in the patient's organism are incredibly severe, requiring the application of intensive care for the patient and including expensive consumables and medications—antibiotics, blockers of pancreatic secretion, artificial pulmonary ventilation, blood transfusions, and other costly bioproducts. Consequences of developed postoperative pancreatitis, in most cases, can lead to a lethal outcome for the patient.

Conflict of interest

The authors declare no conflict of interest.

Author details

Radoslav S. Todorov[1,2]*, Evgeni E. Zhivkov[1,2], Elena Arabadjieva[1,2], Dimitar I. Bulanov[1,2] and Atanas S. Yonkov[1,2]

1 Department of General and Operative Surgery, Medical Faculty, Medical University Sofia Bulgaria, Bulgaria

2 Clinic of General and Liver Pancreatic Surgery, University Hospital Alexandrovska Sofia, Bulgaria

*Address all correspondence to: x_branko@abv.bg

References

[1] Chen JW, Saccone GT, Toouli J. Sphincter of Oddi dysfunction and acute pancreatitis. Gut. 1998;**43**:305

[2] Cohn JA et al. Relation between mutations of the cystic fibrosis gene and idiopathic pancreatitis. The New England Journal of Medicine. 1998;**339**:653

[3] Eckerwall G, Andersson R. Early enteral nutrition in severe acute pancreatitis: A way of providing nutrients, gut barrier protection, immunomodulation, or all of them? Scandinavian Journal of Gastroenterology. 2001;**36**:449

[4] Etemad B, Whitcomb DC. Chronic pancreatitis: Diagnosis, classification, and new genetic developments. Gastroenterology. 2001;**120**:682

[5] Granger J, Remick D. Acute pancreatitis: Models, markers, and mediators. Shock. 2005;**24**(Suppl. 1):45

[6] Halangk W et al. Role of cathepsin B in intracellular trypsinogen activation and the onset of acute pancreatitis. The Journal of Clinical Investigation. 2000;**106**:773

[7] Layer P, Keller J. Pancreatic enzymes: Secretion and luminal nutrient digestion in health and disease. Journal of Clinical Gastroenterology. 1999;**28**:3

[8] Miskovitz P. Role of selectins in acute pancreatitis. Critical Care Medicine. 2001;**29**:686

[9] Opie EL. The theory of retrojection of bile into the pancreas. Review of Surgery. 1970;**27**:1

[10] Sharer N et al. Mutations of the cystic fibrosis gene in patients with chronic pancreatitis. The New England Journal of Medicine. 1998;**339**:645

[11] Spanier BW, Dijkgraaf MG, Bruno MJ. Epidemiology, aetiology and outcome of acute and chronic pancreatitis: An update. Best Practice & Research. Clinical Gastroenterology. 2008;**22**:45

[12] Townsend M Jr, Beauchamp RD, Evers BM, Mattox KL. Exocrine pancreas. In: Steer ML, editor. Sabiston Textbook of Surgery. 18th ed. By Courtney. 2008. pp. 1589-1623. Chapter 55

[13] Doherty GM. Pancreas. In: Doherty GM, editor. Current Diagnosis & Treatment: Surgery. 14e ed. McGraw-Hill Education; 2014. Available from: https://accesssurgery.mhmedical.com/content.aspx?bookid=1202&sectionid=71521584

[14] Popkirov S. Purulent-Septic Surgery. Sofia; 1984. pp. 422-427. ISBN: 954-9806-20-0

[15] Dimitrova V. Textbook of Surgery Clinical Surgery. Book 2 Sofia; 2005. pp. 369-382. ISBN: 978-954-9301-28-1

[16] Cuschieri A, Davies RS. Acute pancreatitis complicating a choledochal cyst. British Medical Journal. 1969;**3**(5672):698. DOI: 10.1136/bmj.3.5672.698

[17] McCutcheon AD. A fresh approach to the pathogenesis of pancreatitis. Gut. 1968;**9**(3):296-310. DOI: 10.1136/gut.9.3.296

[18] Millbourn E. On acute pancreatic affectations following gastric resection for ulcer or cancer and the possibilities of avoiding them. Acta Cbir. Scandinav. 1949;**9**:1-21

[19] Steer ML. How and where does acute pancreatitis begin? Archives of Surgery. 1992;**127**:1350

[20] Cattell RB. The use of a long T-tube in surgery of the biliary tract. Surgical Clinics of North America. 1948;**28**:659-688

[21] Hinshaw DB, Carter R, Baker HW, Wise RA. Postgastrectomy afferent loop obstruction simulating acute pancreatitis. Annals of Surgery. 1960;**151**(4):600-604

[22] Opie EL. The etiology of acute hemorrhagic pancreatitis. Bulletin of the Johns Hopkins Hospital. 1901;**12**:182-192

[23] Lerch MM, Saluja AK, Runzi M, et al. Pancreatic duct obstruction triggers acute necrotizing pancreatitis in the opossum. Gastroenterology. 1993;**104**:853-861

[24] Pfeffer RB, Stasior O, Hinton JW. The clinical picture of the sequential development of acute hemorrhagic pancreatitis in the dog. Surgical Forum. 1957;**8**:248-251

[25] Owyang C, Logsdon CD. New insights into neurohumoral regulation of pancreatic secretion. Gastroenterology. 2004;**127**:957-964

[26] Kornfeld S. Trafficking of lysosomal enzymes in normal and disease states. The Journal of Clinical Investigation. 1986;**77**:1-6

[27] Palade G. Intracellular aspects of the process of protein secretion. Science. 1975;**189**:347-358

[28] Case RM. Pancreatic exocrine secretion: Mechanisms and control. In: Beger HG, Warshaw AW, Buchler MW, et al., editors. The Pancreas. Oxford: Blackwell Science; 1998. pp. 63-100

[29] Case RM, Argent BE. Pancreatic duct cell secretion: Control and mechanisms of transport. In: Go VLW, DiMagno EP, Gardner JD, et al., editors. The Pancreas: Biology, Pathobiology, and Disease. 2nd ed. New York: Raven Press; 1993. pp. 301-350

[30] Steer ML. Pancreas divisum and pancreatitis: Implications and rationale for treatment. In: Beger HG, Buchler M, Ditschuneit H, Malfertheiner P, editors. Chronic Pancreatitis. New York: Springer-Verlag; 1990. pp. 245-252

[31] Hashimoto N, Haji S, Nomura H, Ohyanagi H. Hyperamylasemia after hepatic resection. Hepato-Gastroenterology. 2003;**50**:1472-1473

[32] Abdalla EK, Noun R, Belghiti J. Hepatic vascular occlusion: Which technique? Surgical Clinics of North America. 2004;**84**:563-585

[33] Kubota K, Makuuchi M, Noie T, Kusaka K, Sakamoto Y, Miki K, et al. Risk factors for hyperamylasemia after hepatectomy using the Pringle maneuver: Randomized analysis of surgical parameters. Archives of Surgery. 1998;**133**:303-308

[34] Unalp OV, Aydin U, Yazici P, Nart D, Yenisey C, Kavak T, et al. The effects of the Pringle Maneuver on the pancreas: Can octreotide be protective? JOP : Journal of the Pancreas. 2009;**10**(3):284-291

[35] Peng SY, Wang JW, Lau WY, et al. Conventional versus binding pancreaticojejunostomy after pancreaticoduodenectomy: A prospective randomized trial. Annals of Surgery. 2007;**245**(5):692-698

[36] Peng SY, Mou YP, Liu YB, et al. Binding pancreaticojejunostomy: 150 consecutive cases without leakage. Journal of Gastrointestinal Surgery. 2003;**7**(7):898-900

[37] Winter JM, Cameron JL, Campbell KA, et al. Does pancreatic duct stenting decrease the rate of pancreatic fistula following pancreaticoduodenectomy? Results of a prospective randomized trial. Journal of Gastrointestinal Surgery. 2006;**10**(9):1280-1290

[38] Hosotani R, Doi R, Imamura M. Duct-to-mucosa pancreaticojejunostomy reduces the risk of pancreatic leakage after pancreatoduodenectomy. World Journal of Surgery. 2002;**26**(1):99-104

[39] Suzuki Y, Fujino Y, Tanioka Y, et al. Selection of pancreaticojejunostomy techniques according to pancreatic texture and duct size. Archives of Surgery. 2002;**137**(9):1044-1048

[40] Bassi C, Falconi M, Molinari E, et al. Reconstruction by pancreaticojejunostomy versus pancreaticogastrostomy following pancreatectomy: Results of a comparative study. Annals of Surgery. 2005;**242**(6):767-773

[41] Unal B, Elpek GO, Yildirim S, Gelen T, Erdogan O, Ozkaynak C. Echinococcus multilocularis infestation in the head of the pancreas. Journal of Clinical & Experimental Pathology. 2014;**4**:3

[42] Ocampo C, Oría A, Zandalazini H, Silva W, Kohan G, Chiapetta L, et al. Treatment of acute pancreatic pseudocysts after severe acute pancreatitis. Journal of Gastrointestinal Surgery. 2007;**11**(3):357-363

[43] Hackert T, Hartwig W, Fritz S, Schneider L, Strobel O, Werner J. Ischemic acute pancreatitis: Clinical features of 11 patients and review of the literature. The American Journal of Surgery. 2009;**197**(4):450-454

[44] Michels NA. Blood Supply and Anatomy of the Upper Abdominal Organs, with a Descriptive Atlas. Philadelphia: JB Lippincott; 1955

[45] Skandalakis PN, Colborn GL, Skandalakis LJ, Richardson DD, Mitchell WE Jr, Skandalakis JE. The surgical anatomy of the spleen. The Surgical Clinics of North America. 1993;**73**:747-768

[46] Roder JD, Stein HJ, Böttcher KA, Busch R, Heidecke CD, Siewert JR. Stented versus nonstented pancreaticojejunostomy after pancreatoduodenectomy: A prospective study. Annals of Surgery. 1999;**229**(1):41-48

[47] Yikun Q, Ren S, Li C, Qian S, Liu P. Management of postoperative complications following splenectomy. International Surgery. 2013;**98**(1):55-60

[48] Spector D, Perry Z, Shah S, Kim JJ, Tarnoff ME, Shikora SA. Roux-en-Y gastric bypass: Hyperamylasemia is associated with small bowel obstruction. Surgery for Obesity and Related Diseases. Jan-Feb 2015;**11**(1):38-43. DOI: 10.1016/j.soard.2014.04.030. [Epub 2014 May 16]

[49] Chun KS, Yoon WH. The causes and clinical significance of hyperamylasemia following colorectal surgery. Journal of the Korean Society of Coloproctology. 2002;**18**(5):281-286

[50] Law WL, Dr H, Bailey R, Max E, Butts DR, Smith KW, et al. Single-layer continuous colon and rectal anastomosis using monofilament absorbable suture (Maxon®). Diseases of the Colon & Rectum. 1999;**42**(6):736-740

[51] Cheatham ML. Abdominal compartment syndrome: pathophysiology and definitions. Scandinavian Journal of Trauma, Resuscitation and Emergency Medicine. 2009;**17**:10. DOI: 10.1186/1757-7241-17-10

[52] Hamano H, Kawa S, Horiuchi A, et al. High serul IgG4 concentrations in patients with sclerosing pancreatitis. The New England Journal of Medicine. 2001;**344**:732-738

[53] Chao C-T, Chao J-Y. Furosemide and pancreatitis importance of dose and latency period before reaction. Canadian Family Physician. 2013;**59**(1):43-45

[54] Kota SK, Kota SK, Jammula S, Krishna SVS, Modi KD. Hypertriglyceridemia-induced recurrent acute pancreatitis: A case-based review. Indian Journal of Endocrinology and Metabolism. 2012;**16**(1):141-143. DOI: 10.4103/2230-8210.91211

[55] Yadav D, Pitchumoni CS. Issues in hyperlipidemic pancreatitis. Journal of Clinical Gastroenterology. 2003;**36**(1):54-62

[56] Gan SI et al. Hypertriglyceridemia-induced pancreatitis: A case-based review. World Journal of Gastroenterology. 2006;**12**(44):7197-7202

[57] Loscalzo J et al. Harrison's Principles of Internal Medicine. 21e ed. The McGraw Hill Companies, Inc; 2022. Available from: https://accessmedicine.mhmedical.com/content.aspx?bookid=3095&sectionid=259856983

[58] Alagozlu H et al. Heparin and insulin in the treatment of hypertriglyceridemia-induced severe acute pancreatitis. Digestive Diseases and Sciences. 2006;**51**:931-933

[59] Baillie J. How should post-ERCP pancreatitis be managed? Medscape gastroenterology. Disclosures. 2012

[60] Chang L, Lo S, Stabile BE, Lewis RJ, Toosie K, de Virgilio C. Preoperative versus postoperative endoscopic retrograde cholangiopancreatography in mild to moderate gallstone pancreatitis: A prospective randomized trial. Annals of Surgery. 2000;**231**(1):82-87

[61] Li AB, Tskhaĭ VF. Diagnosis and treatment of postoperative pancreatitis. Khirurgiia (Mosk). 1991;**2**:122-126

[62] Mark PE, Zagola GP. Meta-analysis of parenteral nutrition versus enteral nutrition in patients with acute pancreatitis. BMJ. 2004;**328**:1407-1412

[63] Pedersen BK, Febbraio MA. Muscle as an endocrine organ: Focus on muscle-derived interleukin-6. Physiological Reviews. 2008;**88**(4):1379-1406. DOI: 10.1152/physrev.90100.2007

[64] van der Poll T, Keogh CV, Guirao X, Buurman WA, Kopf M, Lowry SF. Interleukin-6 gene-deficient mice show impaired defense against pneumococcal pneumonia. The Journal of Infectious Diseases. 1997;**176**(2):439-444. DOI: 10.1086/514062

[65] Sathyanarayan G, Garg PK, Prasad H, Tandon RK. Elevated level of interleukin-6 predicts organ failure and severe disease in patients with acute pancreatitis. Journal of Gastroenterology and Hepatology. 2007;**22**(4):550-554

[66] Ohmoto K, Yamamoto S. Serum interleukin-6 and interleukin-10 in patients with acute pancreatitis: Clinical implications. Hepato-Gastroenterology. 2005;**52**(64):990-994

[67] Braat H, Rottiers P, Hommes DW, Huyghebaert N, Remaut E, Remon JP, et al. A phase I trial with transgenic bacteria expressing interleukin-10 in Crohn's disease. Clinical Gastroenterology and Hepatology. 2006;**4**(6):754-759. DOI: 10.1016/j.cgh.2006.03.028

[68] Fedorak RN, Gangl A, Elson CO, Rutgeerts P, Schreiber S, Wild G, et al.

Recombinant human interleukin 10 in the treatment of patients with mild to moderately active Crohn's disease. The interleukin 10 inflammatory bowel disease cooperative study group. Gastroenterology. 2000;**119**(6):1473-1482. DOI: 10.1053/gast.2000.20229

[69] Schreiber S, Fedorak RN, Nielsen OH, Wild G, Williams CN, Nikolaus S, et al. Safety and efficacy of recombinant human interleukin 10 in chronic active Crohn's disease. Crohn's disease IL-10 cooperative study group. Gastroenterology. 2000;**119**(6):1461-1472. DOI: 10.1053/gast.2000.20196

[70] van Deventer SJ, Elson CO, Fedorak RN. Multiple doses of intravenous interleukin 10 in steroid-refractory Crohn's disease. Crohn's disease study group. Gastroenterology. 1997;**113**(2):383-389. DOI: 10.1053/gast.1997.v113.pm9247454

[71] Rongione AJ, Kusske AM, Kwan K, Ashley SW, Reber HA, DW MF. Interleukin 10 reduces the severity of acute pancreatitis in rats. Gastroenterology. 1997;**112**(3):960-967

[72] Pezzilli R, Billi P, Miniero R, Barakat B. Serum interleukin-10 in human acute pancreatitis. Digestive Diseases and Sciences. 1997;**42**(7):1469-1472

[73] Van Laethem JL, Marchant A, Delvaux A, Goldman M, Robberecht P, Velu T, et al. Interleukin 10 prevents necrosis in murine experimental acute pancreatitis. Gastroenterology. 1995;**108**(6):1917-1922

[74] Thompson D, Pepys MB, Wood SP. The physiological structure of human C-reactive protein and its complex with phosphocholine. Structure. 1999;7(2):169-177. DOI: 10.1016/S0969-2126(99)80023-9

[75] Barauskas G, Svagzdys S, Maleckas A. C-reactive protein in early prediction of pancreatic necrosis. Medicina (Kaunas, Lithuania). 2004;**40**(2):135-140

[76] Vissers RJ, Abu-Laban RB, DF MH. Amylase and lipase in the emergency department evaluation of acute pancreatitis. The Journal of Emergency Medicine. 1999;**17**:1027-1037

[77] Lang E, Afilalo M, Dankoff J, Colacone A, Tselios C, Guttman A. The prognostic significance of moderate hyperamylasemia in the evaluation of the emergency department patient. The Journal of Emergency Medicine. 1995;**13**(1):107-112. ISSN: 0736-4679

[78] Morrissey R, Edward Berk J, Fridhandler L, Pelot D. The nature and significance of Hyperamylasemia following operation. Annals of Surgery. 1974;**180**(1):67-71

[79] Calderon B, Carrero JA, Ferris ST, Sojka DK, Moore L, Epelman S, et al. The pancreas anatomy conditions the origin and properties of resident macrophages. JEM. 2015;**212**(10):1497-1512. DOI: 10.1084/jem.20150496

[80] Frulloni L, Patrizi F, Bernardoni L, Hyperenzymemia GCP. Clinical significance and diagnostic approach. JOP. Journal of Pancreas (Online). 2005;**6**(6):536-551

[81] Xiao X, Gaffar I, Guo P, Wiersch J, Fischbach S, Peirish L, et al. M2 macrophages promote beta-cell proliferation by up-regulation of SMAD7. Proceedings of the National Academy of Sciences of the United States of America. 2014;**111**:E1211-E1220. DOI: 10.1073/pnas.1321347111

[82] Kuo I-M, Wang F, Liu K-H, Jan Y-Y. Post-gastrectomy acute pancreatitis in

a patient with gastric carcinoma and pancreas divisum. World Journal of Gastroenterology. 2009;**15**(36):4596-4600. Published online 2009 Sep 28. DOI: 10.3748/wjg.15.4596

[83] Soybel DI, Zinner MJ. Complications following gastric operations. In: Zinner MJ, Schwartz SI, editors. Maingot's Abdominal Operations. 10th ed. Stamford, CT: Appleton and Lange; 1997. pp. 1029-1056

[84] Bo T, Zhihong P, Peiwu Y, Feng Q, Ziqiang W, Yan S, et al. General complications following laparoscopic-assisted gastrectomy and analysis of techniques to manage them. Surgical Endoscopy. 2009;**23**:1860-1865

[85] Kim Z, Kim MJ, Kim JH, Jin SY, Kim YB, Seo D, et al. Prediction of post-operative pancreatic fistula in pancreaticoduodenectomy patients using pre-operative MRI: A pilot study. HPB: The Official Journal of the International Hepato Pancreato Biliary Association. 2009;**11**(3):215-221

[86] Sandrasegaran K, Maglinte DD, Howard TJ, Lappas JC. Surgery for chronic pancreatitis: Cross-sectional imaging of postoperative anatomy and complications. Abdominal Imaging Pictorial Essay. 2005;**184**(4):1118-1127. DOI: 10.2214/ajr.184.4.01841118

[87] Yamauchi FI, Ortega CD, Blasbalg R, Rocha MS, Jukemura J, Cerri GG. Multidetector CT evaluation of the postoperative pancreas. Gastrointestinal Imaging. 2012;**32**(3)743-764. DOI: 10.1148/rg.323105121

[88] Lichanska AM, Hume DA. Origins and functions of phagocytes in the embryo. Experimental Hematology. 2000;**28**:601-611. DOI: 10.1016/S0301-472X(00)00157-0

[89] Mosser DM, Edwards JP. Exploring the full spectrum of macrophage activation. Nature Reviews Immunology. 2008;**8**(12):958-969. DOI: 10.1038/nri2448

[90] Galdiero MR, Garlanda C, Jaillon S, Marone G, Mantovani A. Tumor associated macrophages and neutrophils in tumor progression. Journal of Cellular Physiology. 2012;**228**(7):1404-1412. DOI: 10.1002/jcp.24260

[91] Miyagawa S, Makuuchi M, Kawasaki S, Kakazu T, Hayashi K, Kasai H. Serum amylase elevation following hepatic resection in patients with chronic liver disease. The American Journal of Surgery. 1996;**171**(2):235-238

[92] Tocchi A, Mazzoni G, Liotta G, Lepre L, Costa G, Miccini M. Increased blood amylase levels in the postoperative period after liver resection. Il Giornale di Chirurgia. 1998;**19**(6-7):262-264

[93] Bacchini I, Martino G, Falaschi CF, Viti M, Sammartano C, Mantovani R. Postoperative acute pancreatitis (PAP). Direct Personal Experience Minerva Chir. 1980;**35**:421-427

[94] Lubianskiĭ VG, Nasonov SV. Acute pancreatitis after resection of stomach for low duodenal ulcer. Khirurgiia (Mosk). 2001;**35**:8-11

[95] Vasiliadis K, Fortounis K, Kokarhidas A, Papavasiliou C, Al Nimer A, Stratilati S, et al. Delayed duodenal stump blow-out following total gastrectomy for cancer: Heightened awareness for the continued presence of the surgical past in the present is the key to a successful duodenal stump disruption management. A case report. International Journal of Surgery Case Reports. 2014;**5**(12):1229-1233. Published online 2014 Nov 13. DOI: 10.1016/j.ijscr.2014.11.026

[96] Kim HJ, Kim JW, Kim KH, Jo KW, Hong JH, Baik SK, et al. A case of

afferent loop syndrome treated by endoscopic drainage procedure using nasogastric tube. Korean: The Korean Journal of Gastroenterology. Mar 2007;**49**(3):173-176

[97] Merenda M, Janczak D, Cianciara J, Litarski A. Acute pancreatitis as an early complication after gastric resection. Polski Przegląd Chirurgiczny. 2010;**82**(12):645-650. DOI: 10.2478/v10035-010-0099-5

[98] Kriger AG, Kubishkin VA, Karmazanovskiĭ GG, Svitina KA, Kochatkov AV, Berelavichus SV, et al. The postoperative pancreatitis after the pancreatic surgery. Khirurgiia (Mosk). 2012;**4**:14-19

[99] Surgical treatment of chronic pancreatitis and tumors of the exocrine pancreas R. N. Gaidarsky – dissertation thesis

[100] Sathasivam S, Ritchie A, Brooks AJ, Morris DL. Acute pancreatitis following liver resection: Report of three fatal cases and a review of the literature. ANZ Journal of Surgery. 2004;**74**(8):643-645

[101] Griffith E, Leong H, Nyam S-C. The significance of hyperamylasaemia after colonic resection. Colorectal Disease. 1999;**1**(6):347-350. DOI: 10.1046/j.1463-1318.1999.00094.x

[102] Burne JJ, Boyd TF. Hyperamilasemia in intestinal obstruction and its relationship to pancreatitis. The American Journal of Surgery. 1963;**105**(6):720-729. DOI: 10.1016/0002-9610(63)90484-7. ISSN: 0002-9610

[103] Chand B, Walsh RM, Ponsky J, Brody F. Pancreatic complications following laparoscopic splenectomy. Surgical Endoscopy. 2001;**15**(11):1273-1276. Epub 2001 Sep 4

[104] Kazuyoshi K, Shinichi T, Kyoko N, Makio S. Managenet of pancreatic fistulas after a splenectomy as part of Cytoreductive surgery for ovarian cancer. International Journal of Gynecological Cancer. 2013;**23**(8):1506-1511

[105] Mathew A, Chiemprabha AF, Donelson S, Talavera F, Anand BS, Patel T. Hyperamylasemia: Background, Pathophysiology, Etiology Medscape. 2016. Available from: https://emedicine.medscape.com/article/186389-overview?form=fpf

[106] Baniel J, Leibovitch I, Foster RS, Donohue JP. Hyperamylasemia after post-chemotherapy retroperitoneal lymph node dissection for testis cancer article in with 12 reads. The Journal of Urology. 1995;**154**(4):1373-1375. DOI: 10.1097/00005392-199510000-00032

[107] Burkey SH, Valentine RJ, Jackson MR, Modrall JG, Clagett GP. Acute pancreatitis after abdominal vascular surgery. Journal of the American College of Surgeons. 2000;**191**(4):373-380

[108] Al-Ali BM, Thimary F, Pummer K. Acute pancreatitis as rare complication of the right radical transperitoneal open nephrectomy. Central European Journal of Urology. 2012;**65**(4):219-220. Published online 2012 Dec 11. DOI: 10.5173/ceju.2012.04.art8

[109] De Waele JJ, Hoste E, Blot SI, Decruyenaere J, Colardyn F. Intra-abdominal hypertension in patients with severe acute pancreatitis. Critical Care. 2005;**9**(4):R452-R457. Published online 2005 Jul 6. DOI: 10.1186/cc3754

[110] Ke L, Tong Z-H, Ni H-B, Ding W-W, Sun J-K, Li W-Q, et al. The Effect of Intra-Abdominal Hypertension Incorporating Severe Acute Pancreatitis in a Porcine Model. PLoS One. 2012;7(3):e33125. DOI: 10.1371/journal.pone.0033125

[111] Z'graggen K, Aronsky D, Maurer CA, Klaiber C, Baer HU. Acute postoperative pancreatitis after laparoscopic cholecystectomy. Results of the prospective Swiss Association of Laparoscopic and Thoracoscopic Surgery Study. Archives of Surgery. 1997;**132**(9):1026-1030; discussion 1031

[112] Gloor B, Stahel PF, Müller CA, Worni M, Büchler MW, Uhl W. Incidence and management of biliary pancreatitis in cholecystectomized patients. Results of a 7-year study. Journal of Gastrointestinal Surgery. 2003;**7**(3):372-377

[113] Tejedor L, Serrablo A. Postoperative pancreatic biliary surgical complications. Journal of Gastroenterology and Hepatology Research. 2013;**2**(7):661-671

[114] Bardenheier JA III, Kaminski DL, Willman VL. Pancreatitis after biliary tract surgery. The American Journal of Surgery. 1968;**116**(5):773-776

[115] Tsuzuki T, Shimizu S, Takahashi S, Iio H. Hyperamylasemia after hepatic resection. The American Journal of Gastroenterology. 1993;**88**(5):734-736

[116] Connor S. Defining post-operative pancreatitis as a new pancreatic specific complication following pancreatic resection. HPB: The Official Journal of the International Hepato Pancreato Biliary Association. 2016;**18**(8):642-651. Published online 2016 Jun 20. DOI: 10.1016/j.hpb.2016.05.006

[117] Jin S, Shi XJ, Sun XD, Zhang P, Lv GY, Du XH, et al. The gastric/pancreatic amylase ratio predicts postoperative pancreatic fistula with high sensitivity and specificity. Medicine (Baltimore). 2015;**94**(3):e339. DOI: 10.1097/MD.0000000000000339

[118] Yang J, Huang Q, Wang C. Postoperative drain amylase predicts pancreatic fistula in pancreatic surgery: A systematic review and meta-analysis. International Journal of Surgery. 2015;**22**:38-45. DOI: 10.1016/j.ijsu.2015.07.007. Epub 2015 Jul 26

[119] Rudis J, Ryska M. Pancreatic leakage and acute postoperative pancreatitis after proximal pancreatoduodenectomy. Rozhledy v Chirurgii. 2014;**93**(7):380-385

[120] van Acker GJ, Perides G, Steer ML. Co-localization hypothesis: A mechanism for intra pancreatic activation of digestive enzymes during the early phases of acute pancreatitis. World Journal of Gastroenterology. 2006;**12**(13):1985-1990

[121] Dixit A, Dawra RK, Dudeja V, Saluja AK. Role of trypsinogen activation in genesis of pancreatitis. In: Pancreapedia a Exocrine Pancreas Knowledge Base. 2016. DOI: 10.3998/panc.2016.25

[122] Wang G-J, Gao C-F, Wei D, Wang C, Ding S-Q. Acute pancreatitis and pathogenesis. World Journal of Gastroenterology. 2009;**15**(12):1427-1430

[123] Binker MG, Laura CB I. Acute pancreatitis: The stress factor. World Journal of Gastroenterology. 2014;**20**(19):5801-5807

[124] Yegneswaran B, Kostis JB, Pitchumoni CS. Cardiovascular manifestations of acute pancreatitis. Journal of Critical Care. 2011;**26**(2):225.e11-225.e18. DOI: 10.1016/j.jcrc.2010.10.013. Epub 2010 Dec 23

Chapter 2

Pancreatic Tumour Microenvironment and Microenvironment Targeted Therapeutic Approaches

Demet Kacaroglu

Abstract

Pancreatic cancer is characterised by high metastatic potential and poor survival rates. The major reason for this is the failure of therapeutic agent to reach the target cells due to the dense desmoplastic microenvironment formed in pancreatic tumours. The development of an immunosuppressive tumour microenvironment, due to disruption of matrix morphology, reduces the success rate of immunotherapy, chemotherapy and targeted therapy methods used in the treatment of Pancreatic Adenoductal Carcinoma (PDAC). In this chapter, the components of the pancreatic tumour microenvironment; cancer cells, stromal cells (mesenchymal stem cells, fibroblasts, cancer-associated fibroblasts, pancreatic stellate cells), immune system cells and extracellular components (ECM, cytokines, growth factors, DNA and small RNAs) are explained. This stroma is a vital dynamic structure that regulates tumour growth, metabolism, vascularisation, drug resistance, immune tolerance and metastasis pathways. To comprehend and manage the intense desmoplastic stroma, it is crucial to elucidate the behaviour of the microenvironment components in pancreatic cancer. The microenvironment of PDAC, the most frequent type of pancreatic cancer, and microenvironment-targeted therapeutic approaches are then presented as *in vitro*, *in vivo* and clinical phase studies.

Keywords: pancreatic cancer, tumour microenvironment, tumour immunology, targeted therapy, pancreatic ductal adenocarcinoma

1. Introduction

Pancreatic cancer is one of the most aggressive cancers with a significantly high mortality rate. Although its incidence ranks 10th among cancers, it ranks 4th in cancer-associated deaths in many developed countries [1]. Currently, pancreatic carcinoma ranks 7th in cancer-associated deaths in developed countries and is expected to be the second most lethal cancer in the world by 2030 [2]. Pancreatic cancer is primarily divided into two types: pancreatic adenocarcinoma (85% of cases), which is the most common in the exocrine glands of the pancreas, and pancreatic neuroendocrine tumours (less than 5%), which are less common in the endocrine tissue of the pancreas. Additionally, pancreatic ductal adenocarcinoma (PDAC) is the most prevalent histological subtype of pancreatic cancer (90%) and arises from the progression of precursor lesions known as pancreatic intraepithelial neoplasia [3]. Due to its high metastatic potential, pancreatic cancer has a very aggressive progression, and standard treatments such as chemotherapy, radiotherapy and surgery are not adequate enough to ensure survival [4]. The five-year survival ratio is less than 6% and 50% of patients die within the first six months due to metastasis [5]. Although many conventional approaches such as chemotherapy, surgery and targeted therapy have been attempted for the treatment of pancreatic cancer, no effective results can be obtained [6]. The failure of these therapies to provide success is due to the inability of the therapeutic agent to reach the target cells due to the dense desmoplastic microenvironment formed in pancreatic cancer. Recent studies have shown that not only cancer cells but also the tumour microenvironment contribute to the aggressive prognosis of pancreatic cancer. Approximately 90% of the pancreatic tumour mass consists of desmoplastic stroma, while tumour cells constitute only 10% of the tumour [7]. It is known that the tumour microenvironment formed by extracellular matrix and stromal cells in close contact with tumour cells plays an active role in tumour development, invasion, metastasis, chemoresistance, apoptosis and escape from the immune system [8]. Under normal conditions, the stroma has anti-carcinogenic properties, but when the cells forming the stroma are stimulated by various stimuli and transformed, they begin to support cancer development. Under these conditions, stromal cells change together with cancer cells and differentiate to synthesise various cytokines, chemokines, growth factors and proteases enzymes [9]. Therefore, therapies targeting only tumour cells fail and it is thought that the tumour microenvironment should be targeted together with carcinoma cells in order to apply effective treatment.

The pancreatic cancer microenvironment involves stromal cells, cancer cells, and extracellular components. Cellular components include mesenchymal stem cells (MSCs), fibroblasts, pancreatic stellate cells (PSCs), cancer-associated fibroblasts (CAFs), regulatory T cells (Tregs), myeloid-derived suppressor cells (MDSCs) and tumour-associated macrophages (TAMs). CAFs, endothelial cells, MSCs, PSCs and immune system cells all constitute stromal cells (**Figure 1**). CAFs are one of the most important regulatory cells of the pancreatic tumour microenvironment, differentiated from progenitors of epithelial, endothelial, fibroblast cells and MSCs [10]. These cells and cancer cells secrete extracellular components such as extracellular matrix, MMPs, growth factors and Transforming growth factor beta (TGF-β) to maintain the microenvironment. Since there is a high proportion of extracellular matrix proteins around the cells, it is a physically hard tumour with high interstitial fluid pressure. Extracellular components consist of extracellular matrix (ECM) and cytokines, growth factors, DNA and small RNAs. This stroma is a highly dynamic structure that regulates tumour growth, vascularisation, drug response, immune responses and metastasis [11].

In order to better understand and control the dense desmoplastic microenvironment of PDAC, it is crucial to clarify the behaviour of microenvironmental constituents. In this study, cellular and non-cellular structures in the microenvironment of PDAC are described. The microenvironment, which has a significant potential in targeted cancer therapies, is of high importance for the development of targeted therapeutic approaches. Current *in vivo* and *in vitro* studies targeting the microenvironment are also discussed. This chapter is expected to be useful for molecular cancer biologists and oncologists in their research in this field.

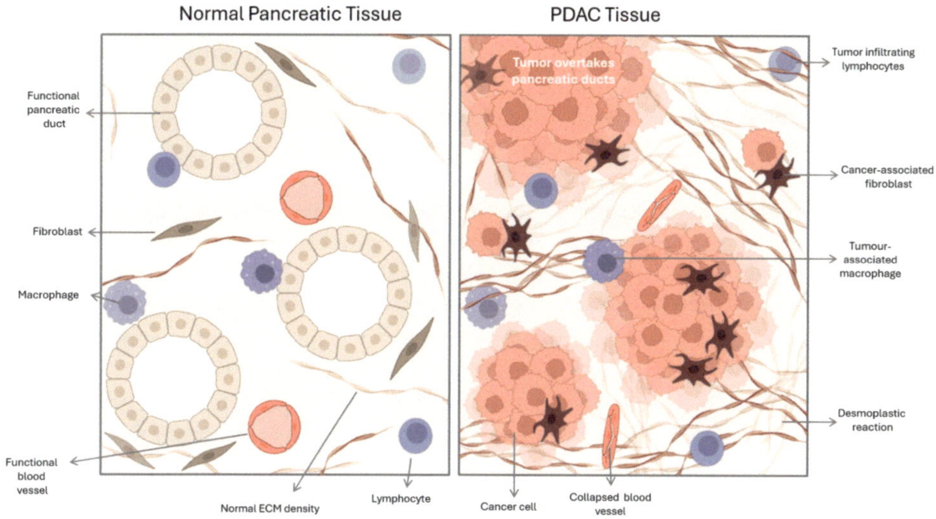

Figure 1.
Histological illustration of the PDAC microenvironment [11].

2. Pancreatic tumour microenvironment and microenvironment targeted therapeutic approaches

The tumour microenvironment is a heterogeneous environment composed of cellular and non-cellular components, and the diversity of these components depends on the type and stage of the tumour. The pancreatic cancer microenvironment has two main features: intense desmoplasia and widespread immunosuppression. These two traits facilitate pancreatic cancer cell proliferation, escape from immune system cells through direct inhibition of antitumour immunity, formation of cancer stem cell niche and metastasis [12]. In pancreatic cancer, there is extensive fibrosis called desmoplasia in the primary tumour sites. Clinical signs of desmoplasia are overexpression of extracellular matrix proteins and widespread transformation of fibroblastic type cells into myofibroblastic phenotype. Stromal cellular components also promote desmoplasia formation by secreting specific molecules such as TGF-β, fibroblast growth factor-2 (FGF-2) and connective tissue growth factor. Desmoplasia also supports the progression of pancreatic cancer and resistance to chemotherapy [13]. During tumour progression from the pre-neoplastic PanIN to the invasive stage, the composition of the microenvironment, the interaction of immune system cells with tumour cells and the metabolic properties of the microenvironment are constantly changing [14].

Desmoplasia creates a hypoxic microenvironment by promoting the function of antiangiogenic factors. Hypoxia due to poor vascularisation induces metabolic reprogramming, inhibition of apoptosis, maintenance of proliferation signalling and metastasis formation. In general, this desmoplastic microenvironment creates a supportive microenvironment for pancreatic cancer cells to develop proliferation, invasion, metastasis, angiogenesis, metabolism, immunosuppression and chemoresistance [12]. Another characteristic feature of the pancreatic microenvironment is the suppression of the activity of the immune system which is called immunosuppression. In pancreatic cancer, the immune system suppresses tumour development and progression by destroying mutated cells and preventing their transformation into tumour cells in the early stages, but in later stages, it promotes suppression of the immune system [15]. As a result of analyses of enzymatic application and cell separation procedures, it has been shown that immune system cells constitute roughly 50% of the tumour tissue. The majority of these cells are immunosuppressive cells like Tregs and MDSCs [7].

Cytokines are low molecular weight proteins that regulate intercellular signalling. Immune system cells, stromal cells, fibroblasts and endothelial cells synthesise cytokines. These secreted cytokines regulate cell proliferation, survival, differentiation, activation of immune system cells, cell migration and cell death. In the tumour microenvironment; interleukins, tumour necrosis factor family, interferons and cytokines in the TGF-β protein family are present. Cytokines with different functions may affect tumour formation by acting directly on tumour cells as a growth-promoting factor or indirectly by stimulating inflammatory cell types [16]. Depending on the tumour microenvironment, cytokines can modulate the antitumour response. However, the balance state of proinflammatory and anti-inflammatory cytokines is impaired in chronic inflammation. Since the concentrations of cytokines, cytokine receptor expression levels and the activation status of surrounding cells change in the same environment, an environment is created to trigger malignancy. In the literature, it has been shown that cytokines such as IL-1, IL-6 and IL-8 secreted from cancer cells and tumour-infiltrating cells support invasion, proliferation and transition to mesenchymal phenotype for the development of tumour microenvironment [17].

Metastasis is a multi-step process in which cancer cells migrate, penetrate, invade and proliferate from the site of the primary tumour to distant sites *via* the blood or lymph circulation. Metastases can sometimes develop long after diagnosis as a result of the slow adaptation of a single cell in the remote microenvironment, but in some tumours metastases occur simultaneously during the growth of the primary tumour. As a matter of fact 91% of PDAC patients are diagnosed with metastatic cancer indicates that the risk of metastasis is very high. As this metastatic process occurs very rapidly, elucidation of the basic processes driving metastatic behaviour is critical in determining how to approach the disease in the clinic [18]. Recent studies have shown that the microenvironment acts a critical role in PDAC progression, suggesting a close relationship between the microenvironment and metastasis. Studies have also recently focused on the tumour microenvironment of pancreatic cancer [12].

2.1 Cellular and non-cellular components

PDAC is a heterogeneous environment composed of cellular and non-cellular components. There is a paracrine interplay cycle between cancer cells and stromal cells that activate each other through various signals. While normal pancreatic stroma prevents or inhibits tumour development, pathologic stromal components have a role in tumour progression [19].

2.1.1 Cellular components

Fibroblasts are the most numerous cells in connective tissue and form the basic structure of tissues with the ECM proteins they secrete. Fibroblasts, which are quiescent under normal conditions, are activated in wound healing and fibrosis conditions and turn into an active cell group called 'myofibroblast'. Myofibroblasts have stress fibres with contractile ability, express α-smooth muscle actin and ED-A domain fibronectin, a variant form of fibronectin. Several studies have shown that fibroblasts are essential players in tumourigenesis. Especially in pancreatic, breast and prostate cancers, they constitute the majority of stromal cells around the tumour [20]. These activated fibroblasts, which are located in the tumour stroma and called 'CAF', show many similar characteristics with these myofibroblasts involved in wound healing and inflammation processes. When tissue damage occurs, fibroblasts in that region transform into myofibroblasts in response to paracrine signals. Induction of myofibroblasts also causes organ fibrosis which induces cancer development. Various cell groups such as smooth muscle cells, endothelial cells, myoepithelial cells or mesenchymal cells are cell groups that form CAFs [21]. These cells affect cancer cells by expressing and secreting insulin-like growth factor-1, hepatocyte growth factor, epidermal growth factor, stromal cell-derived factor-1 and various FGFs. CAFs promote tumour cell proliferation, angiogenesis, escape from apoptosis, chemoresistance and metastasis. CAFs produce various chemokines, cytokines, growth factors, miRNAs and exosomes. CAFs also suppress immune system cells with the cytokines they secrete and cause acceleration of tumour progression [22]. There are various subtypes of CAFs in the tumour microenvironment. Three main types of CAFs have been described in the pancreatic microenvironment according to the location and stage of the tumour. These are myofibroblastic CAFs (myCAFs), inflammatory CAFs (iCAFs) and antigen-presenting CAFs (apCAFs). Identification and regulation of the functional roles of CAFs are essential for pancreatic cancer progression [23].

MSCs are fibroblast-like stromal cells with high regenerative capacity, multiple differentiation capacity and immunomodulatory properties. Because they do not cause an immune response and have anti-inflammatory, angiogenic and antiapoptotic properties, they are widely used in many fields of medicine [24]. In response to the signals received from the environment in which they are located, MSCs regulate the microenvironment by secreting cytokines, chemokines, growth factors, enzymes, exosomes or by direct contact. As research on the cellular biology of MSCs increases, it is being investigated whether they can be used for therapeutic purposes in cancer. In particular, it is thought that naïve MSCs, that is, MSCs that have not interacted with tumour cells, become trained by tumour cells in line with the signals received over time and support tumour cells through many mechanisms [25].

PSCs are resident cells in the pancreas. They have been a focus of research in fibrosis associated with pancreatic cancer and chronic pancreatitis. Normally, PSCs are quiescent and modulate ECM production. However, during tumourigenesis, the stroma and pancreatic cancer cells secrete various stimulating factors such as TGF-β to activate PSCs. Afterward, activated PSCs can create a malign microenvironment and facilitate cancer progression in pancreatic cancer by promoting excessive fibrosis, tumour metastasis, inducing chemotherapy and radiotherapy resistance [26]. The clinical roles of pancreatic stellate cells (PSCs) in pancreatic ductal adenocarcinoma (PDAC) progression are associated with several important processes. PSCs alter the tumour microenvironment by increasing the density of the ECM and triggering the desmoplastic response. PSCs secrete cytokines and growth factors that promote the proliferation and migration of cancer cells. This promotes angiogenesis by increasing tumour vascularization. PSCs may contribute to the development of resistance of tumour cells to therapy. PSCs secrete cytokines such as IL-1, IL-6, colony-stimulating factor 1 (CSF-1) and tumour necrosis factor-α (TNF-α). These cytokines may influence the behaviour of tumour cells. PSCs may enhance the aggressive properties of PDAC by interacting with other stroma cells, such as endothelial cells, immune cells and neuronal cells. These interactions and processes suggest that PSCs play an important role in regulating the malignancy of PDA [27].

Dendritic cells (DCs) are essential regulators of immunity and function as professional antigen-presenting cells when fully activated. Tumour cells have the ability to evade immunosurveillance and create an immunosuppressive microenvironment that inhibits the maturation of DCs. DCs, a key component of the immune system, mainly participate in adaptive immune responses; however, they have a dual function in the tumour microenvironment (TME). On the one hand, mature immunogenic DCs contribute to T cell-mediated antitumour responses through antigen uptake, processing and presentation. On the opposite side, immature or partially differentiated myeloid DCs are unable to induce antitumour immune responses; instead, as regulatory DCs, they contribute to immune suppression and tolerance in TME. Dysfunction of immunogenic DCs leads to failures in immune surveillance and elimination of tumour cells [28]. In several clinical trials on pancreatic cancer, a reduced number of tumour-associated fully activated DCs were observed for the first time. Crucially, abnormal myelopoiesis has been confirmed as the main mechanism causing DC disruptions in cancer, leading to increased production of immature DCs. Moreover, DCs in the peripheral blood circulation are reduced in number and impaired in function in pancreatic cancer patients. By studying circulating and lymphoid and myeloid DCs in unresectable pancreatic cancer patients, it was proposed that high levels of circulating myeloid DCs are associated as a prognostic factor and improve survival in unresectable pancreatic cancer patients. Significantly increased levels of immune modulatory and chemotactic factors (IL-6, TGF-β, IDO, COX-2, CCL2 and CCL20) and immune cell-specific markers from macrophages, myeloid and plasmacytoid DCs were detected in human PDAC tissues [29].

Suppressing the immune response within the tumour microenvironment is a crucial factor in tumour development. MDSCs are known as a cell population that can support primary tumour growth and metastasis by affecting various mechanisms. MDSCs enable tumour cells to evade the immune system by inhibiting the activation of lymphocytes. A high population of MDSCs is frequently observed in pancreatic cancer [30]. PDAC tissue samples have shown that MDSCs are present both in the microenvironmental tissues and in the bone marrow, peripheral blood and spleen. This indicates that MDSC populations proliferate systemically and migrate to the tumour site. However, the mechanisms by which MDSCs are attracted to the microenvironment have not been fully elucidated. GM-CSF, produced by pancreatic tumours, plays an important role in these processes. Disrupting the interaction between GM-CSF-associated tumour cells and MDSCs has been shown to prevent the accumulation of MDSCs and restore the function of CD8+ cytotoxic T cells [29].

The main inflammatory cell population in solid tumours are TAMs, which are derived from blood monocytes or macrophages of local tissues. TAMs can have different activation and polarisation states. M1 macrophages have an anti-tumoural effect, while M2 macrophages perform pro-tumourigenic actions that promote tumour growth. Studies in pancreatic cancer have shown that CD68-positive TAMs are associated with shorter survival, while CD163-positive TAMs are associated with longer survival. However, M2-polarised TAMs have also been found to be concentrated in invasive tumour sites and are associated with poor prognosis. These data suggest that the M1/M2 classification of macrophages may not fully reflect their effects on tumour progression [31]. Factors such as GM-CSF expressed in the tumour or its microenvironment may regulate the maturation of TAMs. TAMs appear to colonise the tumour early, not only in invasive carcinomas but also in proximity to the lowest-grade PanIN lesions. Furthermore, TAMs are key regulators of PanIN progression. In KrasG12D mice, TAMs in PanIN lesions are a major source of IL-6 and promote cancer progression *via* STAT3 signalling. Furthermore, NFκB-activated monocytes have been reported to stimulate the proliferation of pancreatic cancer cells *via* sonic hedgehog production [29].

There are diverse T cell populations that infiltrate the tumour microenvironment. These T cells are known to control the immune response depending on the cytokine profile they secrete. Among these cell groups, cytotoxic CD8+ T cells, which have the ability to kill tumour cells and are associated with favourable prognosis, are supported by CD4+ T cells characterised by the production of interleukin-2 (IL-2) and interferon-gamma (IFN- γ). High expression of these cytokines in the tumour microenvironment is also associated with a good prognosis. Other CD4+ cell groups such as Th2 cells, which produce interleukins such as IL-5, IL-4 and IL-13, which induce B cell responses, are generally thought to be associated with tumour growth [32]. Cytotoxic CD8+ T lymphocytes effectively recognise and attack tumour cells that present tumour-associated antigen peptides with MHC I. CD8+ T cells have the capacity to destroy tumour cells by acting directly on malignant cells through IFN-γ and induction of macrophage tumouricidal activity. Previous studies of many types of cancer prove that tumour-infiltrating CD8+ cells have antitumour activity and a positive impact on clinical outcomes and survival rates [29]. Neo-antigen naïve CD8+ T cells cannot effectively infiltrate into normal peripheral tissues and in the early stages of tumour formation, tumour-specific CD8+ T cells may remain unaware of antigen-expressing cancer cells. As the tumour progresses and adequate tumour antigen is presented in the lymph nodes, tumour-specific T cells may be enabled in the draining lymph node or tumour tissue, often in an inflammatory and stimulus-free context, resulting in anergic, early dysfunctional T cell status (stage 1). The tumour progresses and an immunosuppressive environment develops. The persistent presence of tumour antigens and microenvironmental stimuli lead tumour-specific T cells to a late dysfunctional condition (stage 2) [33].

In many types of cancer, Th1 cells and their produced cytokines contribute significantly to favourable clinical outcomes. However, the roles of other T cell populations in supporting or opposing tumours are not clearly defined. Previous studies on various cancers have determined that IL-17A and Th17 cells have tumour-supportive effects. However, some studies suggest that Th17 cells may also play a protective role against tumours. In mouse models of pancreatic cancer, increased Th17 cells in the tumour microenvironment slowed tumorigenesis and improved survival. This suggests that the role of Th17 cells in PDAC is complex and can exert both protective and detrimental effects depending on the context [34]. Th2 cells are known to have protumorigenic effects and are often associated with poor prognosis and decreased survival in cancers. Th2 immune responses negatively impact survival by promoting tumour-supportive properties in pancreatic cancer and other carcinomas. However, the precise pathological mechanisms and signalling pathways underlying these effects are not yet fully understood. Furthermore, the Th1 immune response in pancreatic cancer patients is indirectly suppressed by tumour cell-derived TGF-β and IL-10, leading to general suppression of the Th1 response [29].

Regulatory T cells are crucial for maintaining immune homeostasis and are immunosuppressive cells. They specifically regulate immune events in the microenvironment and ensure tolerance by inhibiting T-cell activation. Regulatory T cells are abundantly expressed in pancreatic ductal adenocarcinoma (PDAC), where they are recruited to the tumour site by CCL5 produced by Foxp3. Regulatory T cells are stable in challenging environments, such as those with low glucose concentrations. Tregs are classified as either innate or induced, depending on their anatomical position. The former originate from the thymus and migrate to the periphery; the latter develop in the periphery from Foxp3-CD4+ T cells. When the anatomical location is unclear, the term "FoxP3+ Treg cells" is used. Regulatory T cells reshape the immune microenvironment through various mechanisms and promote tumour metastasis [35].

Neutrophils, the most common immune cells in circulation, play a key role in the innate immune system and are found in various cancers. High levels of intratumoural neutrophils and IL-8 are linked to poor outcomes with immune checkpoint inhibitors. The exact role of neutrophils in tumour development is unclear, but they are classified into two types: tumour-suppressive N1 and tumour-supportive N2. N1 neutrophils, activated by TGF-β inhibition, can kill tumour cells and inhibit tumour growth, while N2 neutrophils promote tumour metastasis and angiogenesis through immune-suppressive actions [36].

Natural killer (NK) cells are large granular lymphocytes that are less understood compared to other lymphocytes (T and B cells) in the adaptive immune system. NK cells, which serve as the first line of defence against virally infected and malignant cells, are classified as CD56+ CD3- cells. This classification can be divided into two main populations: immunomodulatory CD56+ CD16- cells, which regulate their functions through cytokine release (especially interferon [IFN]-γ), and cytotoxic CD56+ CD16+ effector cells. Malignant cells often evade detection by T cells by downregulating the expression of surface MHC-1 molecules. This "missing self" signal prevents inhibition by NK cells, leading to cytotoxic activity. In addition, NK cells can be negatively regulated by checkpoint proteins such as programmed death 1 (PD-1) [37].

2.1.2 Non-cellular components

Desmoplastic stroma is composed of the extracellular matrix (ECM) and stromal cells. It is known that the population of fibroblastic cells can constitute up to 90% of the tumour mass in pancreatic cancer, and the size of the stroma can be considered a prognostic factor. The extracellular matrix consists of substances such as collagen, integrin, laminin, fibronectin, glycosaminoglycan, matrix metalloproteinases (MMP) and SPARC. Under normal conditions, the ECM inhibits desmoplasia while maintaining cellular polarity, proliferation and migration. In contrast, the irregular integrin subunits observed in the basal membrane of pancreatic cancer tissue contribute to the survival and invasion of cancer cells. Hyaluronan is highly accumulated, and when it binds to the hyaluronan receptor CD44, subsequent interactions prolong the survival of cancer cells [10].

The ECM is a non-cellular component found in all tissues. Composed of water, proteins and polysaccharides, the composition of the ECM is determined by the needs of the microenvironment. Changes in the structure of the ECM are a result of malignant cell transformation in many cancers. Tumour stroma often contributes to cancer development and tumour progression. However, several recent preclinical and clinical studies have shown that stromal depletion can lead to more aggressive conditions. Therefore, the stroma and ECM play a dual role as both tumour-supportive and tumour-preventive components in the microenvironment. For success in this area, a more complete understanding of the stroma and the TME is required. PDAC consists of collagens, integrins, glycoproteins and proteases that interact with tumour cells through various mechanisms [37].

To summarise the first part; PDAC is one of the cancers with a complex TME composed of rich stromal components. Many features present in the PDAC stroma contribute to the resistance of this tumour to cytotoxic and immunotherapeutic treatments and its propensity to metastasise. At the cellular level, PDAC cells engage in a complex interaction with non-neoplastic cell types such as fibroblasts, endothelial cells and immune cells. These complex interactions fuel the progression and therapeutic resistance of this aggressive cancer. Studies suggest that the polarisation of these cell types, particularly immune system cell and fibroblast populations, determines how PDAC tumours grow, metastasise and respond to therapy. Therefore, current research focuses on how to best target these populations so that tumours can be made to respond to treatment. Taken together, it is now clear that the PDAC TME is composed of numerous and various cell types that commonly associate at all stages of tumour development. This section provides an overview of the TME.

2.2 Microenvironment targeted therapies

Pancreatic cancer treatment mainly consists of four methods: surgical treatments, systemic therapies, radiation therapies and combined therapies. Systemic treatments consist of chemotherapies, targeted therapies and immunotherapies. Depending on the stage of pancreatic cancer, in some cases, only one treatment modality is used, while in other combinations of multiple treatment modalities may be required. Although surgical resection treatment offers a curative treatment in the early stages, cancer recurs in approximately 80% of patients who undergo surgery. The fact that PDAC typically occurs in late stages makes these processes difficult, as it does not show specific findings and symptoms. When detected at an early stage, good results can be achieved. Moreover, since PDAC is highly resistant to these classical treatment modalities, new treatment strategies continue to be explored. In recent years, advances in immunotherapy and targeted therapy have led to a radical change in the classical treatment paradigms for pancreatic cancer. The treatment of pancreatic cancer should be planned with a multidisciplinary team as much as possible, taking into account the general state of health of the person according to the stage of cancer [38].

The microenvironment of pancreatic cancer consists of stromal cells, a dense extracellular matrix, and immune system cells. This stroma is a critical feature that regulates tumour growth, vascularization, drug response, immune modulation and metastasis. The desmoplastic environment in pancreatic cancer restricts the transport of nutrients and oxygen to cancer cells. Moreover, due to the highly hypoxic environment of pancreatic cancer, anti-angiogenic therapy is not an option, as it exacerbates tumour hypoxia, thereby promoting chemotherapy resistance, cancer stem cell proliferation, invasion and metastasis. In the absence of oxygen and nutrients, cancer cells undergo metabolic reprogramming to survive, such as shifting from oxidative phosphorylation to glycolysis, inhibiting fatty acid oxidation and increasing the excretion of lipids and proteins. The acute effect of hypoxia is the transition from oxidative phosphorylation to glycolysis due to the stabilisation of hypoxia-inducible factor 1α (HIF-1α) [39]. We can classify microenvironment targeted therapies as ECM targeted therapies (antifibrotic therapies, hyaluronic acid inhibitors, MMP inhibitors, use of antagonist monoclonal antibodies and small peptides to Hedgehod receptors, CD40 agonists, endothelial cell targeted angiogenesis inhibitors), immune microenvironment targeted therapies (targeting TAMs, MDSCs, TANs, TILs, NKs, DCs) and non-immune stromal cell targeted therapies (targeting MSCs, PSCs, CAFs) (**Figure 2**).

2.2.1 ECM targeted therapies

Hyaluronidase breaks down hyaluronic acid and is beneficial in conditions such as bladder cancer and brain cancer. The long time effects of hyaluronidase on cancer

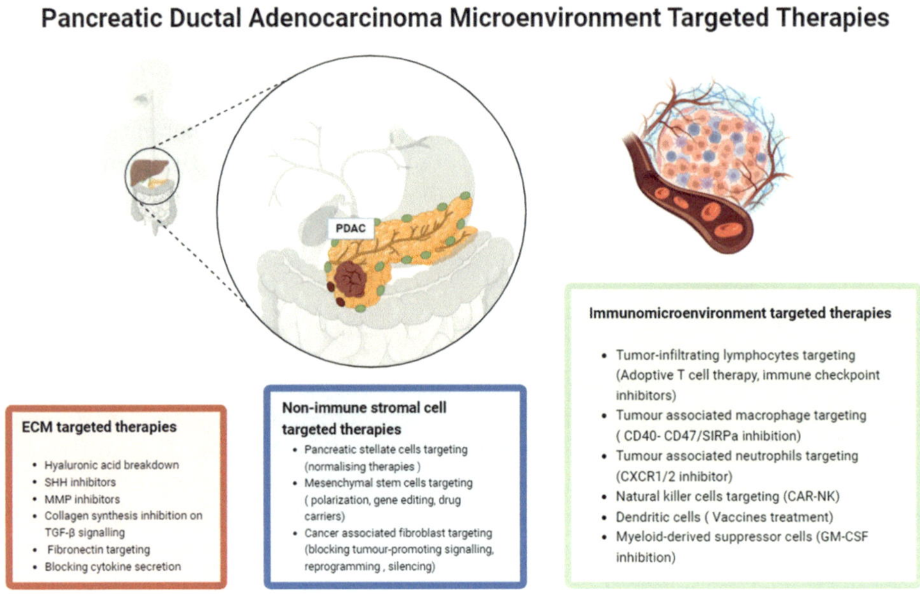

Figure 2.
Microenvironment targeting approaches in PDAC treatments.

treatment are still a subject of research [40]. Hyaluronic acid-targeted therapeutic approaches aim inhibition of hyaluronic acid synthesis, blocking of hyaluronic acid synthesis signalling or degradation of stromal hyaluronic acid to increase the efficacy of chemotherapeutic drugs in PDAC patients [41]. 4-methylumbelliferone (4- MU), used in the therapeutic approach based on hyaluronic acid inhibition, has been observed to inhibit PDAC tumour metastasis and growth in *in vivo* and *in vitro* studies [42]. In PDAC, which is characterised by desmoplastic fibrotic stroma, hyaluronic acid accumulation compresses the capillaries in the stroma, making it difficult for drugs administered into the circulatory system by injection to reach the target. It was observed that tumour growth decreased and survival time increased when the hyaluronidase-based agent PEGPH20, which is used to ensure the breakdown of stromal hyaluronic acid, was given in combination with chemotherapeutic drugs such as doxorubicin and gemcitabine rather than intravenously alone to mice with PDAC model [43].

Overexpression of sonic hedgehog (SHH) ligands provokes cancer initiation and tumour metastasis due to desmoplastic reaction. Expression of Smo protein increases as a result of binding of SHH ligands to PTCH1 receptors. Sarigedib, an agent used for the inhibition of Smo receptors, has been observed to reduce desmoplasia, decrease collagen deposition and increase survival in mice when combined with gemcitabine. On the other hand, in a pilot study on 118 patients in phase II, it was shown that vismodegib, a Smo antagonist, did not produce the expected therapeutic effect in clinical trials. However, therapy methods targeting Hedgehog signalling pathway seem to be a good strategy since they can effect both desmoplastic stroma and tumour mass [44]. It is known that tumour invasion, angiogenesis and metastasis occur with increased expression of MMPs which degrade many components of extracellular matrix by proteolytic cleavage. It is known that Batimastat, a peptidomimetic zinc chelate targeting the zinc-dependent MMP unit in studies in which

MMPs were taken as pharmacological targets for PDAC treatment, failed in the Phase III phase because it increased toxicity in the pancreatic tumour microenvironment. Phase II and Phase III studies using andecaliximab, a monoclonal antibody targeting MMP-9, are ongoing [45].

Several therapeutic strategies have been developed to alleviate excessive collagen deposition in solid tumours, mostly focusing on the production, depletion and cross-linking of collagen. It has been reported that the combination of collagenase enzyme, which reaches the tumour microenvironment without denaturing by using 100 nm diameter targeted liposomes in mouse models of PDAC, with paclitaxel micelles resulted in 87% decreased tumour size. In the same study, it was noteworthy that the number of metastasised tumour cells did not increase as a result of ECM degradation by collagenase enzyme [46]. Regulation of TGF-β signalling during collagen synthesis is a target to inhibit collagen production. Furthermore, the therapeutic effect of the TGF-β monoclonal antibody fresolimumab is being evaluated in various clinical trials (NCT01401062 and NCT02581787) [40]. Vitamin D inhibits collagen secretion in various cell types. The vitamin D receptor (VDR) has been shown to regulate the transcription of pancreatic stellate cells (PSCs) and cancer-associated fibroblasts (CAFs). Treatment with the VDR ligand calcipotriol reprograms the stroma, reduces inflammation and improves the drug response to gemcitabine. Several studies are ongoing regarding the use of paricalcitol in combination with chemotherapies and immunotherapies [47].

Fibronectin-targeted research in cancer treatment focuses particularly on providing precise drug delivery to tumours. Several studies have shown that drugs such as tranilast, metformin and dexamethasone can reduce matrix stiffness. Also, conventional drugs such as hydroxychloroquine, retinoic acid receptor agonists and focal adhesion kinase (FAK) inhibitors have been suggested to have this potential. However, further mechanistic studies are needed to better understand the effects of these drugs in cancer treatment [48, 49].

2.2.2 Immuno microenvironment targeted therapies

The tumour immune microenvironment (TIME) in PDAC consists of tumour cells, immune cells, blood vessels, nerves and extracellular matrix components. Due to the high heterogeneity of TIME in PDAC, identifying its subtypes is crucial for developing clinical perspectives. Studies on subtyping are being updated with molecular genetic, genomic, transcriptomic, proteomic and metabolomic approaches [50]. These advancements will provide a more solid foundation for the future development of immunotherapies targeting various components of TIME.

One of the first things that come to mind when we think of immunotherapy in cancer is immune checkpoint regulators. The discovery of immune checkpoint inhibitors has been a new hope in cancer treatment and therefore immunotherapy is now used in cancer treatment is called the fourth generation of immunotherapy. The aim of these therapies is to re-strengthen the immune system by triggering it to fight against cancer. Currently, while anti-PD-1, anti-CTLA-4 and anti-PD-L1 antibodies reveal the role of precursor CD8+ T cells in patients with malignant melanoma, especially in non-small cell lung cancers, they are used as immunotherapy agents inducing T cell development in renal cell cancers [51]. Although these checkpoint inhibitors have been used effectively in non-small cell lung cancer, malignant melanoma and renal cell cancers. In contrast, no immunotherapeutic modality for pancreatic cancer is yet available for clinical use. Pancreatic cancer is considered to be an immunogenically weak cancer type. In pancreatic cancer, the tumour microenvironment is thought to create an immunosuppressive environment that interferes with the success of immunotherapy. Monotherapy with CTLA-4 or PD1 inhibitors is largely ineffective in pancreatic cancer. Clinical trials testing combinations of chemotherapy, vaccines, radiotherapy and cytokine antagonists in combination with checkpoint inhibitors are ongoing. In theory, clinically used chemotherapeutics such as gemcitabine and/or capecitabine should reduce the immune response. However, clinical studies show that the immune response is largely preserved. Currently, there is a small subgroup of pancreatic cancer patients who can be treated with immunotherapy. Pembrolizumab has been approved by the FDA for the treatment of cancers with microsatellite instability, regardless of cancer type. However, this landmark drug is effective against only 1% of patients with pancreatic cancer [52].

Adoptive T cell therapy involves reinfusing patients' T cells genetically modified to fight tumour cells. This treatment has shown promise, particularly with Chimeric Antigen Receptor-T (CAR-T) cells. CAR-T cells can selectively destroy tumour cells by recognising and targeting specific antigens on their surface [53]. In summary, while CAR-T therapy holds promise for treating PDAC, its effectiveness is currently limited by challenges related to antigen identification, toxicity management and the immunosuppressive nature of the PDAC microenvironment. Continued research and technological advancements are crucial for overcoming these hurdles and improving treatment outcomes [54].

Macrophage-targeted therapies can basically be classified into three aspects: Preventing tumour recruitment of macrophages, restoration of the antitumour capability of macrophages and macrophage reprogramming [55]. Activation of CD40 and CD47/SIRPa signalling is one method to restore normal macrophage function. Recently, Selicrelumab has been studied in the TIME as a treatment that induces T cell activity and proliferation, stimulates DCs, reduces M2 macrophage numbers and decreases tumour fibrosis [56].

Tumour-associated neutrophils (TANs) in PDAC overexpress the genes CXCR1, CXCR2, FCGR3B and S100A8. These are neutrophils that infiltrate tumour tissues and can have various roles depending on their polarisation state. They can promote or inhibit tumour progression. TANs are commonly found in PDAC tumours. Their presence and behaviour can significantly impact tumour progression and patient prognosis. N2 TANs are known to promote tumour growth and metastasis in PDAC by promoting angiogenesis and suppressing antitumour immune responses. High levels of TANs, especially those showing the N2 phenotype, are often associated with poor prognosis and reduced survival in PDAC patients. In order to develop more effective treatments for this aggressive cancer, it is vital to investigate their specific functions and potential therapeutic targeting [57].

DCs are rare in PDAC and are one of the reasons why immunotherapy fails. Strategies to enhance DC function or reprogram to bypass immunosuppressive TME are being investigated. This includes using DC-based vaccines or combining DC therapies with other immunotherapies to increase their efficacy. Developing new approaches to improve DC function and exploit their potential for antitumour immunity is an important area of research [58].

MDSCs are stimulated by the cytokine GM-CSF to differentiate in the microenvironment. Blocking GM-CSF can be considered a knockout strategy. Researchers are investigating ways to target MDSCs to enhance antitumour immunity. Current strategies include depleting MDSCs, inhibiting MDSC function and reprogramming MDSCs. Furthermore, combining MDSC-targeting strategies with other therapies, such as immune checkpoint inhibitors, to increase treatment efficacy is an area of active research [12].

2.2.3 Non-immune stromal cell targeted therapies (PSCs, MSCs, CAFs)

Various strategies targeting PSCs in the tumour stroma have been reported; Blocking PSC Activation, Targeting Fibrosis, Regulating PSC Function. However, the PSC depletion strategy has been shown to result in lower viability in transgenic mice [59]. Therefore, most of the present strategies focus on restorating PSCs or decreasing ECM production. Targeting PSCs and their effects in the tumour microenvironment offers potential avenues to improve treatment strategies for PDAC. Hyaluronic acid degradation, Hedgehog pathway inhibitor, MMP inhibitor retinoic acid derivatives, Target CSF1R, Target VDR, TGF-β signalling inhibitor, Calpains inhibitor, Ang II receptor 1 antagonists, Rho-associated protein kinase inhibitor, CXCR4 antagonist, HGF inhibitor, Glucagon-peptide-1 receptor agonist, Resveratrol, β-catenin/CBP inhibitor, Hsp90 inhibitor and proton pump inhibitor are being investigated for the improvement of PSCs [27].

Mesenchymal stem cells are used for various therapeutic purposes in cancer by modifying them in different ways since their direct effects in cancer therapy vary according to the source, dose and cancer type [60]. MSCs can be designed easily in gene therapies to specifically exhibit antiproliferative, proapoptotic, antiangiogenic agents according to different cancer types [61]. In addition, the exosomes or the exosomes of the MSCs themselves are widely used in targeted therapy by carrying cancer-targeted therapeutic agents such as precursor drugs, cytotoxic agents, viral vectors, immunomodulators or RNAi [62]. Although unmodified MSCs mostly support tumour cells in direct studies, there are also studies showing antitumour effects [63]. It has been shown in studies adipose tissue-derived MSCs contribute to the intensification of tumour stroma by producing dense collagen matrices after arriving in extrapancreatic tissue [64]. MSCs derived from umbilical cord with increased IL-15 expression by lentiviral vector enhanced survival by stimulating Natural Killer cells and CD8+ T cells in pancreatic cancer model [65]. In the *in vivo* cancer model, tumour growth was decreased and survival was increased in the MSC group whose IL-10 expression was increased *via* plasmid vector. However, it was shown that proinflammatory cytokines such as IL-6 and TNF-α helped to increase survival by inhibiting angiogenesis in the IL-10 MDC group [66]. In a study with MSC-derived myofibroblasts, it induced mesenchymal profile *via* NOTCH signalling in pancreatic cancer cells and also caused chemoresistance, and these effects decreased when treated with Jagged-1 siRNA [67]. Studies on the effects of MSCs in the pancreatic cancer tumour microenvironment are much more limited than in many cancer types. In order to develop a targeted therapy approach to the tumour microenvironment in pancreatic cancer, it is important to elucidate the behaviour of MSCs, one of the most key components of the microenvironment, and their transformation into CAFs.

CAF-targeted therapies include mainly three different methods: silencing of CAFs, blocking tumour-promoting signalling of CAFs and reprogramming of CAFs. CAFs expressing fibroblast activation protein (FAP), which causes poor prognosis, are currently being further investigated. DNA vaccines can stimulate tumour-infiltrating lymphocytes specific to the vaccine to destroy CAFs and disrupt tumour tolerance [68]. To enhance the effectiveness of CAF depletion therapies, a detailed characterisation of subtypes is required. Approaches targeting IL-1 and TGF-β have the potential to provide therapeutic effects due to their impact on CAF transformation.

The combination of CAF-targeted therapies with immunotherapies shows promise in animal models and some clinical trials [69].

3. Conclusions

PDAC is characterised by a complicated tumour microenvironment comprising abundant stromal components. Many of the therapeutic failures of chemotherapy, targeted therapy and immunotherapy have been linked to the PDAC microenvironment. Many characteristics inherent in the PDAC stroma contribute to its tendency to metastasise. At the subcellular level, PDAC cells interact in a complex interaction with non-neoplastic cell types such as non-immune cells, ECM compounds and immune cells. These sophisticated interactions fuel the progression and therapeutic resistance of this aggressive PDAC. Researchers propose that the polarisation of these cell types, particularly immune system cell and fibroblast populations, determines how PDAC tumours grow, metastasise and react to the therapy. For this reason, current research focuses on how to best target these populations so that tumours can be made to respond to therapy. In this study, we briefly summarise the components of the PDAC microenvironment, the effects of individual elements on the microenvironment, and targeted therapies. This book chapter provides an overview of the tumour microenvironment in PDAC and offers insights into how targeting the microenvironment can improve patient outcomes.

Author details

Demet Kacaroglu
Lokman Hekim University, Ankara, Turkey

*Address all correspondence to: demet.kacaroglu@lokmanhekim.edu.tr

References

[1] Jelski W, Mroczko B. Biochemical diagnostics of pancreatic cancer - present and future. Clinica Chimica Acta. 2019;**498**:47-51. DOI: 10.1016/j.cca.2019.08.013

[2] Sunami Y, Häußler J, Klee J. Cellular heterogeneity of pancreatic stellate cells, mesenchymal stem cells, and cancer-associated fibroblasts in pancreatic cancer. Cancers (Basel). 2020;**12**(12): 1-15. DOI: 10.3390/cancers12123770

[3] Orth M, Metzger P, Gerum S, et al. Pancreatic ductal adenocarcinoma: Biological hallmarks, current status, and future perspectives of combined modality treatment approaches. Radiation Oncology. 2019;**14**(1):141. DOI: 10.1186/s13014-019-1345-6

[4] Carr RM, Fernandez-Zapico ME. Pancreatic cancer microenvironment, to target or not to target? EMBO Molecular Medicine. 2016;**8**(2):80-82. DOI: 10.15252/emmm.201505948

[5] Rawla P, Sunkara T, Gaduputi V. Epidemiology of pancreatic cancer: Global trends, Etiology and risk factors. World Journal of Oncology. 2019;**10**(1):10-27. DOI: 10.14740/wjon1166

[6] Van Cutsem E, Vervenne WL, Bennouna J, et al. Phase III trial of bevacizumab in combination with gemcitabine and erlotinib in patients with metastatic pancreatic cancer. Journal of Clinical Oncology. 2009;**27**(13):2231-2237. DOI: 10.1200/JCO.2008.20.0238

[7] Feig C, Gopinathan A, Neesse A, Chan DS, Cook N, Tuveson DA. The pancreas cancer microenvironment. Clinical Cancer Research. 2012;**18**(16):4266-4276. DOI: 10.1158/1078-0432.CCR-11-3114

[8] Hanahan D, Weinberg RA. Hallmarks of cancer: The next generation. Cell. 2011;**144**(5):646-674. DOI: 10.1016/J.CELL.2011.02.013

[9] Junttila MR, De Sauvage FJ. Influence of tumour micro-environment heterogeneity on therapeutic response. Nature. 2013;**501**(7467):346-354. DOI: 10.1038/nature1262

[10] Murakami T, Hiroshima Y, Matsuyama R, Homma Y, Hoffman RM, Endo I. Role of the tumor microenvironment in pancreatic cancer. Annals of Gastroenterological Surgery. 2019;**3**(2):130-137. DOI: 10.1002/ags3.12225

[11] Argentiero A, Andriano A, Caradonna IC, de Martino G, Desantis V. Decoding the intricate landscape of pancreatic cancer: Insights into tumor biology, microenvironment, and therapeutic interventions. Cancers. 2024;**16**(13):2438. DOI: 10.3390/cancers16132438

[12] Ren B, Cui M, Yang G, et al. Tumor microenvironment participates in metastasis of pancreatic cancer. Molecular Cancer. 2018;**17**(108):4-15. DOI: 10.1186/s12943-018-0858-1

[13] Incio J, Liu H, Suboj P, et al. Obesity-induced inflammation and desmoplasia promote pancreatic cancer progression and resistance to chemotherapy. Cancer Discovery. 2016;**6**(8):852. DOI: 10.1158/2159-8290.CD-15-1177

[14] Farrow B, Albo D, Berger DH. The role of the tumor microenvironment in the progression of pancreatic cancer. Journal of Surgical Research. 2008;**149**(2):319-328. DOI: 10.1016/J.JSS.2007.12.757

[15] Perdiguero EG, Geissmann F. Cancer immunology, Identifying the infiltrators. Science. 2014;**344**(6186):801-802. DOI: 10.1126/SCIENCE.1255117

[16] Baş Topcu KS. Tümör İlerlemesinde Tümör Mikroçevrenin Rolü. Türk Nöroşirürji Dergisi. 2022;**1**(98):98-104. Available from: https://www.rndsystems.com/product-highlights/ [Accessed: July 6, 2022]

[17] Landskron G, De La Fuente M, Thuwajit P, Thuwajit C, Hermoso MA. Chronic inflammation and cytokines in the tumor microenvironment. Journal of Immunology Research. 2014;**2014**:149185. DOI: 10.1155/2014/149185

[18] Le Large TYS, Bijlsma MF, Kazemier G, van Laarhoven HWM, Giovannetti E, Jimenez CR. Key biological processes driving metastatic spread of pancreatic cancer as identified by multi-omics studies. Seminars in Cancer Biology. 2017;**44**:153-169. DOI: 10.1016/j.semcancer.2017.03.008

[19] Kleeff J, Beckhove P, Esposito I, et al. Pancreatic cancer microenvironment. International Journal of Cancer. 2007;**121**(4):699-705. DOI: 10.1002/ijc.22871

[20] Monteran L, Erez N. The dark side of fibroblasts: Cancer-associated fibroblasts as mediators of immunosuppression in the tumor microenvironment. Frontiers in Immunology. 2019;**10**(AUG):1-15. DOI: 10.3389/fimmu.2019.01835

[21] Mhaidly R, Mechta-Grigoriou F. Fibroblast heterogeneity in tumor micro-environment: Role in immunosuppression and new therapies. Seminars in Immunology. 2020;**48**:101417. DOI: 10.1016/j.smim.2020.101417

[22] Pereira BA, Vennin C, Papanicolaou M, et al. CAF subpopulations: A new reservoir of stromal targets in pancreatic cancer. Trends Cancer. 2019;**5**(11):724-741. DOI: 10.1016/J.TRECAN.2019.09.010

[23] Geng X, Chen H, Zhao L, et al. Cancer-associated fibroblast (CAF) heterogeneity and targeting therapy of CAFs in pancreatic cancer. Frontiers in Cell and Development Biology. 2021;**9**:1766. DOI: 10.3389/FCELL.2021.655152/BIBTEX

[24] Pountos I, Giannoudis PV. Biology of mesenchymal stem cells. Injury. 2005;**36**(Suppl. 3):S8. DOI: 10.1016/j.injury.2005.07.028

[25] Sun Z, Wang S, Zhao RC. The roles of mesenchymal stem cells in tumor inflammatory microenvironment. Journal of Hematology and Oncology. 2014;**7**(1):1-10. DOI: 10.1186/1756-8722-7-14

[26] Jin G, Hong W, Guo Y, Bai Y, Chen B. Molecular mechanism of pancreatic stellate cells activation in chronic pancreatitis and pancreatic cancer. Journal of Cancer. 2020;**11**(6):1505. DOI: 10.7150/JCA.38616

[27] Wu Y, Zhang C, Jiang K, Werner J, Bazhin AV, D'Haese JG. The role of stellate cells in pancreatic ductal adenocarcinoma: Targeting perspectives. Front. Oncologia. 14 Jan 2021;**10**:621937. DOI: 10.3389/fonc.2020.621937

[28] Zhu S, Yang N, Wu J, et al. Tumor microenvironment-related dendritic cell deficiency: A target to enhance tumor immunotherapy. Pharmacological Research. 2020;**159**:104980. DOI: 10.1016/J.PHRS.2020.104980

[29] Wörmann SM, Diakopoulos KN, Lesina M, Algül H. The immune network in pancreatic cancer development and progression. Oncogene.

2013;**33**(23):2956-2967. DOI: 10.1038/onc.2013.257

[30] Greten TF, Manns MP, Korangy F. Myeloid derived suppressor cells in human diseases. International Immunopharmacology. 2011;**11**(7):802-807. DOI: 10.1016/J.INTIMP.2011.01.003

[31] von Itzstein MS, Burke MC, Brekken RA, Aguilera TA, Zeh HJ, Beg MS. Targeting TAM to tame pancreatic cancer. Targeted Oncology. 2020;**15**(5):579-588. DOI: 10.1007/S11523-020-00751-9/FIGURES/1

[32] Goulart MR, Stasinos K, Fincham REA, Delvecchio FR, Kocher HM. T cells in pancreatic cancer stroma. World Journal of Gastroenterology. 2021;**27**(46):7956. DOI: 10.3748/WJG.V27.I46.7956

[33] Philip M, Schietinger A. CD8+ T cell differentiation and dysfunction in cancer. Nature Reviews Immunology. 2021;**22**(4):209-223. DOI: 10.1038/s41577-021-00574-3

[34] Zhou Q, Tao X, Xia S, et al. T lymphocytes: A promising immunotherapeutic target for pancreatitis and pancreatic cancer? Frontiers in Oncology. 2020;**10**:382. DOI: 10.3389/FONC.2020.00382/BIBTEX

[35] Gao Z, Zhang Q, Zhang X, Song Y. Advance of T regulatory cells in tumor microenvironment remodeling and immunotherapy in pancreatic cancer. Eur. Journal of Inflammation. 2022;**20**:1-9. DOI: 10.1177/1721727X221092900/ASSET/IMAGES/LARGE/10.1177_1721727X221092900-FIG 1.JPEG

[36] Jin L, Kim HS, Shi J. Neutrophil in the pancreatic tumor microenvironment. Biomolecules. 2021;**11**(8):1170. DOI: 10.3390/BIOM11081170

[37] Ann Fincham RE, Delvecchio FR, Goulart MR, Sheng Yeong JP, Kocher HM. Natural killer cells in pancreatic cancer stroma. World Journal of Gastroenterology. 2021;**27**(24):3483. DOI: 10.3748/WJG.V27.I24.3483

[38] Anderson EM, Thomassian S, Gong J, Hendifar A, Osipov A. Advances in pancreatic ductal adenocarcinoma treatment. Cancers (Basel). 2021;**13**(21):5510. DOI: 10.3390/cancers13215510

[39] Özbalcı Fİ, Kaçaroğlu D, Gürbüz N. Pankreatik Duktal Adenokarsinomada Ekstrasellüler Matriks Degradasyonu Hedefli Tedavi Yaklaşımları. Sdü Sağlık Bilimleri Dergisi. 2020;**11**(June):260-265. DOI: 10.22312/sdusbed.702977

[40] Whatcott CJ, Han H, Posner RG, Hostetter G, Von Hoff DD. Targeting the tumor microenvironment in cancer: Why hyaluronidase deserves a second look. Cancer Discovery. 2011;**1**(4):291-296. DOI: 10.1158/2159-8290.CD-11-0136

[41] Sato N, Cheng XB, Kohi S, Koga A, Hirata K. Targeting hyaluronan for the treatment of pancreatic ductal adenocarcinoma. Acta Pharmaceutica Sinica B. 2016;**6**(2):101-105. DOI: 10.1016/j.apsb.2016.01.002

[42] Morohashi H, Kon A, Nakai M, et al. Study of hyaluronan synthase inhibitor, 4-methylumbelliferone derivatives on human pancreatic cancer cell (KP1-NL). Biochemical and Biophysical Research Communications. 2006;**345**(4):1454-1459. DOI: 10.1016/j.bbrc.2006.05.037

[43] Wong KM, Horton KJ, Coveler AL, Hingorani SR, Harris WP. Targeting the tumor stroma: The biology and clinical development of Pegylated recombinant human hyaluronidase (PEGPH20). Current Oncology Reports. 2017;**19**(7):47. DOI: 10.1007/s11912-017-0608-3

[44] Aslan M, Shahbazi R, Ulubayram K, Ozpolat B. Targeted therapies for pancreatic cancer and hurdles ahead. Anticancer Research. 2018;**38**(12):6591-6606. DOI: 10.21873/anticanres.13026

[45] Winer A, Adams S, Mignatti P. Matrix metalloproteinase inhibitors in cancer therapy: Turning past failures into future successes. Molecular Cancer Therapeutics. 2018;**17**(6):1147-1155. DOI: 10.1158/1535-7163.MCT-17-0646

[46] Zinger A, Koren L, Adir O, et al. Collagenase nanoparticles enhance the penetration of drugs into pancreatic Tumors. ACS Nano. 2019;**13**(10):11008-11021. DOI: 10.1021/acsnano.9b02395

[47] Perez VM, Kearney JF, Yeh JJ. The PDAC extracellular matrix: A review of the ECM protein composition, tumor cell interaction, and therapeutic strategies. Frontiers in Oncology. 6 Oct 2021;**11**:751311. DOI: 10.3389/fonc.2021.751311

[48] Lo KM, Lan Y, Lauder S, et al. huBC1-IL12, an immunocytokine which targets EDB-containing oncofetal fibronectin in tumors and tumor vasculature, shows potent anti-tumor activity in human tumor models. Cancer Immunology, Immunotherapy. 2007;**56**(4):447-457. DOI: 10.1007/s00262-006-0203-1

[49] Huang J, Zhang L, Wan D, et al. Extracellular matrix and its therapeutic potential for cancer treatment. Signal Transduction and Targeted Therapy. 23 Apr 2021;**6**(1):153. DOI: 10.1038/s41392-021-00544-0

[50] Huang X, Zhang G, Liang T. Subtyping for pancreatic cancer precision therapy. Trends in Pharmacological Sciences. 2022;**43**(6):482-494. DOI: 10.1016/j.tips.2022.03.005

[51] Topalian SL, Hodi FS, Brahmer JR, et al. Five-year survival and correlates among patients with advanced melanoma, renal cell carcinoma, or non-small cell lung cancer treated with Nivolumab. JAMA Oncology. 2019;**5**(10):1411-1420. DOI: 10.1001/jamaoncol.2019.2187

[52] Sarantis P, Koustas E, Papadimitropoulou A, Papavassiliou AG, Karamouzis MV. Pancreatic ductal adenocarcinoma: Treatment hurdles, tumor microenvironment and immunotherapy. World Journal of Gastrointestinal Oncology. 2020;**12**(2):173-181. DOI: 10.4251/wjgo.v12.i2.173

[53] Bejarano L, Jordão MJC, Joyce JA. Therapeutic targeting of the tumor microenvironment. Cancer Discovery. 2021;**11**(4):933-959. DOI: 10.1158/2159-8290.CD-20-1808

[54] Bear AS, Vonderheide RH, O'Hara MH. Challenges and opportunities for pancreatic cancer immunotherapy. Cancer Cell. 2020;**38**(6):788-802. DOI: 10.1016/j.ccell.2020.08.004

[55] Barry F, Murphy M. Mesenchymal stem cells in joint disease and repair. Nature Reviews Rheumatology. 2013;**9**(10):584-594. DOI: 10.1038/nrrheum.2013.109

[56] Liu M, O'Connor RS, Trefely S, Graham K, Snyder NW, Beatty GL. Metabolic rewiring of macrophages by CpG potentiates clearance of cancer cells and overcomes tumor-expressed CD47–mediated 'don't-eat-me' signal. Nature Immunology. 2019;**20**(3):265-275. DOI: 10.1038/s41590-018-0292-y

[57] Quail DF, Amulic B, Aziz M, et al. Neutrophil phenotypes and functions in cancer: A consensus statement. Journal of Experimental Medicine.

23 Apr 2022;**6**(1):153. DOI: 10.1084/jem.20220011

[58] Lau SP, van Montfoort N, Kinderman P, et al. Dendritic cell vaccination and CD40-agonist combination therapy licenses T cell-dependent antitumor immunity in a pancreatic carcinoma murine model. Journal for Immunotherapy of Cancer. Jul 2020;**8**(2):e000772. DOI: 10.1136/jitc-2020-000772

[59] Özdemir BC, Pentcheva-Hoang T, Carstens JL, et al. Depletion of carcinoma-associated fibroblasts and fibrosis induces immunosuppression and accelerates pancreas cancer with reduced survival. Cancer Cell. 2014;**25**(6):719-734. DOI: 10.1016/j.ccr.2014.04.005

[60] Pawitan JA, Bui TA, Mubarok W, et al. Enhancement of the therapeutic capacity of mesenchymal stem cells by genetic modification: A systematic review. Frontiers in Cell and Development Biology. 30 Oct 2020;**8**:587776. DOI: 10.3389/fcell.2020.587776

[61] Shah K. Mesenchymal stem cells engineered for cancer therapy. Advanced Drug Delivery Reviews. 2012;**64**(8):739-748. DOI: 10.1016/J.ADDR.2011.06.010

[62] Xunian Z, Kalluri R. Biology and therapeutic potential of mesenchymal stem cell-derived exosomes. Cancer Science. 2020;**111**(9):3100. DOI: 10.1111/CAS.14563

[63] Rahmatizadeh F, Aziz SGG, Khodadadi K, et al. Bidirectional and opposite effects of Naïve mesenchymal stem cells on tumor growth and progression. Advanced Pharmaceutical Bulletin. 2019;**9**(4):539. DOI: 10.15171/APB.2019.063

[64] Okumura T, Ohuchida K, Kibe S, et al. Adipose tissue-derived stromal cells are sources of cancer-associated fibroblasts and enhance tumor progression by dense collagen matrix. International Journal of Cancer. 2019;**144**(6):1401-1413. DOI: 10.1002/IJC.31775

[65] Jing W, Chen Y, Lu L, et al. Human umbilical cord blood-derived mesenchymal stem cells producing IL15 eradicate established pancreatic tumor in syngeneic mice. Molecular Cancer Therapeutics. 2014;**13**(8):2127-2137. DOI: 10.1158/1535-7163.MCT-14-0175

[66] Zhao C, Pu Y, Zhang H, et al. IL10-modified human mesenchymal stem cells inhibit pancreatic cancer growth through angiogenesis inhibition. Journal of Cancer. 2020;**11**(18):5345-5352. DOI: 10.7150/jca.38062

[67] Kabashima-Niibe A, Higuchi H, Takaishi H, et al. Mesenchymal stem cells regulate epithelial-mesenchymal transition and tumor progression of pancreatic cancer cells. Cancer Science. 2013;**104**(2):157-164. DOI: 10.1111/cas.12059

[68] Duperret EK, Trautz A, Ammons D, et al. Alteration of the tumor stroma using a consensus DNA vaccine targeting fibroblast activation protein (FAP) synergizes with antitumor vaccine therapy in mice. Clinical Cancer Research. 2018;**24**(5):1190-1201. DOI: 10.1158/1078-0432.CCR-17-2033

[69] Stouten I, van Montfoort N, Hawinkels LJAC. The tango between cancer-associated fibroblasts (CAFs) and immune cells in affecting immunotherapy efficacy in pancreatic cancer. International Journal of Molecular Sciences. 13 May 2023;**24**(10):8707. DOI: 10.3390/ijms24108707

Chapter 3

Beyond the Inflammation: Surgical Role in Pancreatitis

Vania Myralda Giamour Marbun and Karl Heinz Leonhardt Rowika

Abstract

Surgery was traditionally avoided in pancreatitis; however, aggressive interventions are now performed to manage its sequelae and complications. Key factors influencing the success of surgical management include indications, contraindications, timing, approach, and surgical goals. Carefully selecting cases and procedures is crucial for achieving favorable outcomes after the intervention is performed for managing pancreatitis. Understanding these elements is essential to optimizing patient care and eventually enhancing recovery. This chapter will explore all factors related to the surgical management of pancreatitis, providing insights into the evolving role of surgery in treating this complex condition and improving patient prognoses through targeted surgical interventions.

Keywords: pancreatitis, surgery, surgical intervention, revised Atlanta classification, complications, debridement, necrosectomy, drainage, pancreatectomy

1. Introduction

Pancreatitis has been a subject of ongoing debate, particularly regarding the role of surgical intervention. In 1886, Senn endorsed surgical treatment for acute and infected cases, while Fitz cautioned in 1889 that early surgical intervention could lead to clinical exacerbation [1]. In the past three decades, there has been a notable shift toward conservative management; however, surgical intervention remains a consideration for specific cases of pancreatitis [1–3]. Thus, surgeons must evaluate the appropriate timing and indications for surgery to determine its potential benefits for patients with this condition.

2. Acute pancreatitis

2.1 Revised Atlanta classification

Pancreatitis can be characterized through various frameworks. In 1992, a symposium in Atlanta sought to establish a global consensus and classification system for acute pancreatitis, specifically for adults over 18 years of age. However, some terminology in this classification led to confusion, prompting a revision in 2012 [4–6]. This revision aimed to align with contemporary understandings of the disease, clarify ambiguities, enhance clinical severity assessment, standardize data reporting, facilitate objective evaluation of novel treatments, and improve communication among healthcare providers. The revised classification categorizes acute pancreatitis into two types: interstitial edematous pancreatitis and necrotizing pancreatitis. Additionally, it classifies severity into three categories and outlines the imaging characteristics of peripancreatic collections that may arise as complications (**Figure 1**; **Table 1**).

2.1.1 Interstitial oedematous pancreatitis (IOP)

According to the Revised Atlanta classification, one of the mildest forms of acute pancreatitis is interstitial edematous pancreatitis, which is characterized by diffuse enlargement that is often localized and accompanied by homogeneous enhancement. This condition generally resolves within a week. Furthermore, mild stranding or haziness may be observed in the peripancreatic fat.

Contrast enhanced CT scan (CECT) criteria:

- Pancreatic parenchyma enhancement by intravenous contrast agent
- No findings of peripancreatic necrosis

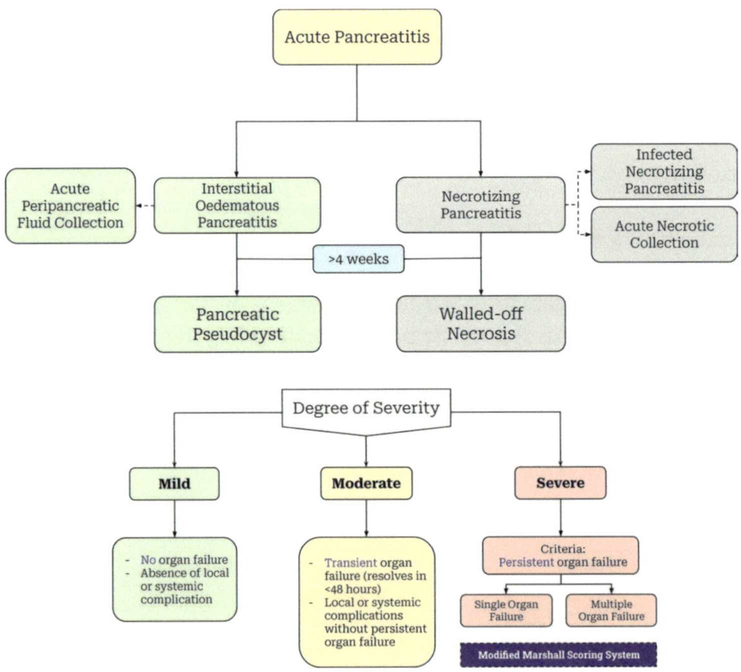

Figure 1.
Revised Atlanta classification.

Modified Marshall scoring system for organ dysfunction					
Organ System	**Score**				
	0	**1**	**2**	**3**	**4**
Respiratory (PaO2/ FiO2)	>400	301-400	201-300	101-200	≤101
Renal					
Serum creatinine mg/dl	<1.4	1.4 - 1.8	1.9 - 3.6	3.6 - 4.9	>4.9
Cardiovascular (systolic blood pressure mmHg) without inotropic support	>90	<90, fluid responsive	<90, not fluid responsive	<90, pH <7.3	<90, pH <7.2
For non-ventilated patients, the FiO2 can be estimated from below:					

Supplemental oxygen (L/min)	FiO2 (%)
Room air	21
2	25
4	30
6-8	40
9-10	50

A score of 2 or more in any system, the FiO2 defines the presence of organ failure.
A score for patients with pre-existing chronic renal failure depends on the extent of further deterioration of baseline renal function. No formal correction exists for a baseline serum creatinine ≥1,4 mg/dl

Table 1.
Modified Marshall scoring system for organ dysfunction.

2.1.2 Acute Peripancreatic fluid collection (APFC)

One week after the onset of IOP, fluid collections may form around the pancreas without any signs of necrosis. This phenomenon can occur within the first 4 weeks of the condition. It is essential to highlight that these fluid collections do not exhibit the characteristics associated with a pseudocyst.

CECT criteria:

- Occurs in IOP
- Homogeneous collection with fluid density
- Confined by normal peripancreatic fascial planes
- No definable wall encapsulating the collection
- Adjacent to the pancreas (no intrapancreatic extension)

2.1.3 Pancreatic pseudocyst

A pseudocyst represents a stage in which acute pancreatitis leads to the formation of an encapsulated fluid collection characterized by a well-defined inflammatory wall, typically exhibiting minimal or no necrosis. This condition generally arises more than 4 weeks after the initial onset of pancreatitis.

CECT criteria:

- Well-circumscribed (oval or round)
- Homogeneous fluid density
- No nonliquid component
- Well-defined wall (**Figure 2**)

2.1.4 Necrotizing pancreatitis

It is characterized by compromised pancreatic perfusion resulting in signs of necrosis that develop over several days. This condition typically begins with a patchy pattern that progresses to a non-enhancing area within the pancreatic parenchyma. The pathophysiology of necrotizing pancreatitis involves the activation of pancreatic enzymes leading to local tissue damage and inflammation, which can result in vascular compromise and necrosis of pancreatic tissue. Additionally, systemic inflammatory responses may occur, contributing to complications such as organ failure and the development of infected necrosis.

CECT criteria:

- Lack of pancreatic parenchymal enhancement by intravenous contrast and/or
- Presence of findings of peripancreatic necrosis

2.1.5 Infected necrotizing pancreatitis

An infection could develop but rarely happens during the first week. Infection can be presumed when there is extraluminal gas in the pancreatic and/or peripancreatic tissue.

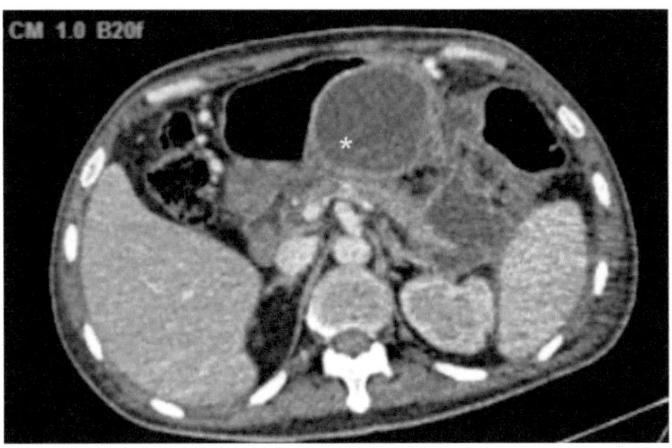

Figure 2.
Collection of fluid in the peripancreatic area. The yellow asterisk (*) shows well-circumscribed fluid collection posterior to the stomach.

Infection can be suspected when there is an extraluminal gas in the pancreatic and/or peripancreatic tissue, or a fine-needle aspiration is positive for bacteria and/or fungi.

CECT criteria:

- Extraluminal gas in the pancreatic and/or peripancreatic tissue (**Figure 3**)

2.1.6 Acute necrotic collection

Fluid collections may accumulate around the pancreas even in the context of necrotizing pancreatitis, affecting both the pancreatic parenchyma and the peripancreatic regions. These collections are characterized by the combination of necrotic tissue and fluid components that surround the necrotic area.

CECT criteria:

- Only in necrotizing pancreatitis
- Heterogeneous and nonliquid densities of varying degrees in different locations
- No definable wall
- Location - intrapancreatic and/or extrapancreatic

2.1.7 Walled-off necrosis

This condition refers to an encapsulated collection of pancreatic and/or peripancreatic necrosis that typically occurs more than 4 weeks after the onset of necrotizing pancreatitis.

CECT criteria:

- Heterogeneous collection with liquid and nonliquid density with varying degrees of loculations

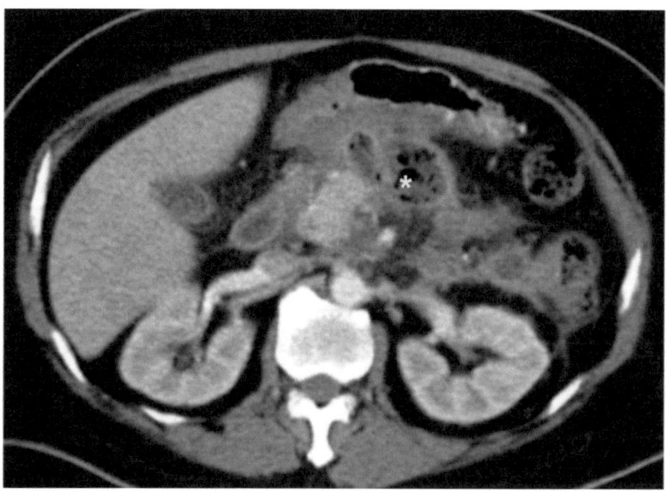

Figure 3.
Infected necrotizing pancreatitis. The yellow asterisk (*) shows extraluminal gas in the peripancreatic tissue.

- Well-defined wall
- Located in intra and/or extrapancreatic
- Maturation requires 4 weeks after onset (**Figure 4**)

2.2 Indications for surgery

2.2.1 Infected necrotizing pancreatitis

Necrotizing pancreatitis can occur in either a sterile or infected state. While infections are relatively rare within the first week after onset, prompt identification by combining clinical, radiology, and laboratory examination (**Table 2**), is essential, as it may require the implementation of aggressive therapeutic strategies alongside the administration of antibiotics.

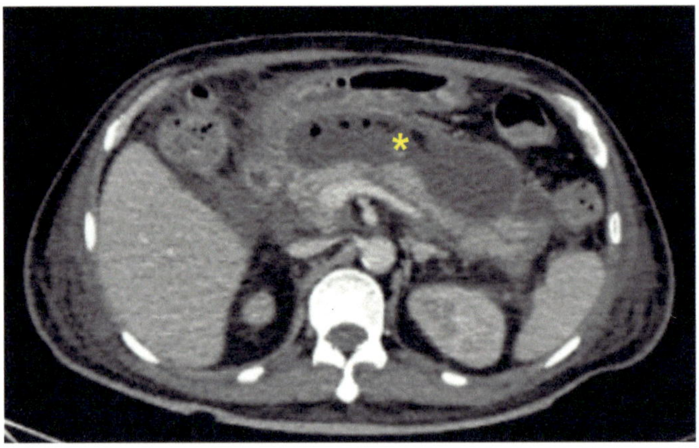

Figure 4.
Walled-off Necrotic. The yellow asterisk (*) shows a well-defined wall filled with a collection of fluid with various degrees of density.

Findings
Clinical Clinical deterioration, especially persistent for more than 10 days Fever
Radiology Gas within necrotic debris on abdominal imaging Extraluminal gas in the pancreatic and/or peripancreatic tissues on CECT Gas bubbles due to fistula to the colon, small bowel, or stomach
Laboratory [7] Increased CRP Increased procalcitonin Increased creatinine Positive for bacteria and/or fungi on Gram stain and culture - analysis from abscess drainage / fine needle aspiration

Table 2.
Findings in infected necrotizing pancreatitis.

DOI: http://dx.doi.org/10.5772/intechopen.1008541

Numerous publications advocate for conservative management, even in cases of infected pancreatitis. However, it is crucial to emphasize that when a patient's clinical condition deteriorates, surgical intervention becomes necessary to manage the worsening condition effectively [8, 9]. This highlights the importance of ongoing clinical evaluation and timely intervention in treating pancreatitis.

Although many publications have recommended delaying intervention for at least 4 weeks following the onset of symptoms to reduce the risk of postoperative complications, recent developments in minimally invasive techniques have made this recommendation less relevant [8, 10]. The timing of drainage is not a crucial factor when choosing a minimally invasive approach; thus, it is acceptable to conduct the procedure promptly upon confirmation of infection in necrotizing pancreatitis.

The "step-up approach" is the most widely accepted management strategy for infected necrotizing pancreatitis [11]. This approach begins with the administration of antibiotics, followed by percutaneous drainage. If these interventions fail, the subsequent step involves performing a minimally invasive necrosectomy (**Figure 5**) [8–10].

One of the most common initial interventions is percutaneous drainage, which targets fluid surrounding the inflamed pancreas. One key factor of successful intervention is the presence of debris. Success is also related to the volume, localization, and distribution of the fluid collection and peripancreatic necrosis.

2.2.2 Abdominal compartment syndrome

Abdominal compartment syndrome (ACS), which occurs in approximately 15–30% of acute pancreatitis, represents a significant and potentially fatal complication of necrotizing pancreatitis, with reported mortality rates ranging from 25–83% [12, 13]. This syndrome occurs due to decreased abdominal compliance, which is

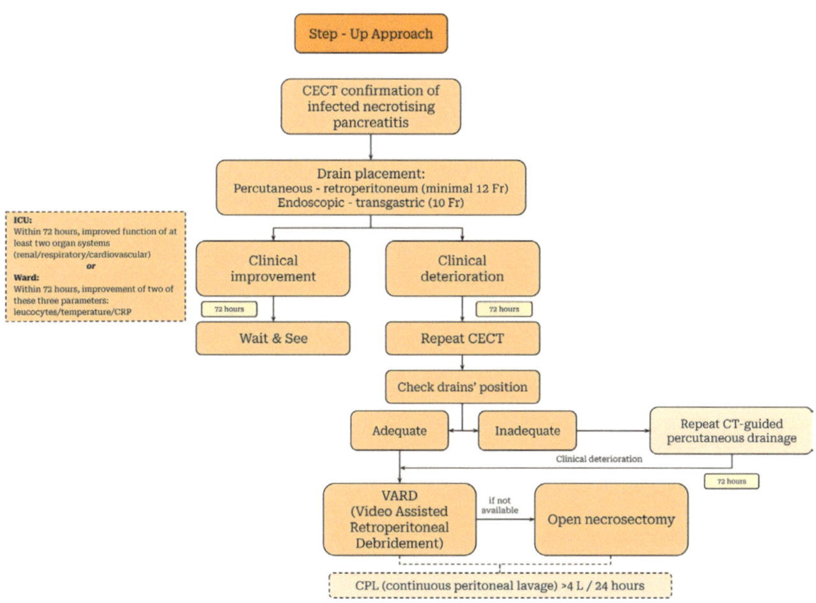

Figure 5.
Algorithm of "step-up approach".

attributed to pain and edema of the abdominal wall. The management of this condition requires timely recognition and intervention to mitigate its serious consequences (**Figure 6**; **Table 3**).

2.2.3 Vascular complications

2.2.3.1 Hemorrhage

Hemorrhage in acute pancreatitis may occur in both the peripancreatic region and distant organs. The identified causes of hemorrhage around the pancreas include (a) an erosion of adjacent vascular walls; (b) the formation of pseudoaneurysms, and (c) complications arising from surgical interventions such as debridement or necrosectomy. Autolytic pancreatic enzymes can digest surrounding visceral and vascular structures, resulting in various vascular complications.

These complications may involve both venous and arterial systems; however, direct bleeding is primarily associated with arterial involvement, whereas venous complications can lead to bleeding and thrombosis. The arteries most commonly affected in proximity to the pancreas include the splenic artery, left gastric artery, gastroduodenal artery, and pancreaticoduodenal artery [15, 16]. The hepatic and

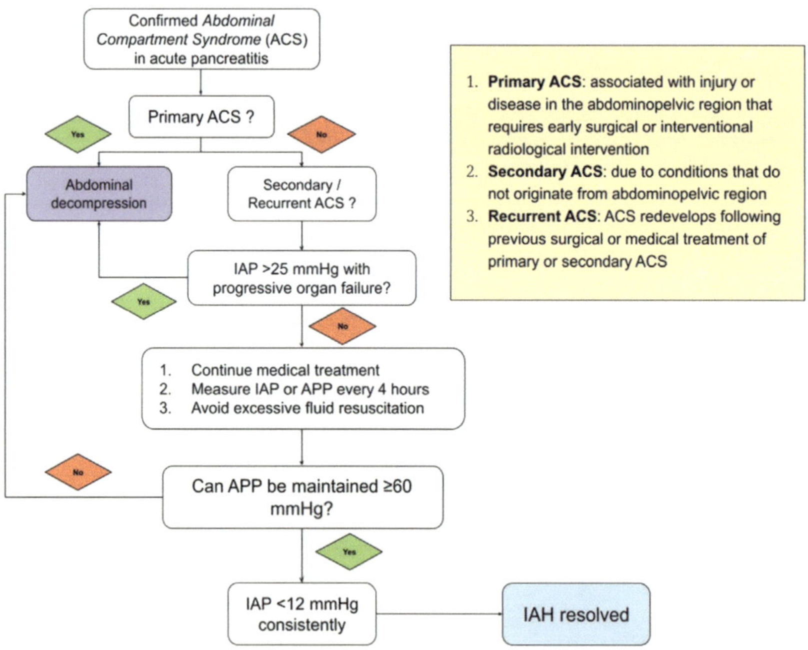

Figure 6.
Algorithm of management of ACS [14].

Important clinical findings
1. Intra-abdominal pressure ≥ 20 mmHg with failure of at least one organ system 2. Significant clinical deterioration

Table 3.
Findings in ACS.

mesenteric arteries may also be affected; however, such involvement is more commonly a consequence of postoperative leakage from pancreaticojejunostomy or iatrogenic injury during dissection or lymphadenectomy [17].

Pang proposed a classification system for peripancreatic pseudoaneurysms specifically pertaining to arterial involvement, aimed at providing a logical framework for managing this lethal complication.

As part of Pang's classification, the artery responsible for the hemorrhage must be identified to guide the initial hemostatic treatment. Embolization of the splenic, gastroduodenal, and pancreaticoduodenal arteries is associated with a low incidence of ischemic complications. Conversely, embolization of the common hepatic artery poses a risk of liver infarction, which may result in further clinical deterioration.

Embolization is considered the first-line treatment for pseudoaneurysms; however, definitive open surgical intervention may be necessary when embolization is unavailable or ineffective or when the patient's hemodynamic status is compromised (**Table 4**) [15–17].

Additionally, identifying the presence of exposure to the gastrointestinal tract and pancreatic juice is crucial for determining the most appropriate course of definitive action, whether through endoscopic or surgical intervention [17].

Hemorrhage may also occur in viscous organs as a result of an intraluminal pseudoaneurysm (IL-PSA) or the development of esophagogastric varices due to thrombosis in the splanchnic veins. Determining intraluminal PSA as the source of ongoing gastrointestinal bleeding (GIB) in severe acute pancreatitis is vital, given its considerably more adverse effects compared to GIB due to peptic ulcers or variceal rupture. Hemosuccus pancreaticus is bleeding from the ampulla of Vater as a result of ruptured parenchymal vascularization caused by the inflammation of the wall of the pancreatic duct, which requires embolization as the first-line treatment [18].

2.2.3.2 Thrombosis

Venous thrombosis is observed in 50% of cases of moderate to severe acute pancreatitis, predominantly affecting the spleno-porto-mesenteric complex, with the splenic vein being the most commonly involved vessel [16, 19]. The anatomical positioning of the splenic vein, located posterior to the body and tail of the pancreas, predisposes it to direct compression during episodes of inflammation, ultimately leading to thrombosis.

Isolated splanchnic vein thrombosis (SVT) can spontaneously recanalize with appropriate management of the underlying disease, often without antithrombotic

Pang classification of peripancreatic arterial pseudoaneurysm					
Type of artery		**Communication of GIT**		**Exposure to pancreatic juice**	
Type I	Minor artery >5 mm away from a major artery	A	No communication	1	No exposure
Type II	Major artery which may be sacrificed	B	Communication	2	Exposure
Type III	Major artery which cannot be sacrificed				

Table 4.
Pang classification of peripancreatic arterial pseudoaneurysm.

therapy. However, a watchful-waiting approach should be adopted to monitor any dynamic changes in the thrombosis [19, 20]. Approximately two-thirds of all cases of SVT may result in bowel and liver failure. Surgical intervention should be performed based on the clinical manifestations presented [16].

Arterial thrombosis is an uncommon complication of acute pancreatitis, with only a limited number of publications in medical literature addressing its management. Documented cases vary, ranging from extensive thrombus formation involving the celiac trunk and mesenteric artery to cardiac complications. Surgical intervention is indicated based on the specific complications and the involved organs, such as splenic necrosis, gastric necrosis, or bowel ischemia [16].

2.2.4 Fistula

A pancreatic fistula may develop as a result of the direct erosion of adjacent organs due to the leakage of activated exocrine enzymes from necrotizing pancreatitis. This enzymatic leakage can lead to autodigestion of the tissues, forming internal fistulas to organs such as the duodenum, stomach, pleural cavity, and pericardial space, as well as external fistulas presenting through the skin [21, 22].

Surgical intervention may be indicated in patients with persistent external fistulas, with the goal of redirecting drainage to the intestine. The surgical procedure is selected based on the anatomical location of the fistula. Fistulas originating from the head or body of the pancreas can be treated through lateral pancreaticojejunostomy. In contrast, those located in the tail of the pancreas can be effectively managed by distal pancreatectomy. Meanwhile, surgical intervention for internal fistulas should be considered when conservative management and interventional therapies have failed to achieve adequate resolution of the condition.

2.2.5 Pseudocyst

Pseudocyst is a form of long-time acute pancreatitis with acute peripancreatic fluid collection. Surgical intervention involves draining the fluid collection internally to the surrounding gastrointestinal tract through the anastomosis of the cyst to the gastric, duodenum, or jejunum.

The primary indications for surgical intervention included symptomatic pancreatic pseudocysts, presenting with manifestations such as satiety, nausea and vomiting, abdominal pain, and upper gastrointestinal bleeding, as well as complicated pancreatic pseudocysts involving factors such as compression of large vessels, gastric or duodenal outlet obstruction, stenosis of the common bile duct due to compression, and concurrent infection and hemorrhage. Persistent pseudocysts exceeding 6 cm are also considered for surgical management (**Table 5**) [24, 25].

Surgical intervention can be approached through various procedures: external drainage, internal drainage, and excision [20, 22–25]. External drainage is particularly indicated for ruptured or infected pseudocysts in patients with inoperable status. The choice of internal drainage procedure depends on the location of the pseudocyst. Roux-en-Y cysto-jejunostomy is a versatile option that can be employed regardless of the lesion's location. Cystogastrostomy is suitable for pseudocysts that are directly adherent to the posterior wall of the stomach. Additionally, cysto-duodenostomy is a viable procedure for pseudocysts situated in the head or uncinate process of the pancreas [23].

Type	Description of pancreatic pseudocyst by Pan et al. [23]
I	<5 cm and without complications, symptoms, and neoplasia
II	Suspected cystic neoplasia
III	The location of the pancreatic pseudocyst is uncinate
IIIa	Pseudocyst communication with the pancreatic duct
IIIb	Without communication between the pseudocyst and pancreatic duct
IV	The location of the pseudocyst is head, neck, and body
IVa	Exist communication between pseudocyst and pancreatic duct
IVb	Distance from the cyst to the gastrointestinal wall is <1 cm
IVc	Neither 1 nor 2
V	The location of the pseudocyst is the tail
Va	Splenic vein involvement or upper gastrointestinal bleeding
Vb	Distance from the cyst to the gastrointestinal wall is <1 cm, without splenic vein involvement or upper gastrointestinal bleeding

Table 5.
Pan classification of pancreatic pseudocyst.

2.2.6 Gallstone pancreatitis

According to the Japanese Guidelines, the recommendation for endoscopic intervention in gallstone pancreatitis is specifically applicable to patients exhibiting concurrent cholangitis [26]. Furthermore, laparoscopic cholecystectomy is recommended to be conducted promptly upon the resolution of abdominal pain related to pancreatitis or during the same hospital stay [26–29].

3. Chronic pancreatitis

Once pancreatitis has reached a certain condition, it progresses into irreversible destruction, worsening small and large ductal disease, calcification, and fibrosis. Ultimately leading to a loss of functional parenchyma and subsequent chronic pain, endocrine and/or exocrine insufficiency, and increased susceptibility to developing pancreatic ductal adenocarcinoma (PDAC).

3.1 Indications for surgery

A multidisciplinary approach is crucial for the comprehensive management of chronic pancreatitis. Numerous pathognomonic symptoms require thorough evaluation and intervention, including surgical options, thereby supporting the hypothesis that chronic pancreatitis may be regarded as a surgical disease [30–33]. Surgical procedures for managing chronic pancreatitis include (1) drainage, (2) partial resection, and (3) a combination of both techniques. The selection of these procedures is guided by the underlying pathogenesis of the related symptoms.

3.1.1 Pain

Chronic pancreatitis can be associated with pain arising from multiple etiologies, including mechanical factors, inflammation, neuropathic involvement, and visceral hyperalgesia. Among these, two predominant mechanisms warrant particular attention regarding surgical intervention: ductal hypertension and neurovascular damage. Furthermore, longstanding theories indicate that the head of the pancreas, when presenting as an inflammatory pseudotumor, may function as the "pacemaker" of significant pain in chronic pancreatitis [32–35].

In the context of minimally invasive techniques, the selection of intervention remains a subject of debate. Endoscopic pancreatic duct drainage may alleviate pain, offering a less invasive alternative for patients. However, recent studies indicate that surgical approaches may provide superior and more sustained pain relief. Therefore, careful patient selection is critical to optimize outcomes [34, 35].

3.1.2 Insufficiency of endocrine and exocrine function

The consequences of chronic pancreatitis include exocrine and endocrine insufficiency. The pancreas experiences irreversible inflammation and fibrosis, compromising its endocrine and exocrine functions. Exocrine insufficiency arises from the destruction of acinar cells, leading to a diminished production of digestive enzymes essential for nutrient digestion and absorption, potentially causing malnutrition which increases the mortality rate. Endocrine insufficiency emerges due to the damage to pancreatic islets, impairing insulin, and glucagon production, often culminating in diabetes mellitus. This dual impairment disrupts critical metabolic and digestive processes, significantly impacting the quality of life and necessitating comprehensive management strategies to mitigate its systemic effects.

3.1.3 Biliary strictures

Biliary strictures are present in 3–46% of individuals with chronic pancreatitis, and the majority of these cases can be effectively managed through endoscopic intervention before considering surgical options. The anatomical location of the stricture plays a vital role in surgical planning, influencing the decision regarding the necessity of duodenal resection.

3.1.4 Pancreatic duct stones (pancreaticolithiasis)

Stones within the pancreatic duct (**Figure** 7) are not a causative factor but rather a sequela of chronic pancreatitis. The removal of these stones should be undertaken during surgical drainage procedures, such as latero-lateral pancreaticojejunostomy.

3.1.5 Inflammatory head mass (pseudotumor)

The presence of a mass in the head of the pancreas requires consideration for resection of the pancreatic head, with the option to preserve the duodenum depending on the specific clinical circumstances. In cases where the suspicion of malignancy arises, a pancreaticoduodenectomy, a complete removal of both the pancreatic head and the duodenum, should be performed [21, 33].

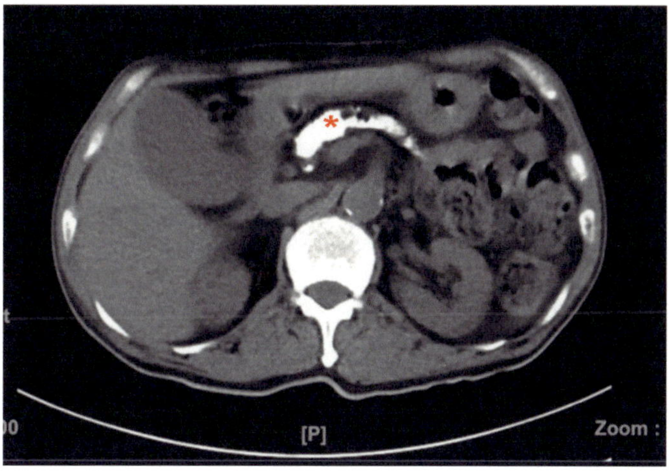

Figure 7.
Pancreatolithiasis. The red asterisk (*) shows stones inside the MPD.

3.2 Types of surgery

Numerous surgical procedures are available for the treatment of chronic pancreatitis, owing to the significant variability in its anatomical presentation. **Table 6** outlines various surgical options for managing the disease, categorized by its morphological characteristics and clinical indications.

3.2.1 Frey procedure

Charles F. Frey and G. Jeffrey Smith published this procedure in 1987 to describe a new technique of surgical drainage for chronic pancreatitis with a multiply structured main pancreatic duct, a pancreatolithiasis in an enlarged (>3,5 cm) fibrotic pancreatic

Pancreatic morphology and clinical indications	**Operation**
Main duct dilatation without inflammatory head mass	Frey procedure
Main duct dilatation with inflammatory head mass	
• Any concern for malignancy	Pancreatoduodenectomy
• No concern for malignancy	Frey procedure
Main duct dilatation and very high stone burden in the head of the pancreas	Pancreatoduodenectomy with lateral pancreaticojejunostomy
Left-sided pancreatitis with main duct disruption ("disconnected duct syndrome")	Distal pancreatectomy
Duodenal obstruction	Pancreatoduodenectomy
Common bile duct obstruction	Pancreatoduodenectomy
Hemosuccus pancreaticus	Pancreatoduodenectomy or distal pancreatectomy[a]

[a]*In the acute bleeding phase, angiographic embolization is preferred: if embolization is definitive, surgery may not be required.*

Table 6.
Type of surgeries in chronic pancreatitis according to pancreatic morphology and clinical indications.

head and uncinate process, and a dilated (≥5 mm) obstructed main pancreatic duct (MPD) in the body and tail of the pancreas [36, 37].

The key procedural steps (**Figure 8**) in this procedure include (1) complete opening of the MPD in the body and tail of the pancreas, followed by drainage into the Roux limb; (2) coring out of the head of the pancreas, preserving a rim of pancreatic tissue along the inner aspect of the first to third portions of the duodenum, while retaining 1 to 1.5 cm of the MPD within the head; (3) extension and suturing of the Roux-en-Y limb to the preserved rim of pancreatic tissue on the inner duodenal surface as well as the duct in the body and tail; and (4) maintenance of a remnant of the posterior aspect of the pancreas between the pancreas and the inferior vena cava to prevent the leakage of pancreatic secretions and jejunal contents into the retroperitoneal space [36].

3.2.2 Beger procedure/duodenum-preserving pancreatic head resection

The Beger procedure, also known as duodenum-preserving pancreatic head resection (DPPHR) (**Figure 9**), is a surgical approach designed to treat severe chronic

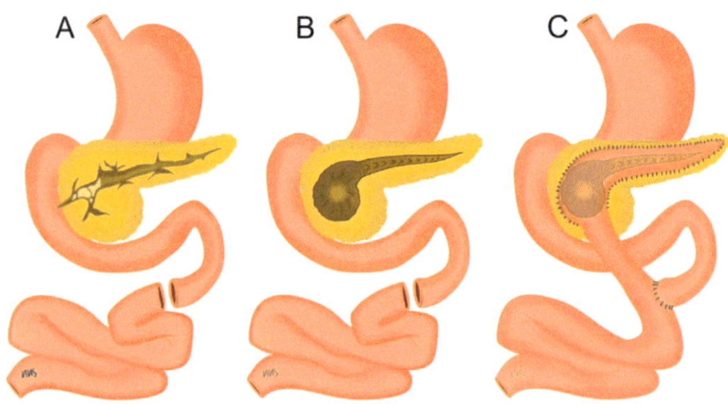

Figure 8.
Frey procedure. (A) Chronic pancreatitis with stricture and stone. (B) Coring out the head of the pancreas and complete opening of the MPD. (C) Roux-en-Y lateral pancreaticojejunostomy.

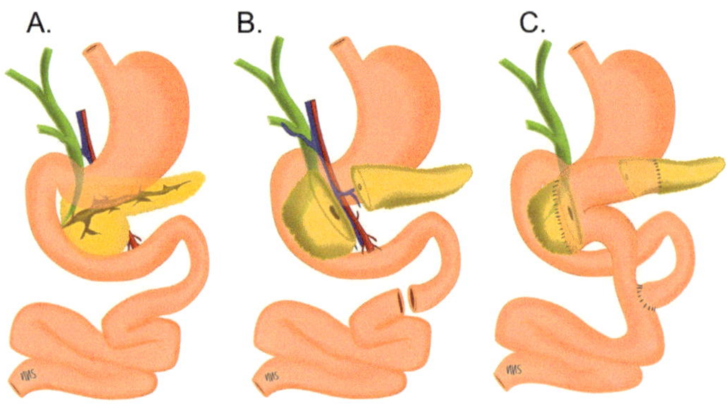

Figure 9.
Beger procedure. (A) Chronic pancreatitis with the enlarged head of the pancreas and dilated bile duct due to compression. (B) Transection of the head of the pancreas started from the duodenal side of the portal vein. (C) Roux-en-Y anastomosis of the remnant left pancreas to the jejunum, with anastomosis of duct-to-mucosa first. Jejunum is also sutured to the remnant head of the pancreas without anastomosis to the duct. If the resection of the pancreatic head does not successfully relieve the bile duct obstruction, an additional anastomosis may be required to restore bile flow.

pancreatitis associated with inflammatory enlargement of the pancreatic head. This technique involves excision of the affected portion while preserving important structures such as the duodenum, stomach, and bile duct, offering a less extensive alternative to procedures like the Whipple operation. Treating the inflammatory mass can simultaneously relieve symptoms such as bile duct obstruction and duodenal stenosis while preserving pancreatic endocrine and exocrine functions [38, 39].

The surgical procedure begins with a laparotomy, allowing access to the pancreas. The pancreatic head is carefully isolated, and any inflammatory or fibrotic tissue is excised to decompress adjacent structures, including the common bile duct, portal vein, and duodenum. The pancreas is dissected at the level of the portal vein, with the pancreatic head meticulously excised while preserving the duodenum, leaving a thin layer of pancreatic tissue intact to maintain its structure. If bile duct obstruction is present, the bile duct may be opened, and an internal anastomosis is performed with the resected pancreatic head to restore biliary flow. Reconstruction is then completed with two key anastomoses: the first connects the pancreatic tail remnant to a Roux-en-Y jejunal loop, and the second links the excavated pancreatic head to the same jejunal loop, ensuring effective drainage and restoration of pancreatic and biliary function [38, 39].

3.2.3 Puestow procedure and its modification

In 1958, Puestow and Gillesby introduced lateral (longitudinal) pancreatico-jejunostomy as a surgical intervention for symptomatic chronic pancreatitis in patients with pancreatic ductal obstruction and a dilated MPD. For this procedure to be feasible, the MPD must have a diameter of at least 6 mm in the body of the pancreas. This procedure involves several primary steps: (1) a resection of the tail of the pancreas, splenectomy, and transversal incision until the duct is exposed; (2) a longitudinal incision along the MPD to facilitate drainage of its contents and relieve pressure caused by obstruction or inflammation; and (3) implantation of the tail of the pancreas into the Roux-en-Y limb of the jejunum [40, 41].

This approach, while effectively decompressing the pancreatic duct, posed challenges in patients with significant adhesions or portal hypertension, as splenectomy could exacerbate these conditions and increase the risk of vascular complications. The modification of the Puestow-Gillesby procedure was essential due to its complexity and associated risks, particularly the removal of the spleen and tail of the pancreas, which could lead to the loss of valuable pancreatic tissue and potential complications [42, 43].

The Partington-Rochelle modification, introduced in 1960, simplified the Puestow-Gillesby procedure by eliminating the need for distal pancreatectomy and splenectomy. This technique preserves the spleen and tail of the pancreas, thereby retaining endocrine function and reducing the risk of complications associated with splenectomy. Instead, the modification involved creating a direct anastomosis between the longitudinally incised pancreatic duct and a Roux-en-Y jejunal loop without resection of the pancreatic tissue. By focusing on ductal decompression while minimizing the extent of surgical dissection, this approach offered a safer and more efficient solution for patients with chronic pancreatitis [42, 43].

The primary steps of the Partington-Rochelle procedure involve (1) exposing the anterior surface of the pancreas to access the dilated pancreatic duct; (2) a longitudinal incision is made along the duct extending toward the head and tail (depending on the extent of the obstruction); (3) a Roux-en-Y jejunal limb is

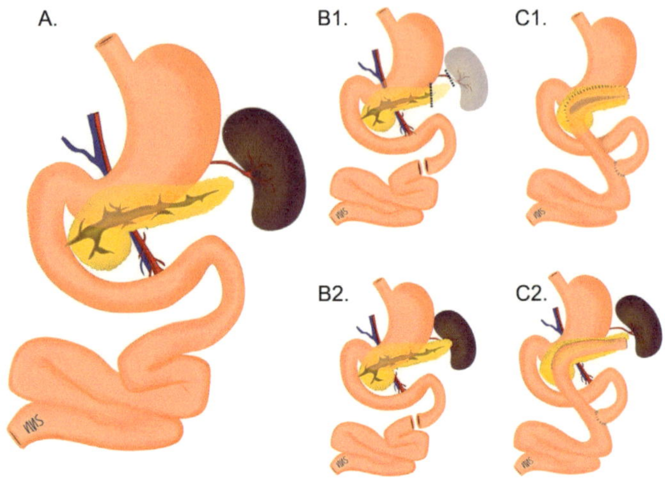

Figure 10.
Puestow procedure and its modification. (A) Chronic pancreatitis. (B1) Puestow-Gillesby procedure; resection of the tail of the pancreas, splenectomy, and complete opening of the MPD. (B2) Partington-Rochele-modified Puestow procedure; no resection of the tail of the pancreas and spleen-preserving. [C1 = C2] Roux-en-Y lateral pancreaticojejunostomy.

prepared and positioned adjacent to the opened duct; and (4) the jejunum is then longitudinally incised to match the duct opening, and the anastomosis is secured with sutures, ensuring proper alignment for effective drainage. This modification not only facilitates drainage but also preserves pancreatic tissue and reduces operative risks (**Figure 10**) [42, 43].

3.2.4 Other resection

Several surgical procedures can be performed for the management of chronic pancreatitis, depending on the morphological changes observed, including proximal, distal, and total pancreatectomy (**Table 7**) [21, 33, 44].

	Indications	**Contraindications**
Proximal pancreatectomy	• Small-duct disease • Biliary obstruction • Gastrointestinal obstruction • Pancreatic obstruction • Symptomatic pseudocyst	• Anatomic concerns • Celiac axis stenosis requiring revascularization • Portal vein thrombosis/stenosis with venous collateralization
Distal pancreatectomy	• Disconnected duct • Symptomatic pseudocyst	• Degree of peripancreatic inflammation • Encasement/abutment of major vascular structures
Total pancreatectomy	• Diffuse small-duct disease • Symptomatic hereditary pancreatitis	• Ongoing toxic exposures • Smoking/nicotine dependence • Alcohol abuse

Table 7.
Resection of the pancreas for chronic pancreatitis.

4. Conclusions

The surgical management of pancreatitis has evolved, transitioning from a primarily conservative approach to a more targeted and interventional strategy guided by classifications such as the Revised Atlanta Classification. Minimally invasive approaches are favored for acute complications, while chronic pancreatitis requires a multidisciplinary approach with tailored surgical options balancing minimally invasive techniques and more extensive procedures to optimize patient outcomes.

Acknowledgements

ChatGPT for its assistance in correcting grammar and rephrasing English sentences

Nafilla Nesantya Sabatini, MD for her exceptional skills and dedication in creating detailed drawings and sketches of surgical procedures. Her quick responsiveness and artistry have greatly enhanced the visual understanding and educational value of this work.

Clarissa Agdelina, MD for her invaluable assistance and outstanding efforts in locating hard-to-find journals that were not available online. Her resourcefulness has been crucial in supporting this chapter.

Conflict of interest

The authors declare no conflict of interest.

Author details

Vania Myralda Giamour Marbun[1*] and Karl Heinz Leonhardt Rowika[2]

1 Cipto Mangunkusumo Hospital, Jakarta, Indonesia

2 Faculty of Medicine, University of Indonesia, Jakarta, Indonesia

*Address all correspondence to: vania.myralda@gmail.com

References

[1] Ranson JHC. The role of surgery in management of acute pancreatitis. Annals of Surgery. 1990;**211**(4):382-393

[2] Heckler M, Hackert T, Hu K, HalloranCM,BüchlerMW,NeoptolemosJP. Severe acute pancreatitis: Surgical indications and treatment. Langenbeck's Archives of Surgery. 2021;**406**(3):521-535

[3] Alzerwi N. Surgical management of acute pancreatitis: Historical perspectives, challenges, and current management approaches. World Journal of Gastrointestinal Surgery. 2023;**15**(3):307-322

[4] Thoeni RF. The revised Atlanta classification of acute pancreatitis: Its importance for the radiologist and its effect on treatment. Radiology. 2012;**262**(3):751-764

[5] Banks PA, Bollen TL, Dervenis C, Gooszen HG, Johnson CD, Sarr MG, et al. Classification of acute pancreatitis—2012: Revision of the Atlanta classification and definitions by international consensus. Gut. 2013;**62**(1):102-111

[6] Foster BR, Jensen KK, Bakis G, Shaaban AM, Coakley FV. Revised Atlanta classification for acute pancreatitis: A pictorial essay. Radiographics. 2016;**36**(3):675-687

[7] Wiese ML, Urban S, Von Rheinbaben S, Frost F, Sendler M, Weiss FU, et al. Identification of early predictors for infected necrosis in acute pancreatitis. BMC Gastroenterology. 2022;**22**(1):405

[8] Boxhoorn L, Van Dijk SM, Van Grinsven J, Verdonk RC, Boermeester MA, Bollen TL, et al. Immediate versus postponed intervention for infected necrotizing pancreatitis. The New England Journal of Medicine. 2021;**385**(15):1372-1381

[9] Mahapatra SJ, Garg PK. Navigating the stormy sea of infected necrotizing pancreatitis: Are we there yet? Well almost! Gastroenterology. 2022;**163**(3):578-581

[10] Rasslan R, Novo FDCF, Bitran A, Utiyama EM, Rasslan S. Management of infected pancreatic necrosis: State of the art. Revista do Colégio Brasileiro de Cirurgiões. 2017;**44**(5):521-529

[11] Besselink MG, Van Santvoort HC, Nieuwenhuijs VB, Boermeester MA, Bollen TL, Buskens E, et al. Minimally invasive "step-up approach" versus maximal necrosectomy in patients with acute necrotising pancreatitis (PANTER trial): Design and rationale of a randomised controlled multicenter trial [ISRCTN13975868]. BMC Surgery. 2006;**6**(1):6

[12] Siebert M, Le Fouler A, Sitbon N, Cohen J, Abba J, Poupardin E. Management of abdominal compartment syndrome in acute pancreatitis. Journal of Visceral Surgery. 2021;**158**(5):411-419

[13] Zarnescu NO, Dumitrascu I, Zarnescu EC, Costea R. Abdominal compartment syndrome in acute pancreatitis: A narrative review. Diagnostics. 2022;**13**(1):1

[14] The Pediatric Guidelines Sub-Committee for the World Society of the Abdominal Compartment Syndrome, Kirkpatrick AW, Roberts DJ, De Waele J, Jaeschke R, Malbrain MLNG, et al. Intra-abdominal hypertension and the abdominal compartment syndrome:

Updated consensus definitions and clinical practice guidelines from the world society of the abdominal compartment syndrome. Intensive Care Medicine. 2013;**39**(7):1190-1206

[15] Gupta V, Krishna P, Kochhar R, Yadav TD, Bargav V, Bhalla A, et al. Hemorrhage complicating the course of severe acute pancreatitis. Annals of Hepato-Biliary-Pancreatic Surgery. 2020;**24**(3):292-300

[16] Kalas MA, Leon M, Chavez LO, Canalizo E, Surani S. Vascular complications of pancreatitis. World Journal of Clinical Cases. 2022;**10**(22):7665-7673

[17] Pang TCY, Maher R, Gananadha S, Hugh TJ, Samra JS. Peripancreatic pseudoaneurysms: A management-based classification system. Surgical Endoscopy. 2014;**28**(7):2027-2038

[18] Tarar ZI, Khan HA, Inayat F, Goraya MHN, Raza M, Ibrahim F, et al. Hemosuccus pancreaticus: A comprehensive review of presentation patterns, diagnostic approaches, therapeutic strategies, and clinical outcomes. Journal of Investigative Medicine High Impact Case Reports. 2022;**10**:23247096211070388

[19] Pancreas Study Group, Chinese Society of Gastroenterology, Chinese Medical Association. Practice guidance for diagnosis and treatment of pancreatitis-related splanchnic vein thrombosis (Shenyang, 2020). Journal of Digestive Diseases. 2021;**22**(1):2-8

[20] Nawacki Ł, Matykiewicz J, Stochmal E, Głuszek S. Splanchnic vein thrombosis in acute pancreatitis and its consequences. Clinical and Applied Thrombosis/Hemostasis. 2021;**27**:10760296211010260

[21] Beger HG, Büchler MW, Neoptolemos JP, editors. The Pancreas: An Integrated Textbook of Basic Science, Medicine, and Surgery. 3rd ed. Hoboken, N.J. Chichester, West Sussex: Wiley Blackwell; 2018. 1 p. [Wiley online library]

[22] Liu Z, Ke H, Xiong Y, Liu H, Yue M, Liu P. Gastrointestinal fistulas in necrotizing pancreatitis receiving a step-up approach incidence, risk factors, outcomes and treatment. Journal of Inflammation Research. 2023;**16**:5531-5543

[23] Pan G, Wan MH, Xie KL, Li W, Hu WM, Liu XB, et al. Classification and management of pancreatic pseudocysts. Medicine. 2015;**94**:24

[24] Tan JH, Chin W, Shaikh AL, Zheng S. Pancreatic pseudocyst: Dilemma of its recent management (review). Experimental and Therapeutic Medicine. 2021;**21**(2):159

[25] AgalianosC,PassasI,SiderisI,DavidesD, Dervenis C. Review of management options for pancreatic pseudocysts. Translational Gastroenterology and Hepatology. 2018;**3**:18-18

[26] Kimura Y, Takada T, Kawarada Y, Hirata K, Mayumi T, Yoshida M, et al. JPN guidelines for the management of acute pancreatitis: Treatment of gallstone-induced acute pancreatitis. Journal of Hepato-Biliary-Pancreatic Surgery. 2006;**13**(1):56-60

[27] Wilson CT, De Moya MA. Cholecystectomy for acute gallstone pancreatitis: Early vs delayed approach. Scandinavian Journal of Surgery. 2010;**99**(2):81-85

[28] Kundumadam S, Fogel EL, Gromski MA. Gallstone pancreatitis: General clinical approach and the role of endoscopic retrograde

cholangiopancreatography. The Korean Journal of Internal Medicine. 2021;**36**(1):25-31

[29] Isogai M. Pathophysiology of severe gallstone pancreatitis: A new paradigm. World Journal of Gastroenterology. 2024;**30**(7):614-623

[30] Beyer G, Habtezion A, Werner J, Lerch MM, Mayerle J. Chronic pancreatitis. The Lancet. 2020;**396**(10249):499-512

[31] Ashraf H, Colombo JP, Marcucci V, Rhoton J, Olowoyo O. A clinical overview of acute and chronic pancreatitis: The medical and surgical management. Cureus. 2021;**13**(11):e19764

[32] Bouwense SAW, Kempeneers MA, van Santvoort HC, Boermeester MA, van Goor H, Besselink MG, et al. Surgery in chronic pancreatitis: Indication, timing and procedures. Visceral Medicine. 2019;**35**(2):110-118

[33] Zafar HB. Surgical management of chronic pancreatitis: A systemic review. Cureus. 2023;**15**(3):e35806

[34] Skube ME, Beilman GJ. Surgical treatment of pain in chronic pancreatitis. Current Opinion in Gastroenterology. 2018;**34**(5):317-321

[35] Issa Y, Boermeester MA. Management of chronic pancreatitis: More pain than gain? The British Journal of Surgery. 2021;**108**(12):1397-1399

[36] Frey CF, Smith GJ. Description and rationale of a new operation for chronic pancreatitis. Pancreas. 1987;**2**(6):701-707

[37] Ray S, Basu C, Dhali A, Dhali GK. Frey procedure for chronic pancreatitis: A narrative review. Annals of Medicine and Surgery (Lond). 4 Aug 2022;**80**:104229

[38] Beger HG, BüCHLER M, Bittner RR, Oettinger W, Roscher R. Duodenum-preserving resection of the head of the pancreas in severe chronic pancreatitis: Early and late results. Annals of Surgery. 1989;**209**(3):273-278

[39] Beger HG, Schlosser W, Friess HM, Büchler MW. Duodenum-preserving head resection in chronic pancreatitis changes the natural course of the disease: A single-center 26-year experience. Annals of Surgery. 1999;**230**(4):512

[40] Puestow CB. Retrograde surgical drainage of pancreas for chronic relapsing pancreatitis. Archives of Surgery. 1958;**76**(6):898

[41] Fragulidis GP, Vezakis A, Dellaportas D, Sotirova I, Koutoulidis V, Kontis E, et al. Puestow modified procedure in the era of advanced endoscopic interventions for the management of chronic lithiasic pancreatitis. A two cases report. International Journal of Surgery Case Reports. 2015;**15**:85-88

[42] Partington PF, Rochelle REL. Modified Puestow procedure for retrograde drainage of the pancreatic duct*. Annals of Surgery. 1960;**152**(6):1037-1043

[43] Ceppa EP, Pappas TN. Modified Puestow lateral pancreaticojejunostomy. Journal of Gastrointestinal Surgery. 2009;**13**(5):1004-1008

[44] Andersen DK, Frey CF. The evolution of the surgical treatment of chronic pancreatitis. Annals of Surgery. 2010;**251**(1):18-32

Chapter 4

Emergency Management of Patients with Acute Pancreatitis

Nazir Najeeb Kapadia

Abstract

Abdominal pain is one of the common presentations presented to the emergency department. Acute pancreatitis is one of the lethal causes in that list of differential diagnoses of patients with abdominal pain. Identifying and managing such patients in a timely fashion is of utmost importance. Emergency diagnosis and management can be critical in predicting mortality, and the help of scores can guide physicians in prompt management. This chapter will help the readers recognize the presentation, diagnosis/early recognition, and severity of acute pancreatitis in patients. Furthermore, the chapter will focus on the emergency management of such critical patients and deciding their disposition.

Keywords: acute pancreatitis, emergency management, mortality scores, Ranson score, BISAP score

1. Introduction

One of the most common pathologies diagnosed in patients presenting with abdominal pain coming to the emergency department (ED) is acute pancreatitis (AP), which is a major surgical challenge, with the most common triggering factor being gallstones [1]. It is the inflammation of the pancreas in which there is sudden activation of pancreatic enzymes, which self-digest and self-destruct the pancreas itself (**Figure 1**). It is self-limiting in the majority of cases and requires only symptomatic treatment, but severe disease is present in 20–30% of cases that can progress to systemic inflammation and cause life-threatening necrosis of the pancreas, multi-organ failure, and can potentially lead to death [2].

AP can lead to significant morbidity and mortality. It is characterized by abdominal pain, elevated pancreatic enzymes, and systemic complications that may arise rapidly [3]. The incidence of AP has been rising, particularly in Western countries, with estimates suggesting an occurrence of 34 cases per 100,000 population annually [4]. The two most common etiologies are gallstones and chronic alcohol consumption, though other causes such as medications, trauma, and metabolic disorders also play a role [5].

The management of AP in the emergency setting is critical, as early intervention can significantly impact patient outcomes. Timely assessment and treatment can prevent

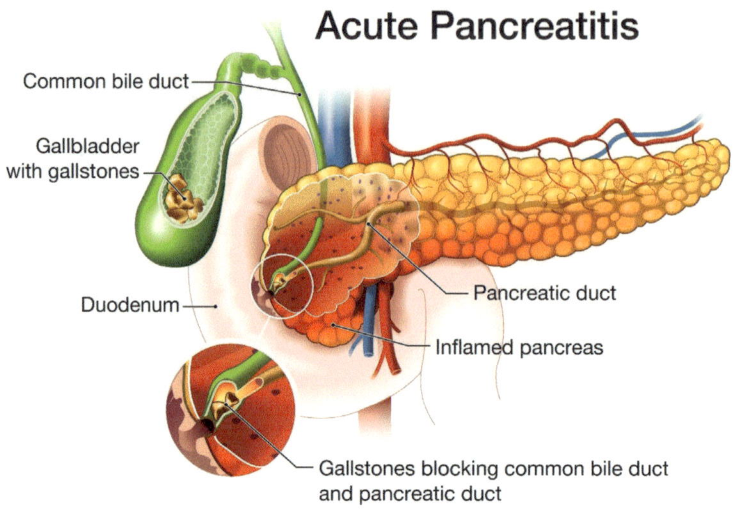

Figure 1.
Illustration of acute pancreatitis: This diagram highlights the inflamed pancreas, the role of gallstones in obstructing the common bile and pancreatic ducts, and the relationship between the pancreas, gallbladder, and duodenum.

the progression of the disease, reduce complications, and improve survival rates. The initial approach generally involves supportive care, including fluid resuscitation, pain management, and nutritional support [6]. Given the varied presentations and potential complications of AP, healthcare providers must be well-versed in the latest guidelines and evidence-based practices to deliver effective emergency management.

A clinically-based classification system, the Atlanta Classification, is widely used and accepted universally [7]. Quick, accurate, and early evidence-based risk stratification of patients allows early initiation of intensive care therapy for patients with severe AP to prevent adverse outcomes, like severe disease and mortality [7]. Therefore, a tool that reliably stratifies risk in predicting the severity and prognoses of AP is of great importance when it comes to managing AP patients [1].

2. Pathophysiology of acute pancreatitis

AP is a complex clinical condition characterized by the sudden onset of inflammation in the pancreas (**Figure 2**). The pathophysiology involves a series of interrelated processes that lead to pancreatic injury and systemic complications.

2.1 Mechanisms of injury

1. Acinar cell injury: The initial event in AP typically occurs within the pancreatic acinar cells. This results in acinar cell damage and the release of digestive enzymes into the pancreatic interstitium, causing autodigestion of pancreatic tissue [8].

2. Inflammatory response: Following acinar cell injury, a local inflammatory response is triggered. This involves the recruitment of inflammatory cells, including neutrophils and macrophages, to the site of injury. The release of pro-inflammatory cytokines, such as tumor necrosis factor-alpha and interleukin-6, further

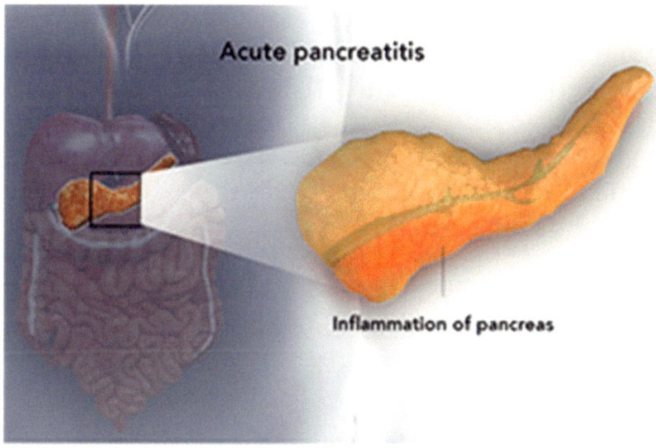

Figure 2.
Acute pancreatitis: This image illustrates the pancreas and highlights the area of inflammation, emphasizing the condition's impact on digestive health.

amplifies the inflammatory response and can lead to systemic inflammatory response syndrome if the response is excessive [8].

2.2 Systemic complications

In severe cases, the inflammatory response can extend beyond the pancreas, leading to complications such as multiple organ dysfunction syndrome. The systemic release of inflammatory mediators can cause vascular permeability changes, leading to edema and potentially resulting in shock and organ failure [8, 9].

2.3 Role of gut microbiota

Emerging research suggests that alterations in gut microbiota may influence the severity of acute pancreatitis. Dysbiosis can exacerbate the inflammatory response and contribute to the development of complications, indicating a potential area for therapeutic intervention [10].

Understanding the pathophysiology of AP is crucial for developing effective management strategies. The interplay between local pancreatic injury, inflammatory responses, and systemic complications underscores the complexity of this condition and the need for timely intervention to mitigate its effects.

3. Clinical presentation of acute pancreatitis

AP is characterized by a range of clinical symptoms and signs that can vary in severity.

3.1 Symptoms

1. Abdominal pain: The hallmark symptom of AP is severe abdominal pain, typically located in the epigastric region. This pain may radiate to the back and is often described as a constant, sharp, or stabbing sensation [11].

2. Nausea and vomiting: Most patients experience nausea and vomiting, which can be persistent and may not provide relief from the abdominal pain. This symptom often accompanies the onset of pain [11].

3. Fever: A low-grade fever may be present, reflecting the inflammatory process occurring within the pancreas. In more severe cases, high fever may indicate complications such as infection [11].

4. Jaundice: In cases where gallstones are the underlying cause, patients may present with jaundice due to bile duct obstruction. This can lead to elevated bilirubin levels and associated symptoms [11].

5. Abdominal distension: Physical examination may reveal abdominal distension, which can be due to fluid accumulation or ileus (a temporary cessation of bowel activity).

3.2 Signs

1. Tachycardia and hypotension: Patients may exhibit signs of systemic involvement, including tachycardia (increased heart rate) and hypotension (low blood pressure), particularly in cases of severe AP or when complications arise [11].

2. Guarding and rigidity: On examination, patients may exhibit abdominal guarding or rigidity, indicating peritoneal irritation. This can be a sign of complications such as pancreatitis-related necrosis or abscess formation [11].

3. Gray Turner's sign and Cullen's sign: These are rare but significant signs of hemorrhagic pancreatitis. Gray Turner's sign refers to bruising of the flanks, while Cullen's sign refers to periumbilical bruising (**Figure 3**). Both indicate severe pancreatic inflammation and potential necrosis [11].

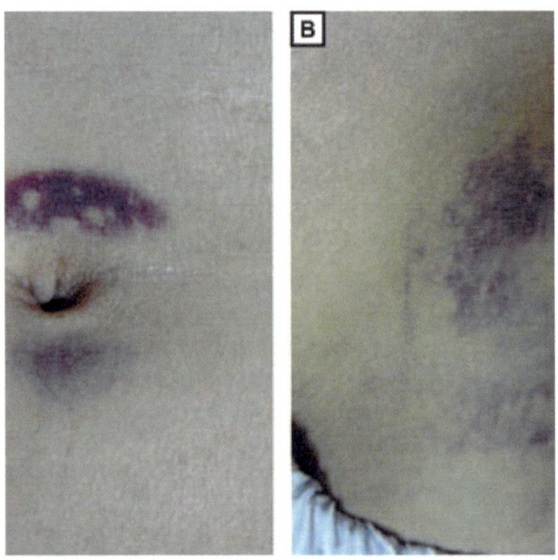

Figure 3.
Cutaneous manifestations of acute pancreatitis: The image shows areas of bruising (ecchymosis) around the abdomen, which indicates severe pancreatitis and associated complications.

4. Respiratory distress: In severe cases, patients may develop respiratory distress due to pleural effusions or acute respiratory distress syndrome, which can complicate the clinical picture [11].

A combination of severe abdominal pain, gastrointestinal symptoms, and systemic signs of inflammation characterizes the clinical presentation of AP. Early recognition and management of these symptoms are crucial to improving patient outcomes and preventing complications.

4. Initial assessment and diagnosis of acute pancreatitis

The initial assessment and diagnosis of AP are critical for effective management and treatment. This process involves a combination of clinical evaluation, laboratory tests, and imaging studies.

4.1 Clinical evaluation

1. History taking: A thorough medical history is essential. Key points to inquire about include:

    - Onset, duration, and character of abdominal pain (typically severe and located in the epigastric region).

    - Associated symptoms such as nausea, vomiting, fever, and changes in bowel habits.

    - Risk factors including alcohol consumption, gallstone disease, recent surgeries, and medication use [12].

2. Physical examination: The physical examination should focus on:

    - Abdominal tenderness, guarding, and rigidity.

    - Signs of systemic involvement, such as tachycardia and hypotension.

    - Specific signs like Gray Turner's sign or Cullen's sign may indicate hemorrhagic pancreatitis [12].

4.2 Laboratory tests

1. Serum amylase and lipase: The diagnosis of AP typically requires at least two of the following three criteria:

    - Elevated serum lipase or amylase levels, with lipase being more specific for pancreatic injury. Levels are usually three times the upper limit of normal [12].

    - Amylase is the marker in the first 24 hours, whereas lipase gets an elevation after 24 hours, with lipase being more specific for acute pancreatitis.

2. Additional blood tests: Other laboratory tests may include:

    - Complete blood count (CBC) to assess for leukocytosis.
    - Liver function tests to evaluate for biliary obstruction.
    - Electrolytes, blood urea nitrogen (BUN), and creatinine to assess renal function [12].

4.3 Imaging studies

1. Ultrasound: Abdominal ultrasound is often the first imaging modality used. It can help identify gallstones, biliary duct obstruction, and fluid collections around the pancreas [12].

2. Computed tomography (CT): If the diagnosis is uncertain or if there are complications suspected, a CT scan of the abdomen is performed. CT is particularly useful for assessing the severity of pancreatitis and identifying complications such as necrosis or abscess formation [12].

3. Magnetic resonance imaging (MRI): MRI may be used in specific cases, especially when there is a need to evaluate the biliary tree or when CT is contraindicated [12].

4.4 Diagnosis

The diagnosis of AP is confirmed when at least two of the following criteria are met:

- Characteristic abdominal pain.
- Elevated serum lipase or amylase levels.
- Imaging findings consistent with pancreatitis [12].

The initial assessment and diagnosis of AP involve a comprehensive approach that includes a detailed history, physical examination, laboratory tests, and imaging studies. Timely and accurate diagnosis is essential for effective management and to prevent complications.

5. Emergency management protocols of acute pancreatitis

The emergency management of AP is crucial for minimizing complications and improving patient outcomes. The management protocols are based on the severity of the condition and involve a multidisciplinary approach. Emergency management always starts with an ABC approach to managing a patient in the emergency department. Addressing a pattern of airway, breathing, and circulation to address the thing that can kill first, also this approach helps clinicians not to miss out on anything more crucial to be managed in the golden hour. Here are the key components of emergency management:

5.1 Initial assessment and stabilization

- Vital signs monitoring: Continuous monitoring of vital signs is essential to detect any signs of shock or respiratory distress early.

- Fluid resuscitation: Aggressive intravenous (IV) fluid resuscitation is critical, especially in the first 24–48 hours. Crystalloids (e.g., normal saline or lactated Ringer's solution) are typically used to maintain hemodynamic stability and prevent hypovolemia [13].

5.2 Pain management

- Analgesics: Pain control is a priority. Opioids are commonly used for severe pain management. The choice of analgesic should be tailored to the patient's needs, considering the potential for side effects.

5.3 Nutritional support

- NPO status: Patients are usually kept nil per oral (NPO) initially to allow the pancreas to rest. This is typically maintained for 24–48 hours, depending on the severity of the pancreatitis and the patient's clinical status.

- Enteral nutrition: If the patient is stable and there are no contraindications, early enteral nutrition (*via* a nasogastric tube or jejunal feeding) is recommended to promote gut integrity and reduce the risk of infection [13].

5.4 Management of complications

- Monitoring for complications: Regular assessment for complications such as necrotizing pancreatitis, abscess formation, or organ failure is essential. This may involve repeat imaging studies and laboratory tests [13].

- Infectious complications: If infection is suspected, broad-spectrum antibiotics may be initiated, particularly in cases of necrotizing pancreatitis.

5.5 Disposition

- Patients with AP usually require admission and the level of care depends on the severity of disease.

5.6 Surgical interventions

- Indications for surgery: Surgical intervention may be necessary in cases of severe AP with complications such as infected necrosis or abscesses. The timing of surgery is critical and should be based on the patient's clinical condition and the extent of pancreatic necrosis [13].

- Drainage procedures: Percutaneous drainage of fluid collections may be performed as a minimally invasive approach before considering more extensive surgical options.

5.7 Special considerations

- Management of underlying causes: Identifying and addressing the underlying cause of AP (e.g., gallstones and alcohol use) is essential for preventing recurrence. This may involve surgical intervention for gallstones or counseling for alcohol cessation [13].

Emergency management of AP requires a systematic approach that includes stabilization, pain management, nutritional support, monitoring for complications, timely surgical intervention and disposition of patient when necessary. Adhering to these protocols can significantly improve patient outcomes and reduce the risk of severe complications.

6. Mortality scores used in emergency department for acute pancreatitis

AP is a potentially life-threatening condition that requires prompt assessment and management in the ED. Various scoring systems have been developed to predict mortality and morbidity associated with acute pancreatitis, helping clinicians make informed decisions regarding patient care. Here are some of the key mortality scores utilized in the ED setting:

6.1 Ranson's criteria

Ranson's criteria is one of the earliest scoring systems developed for assessing the severity of acute pancreatitis. It includes a set of clinical and laboratory parameters measured at admission and during the first 48 hours. The criteria consist of 11 factors, with a higher score indicating a greater risk of mortality. Specifically, a score of 3 or more is associated with a significant increase in mortality risk [14].

6.2 Acute physiology and chronic health evaluation II (APACHE II)

The APACHE II score is a widely used scoring system that assesses the severity of illness in critically ill patients, including those with acute pancreatitis. It incorporates various physiological measurements, laboratory results, and patient age. A higher APACHE II score correlates with increased mortality risk, making it a valuable tool for risk stratification in the ED [14].

6.3 Bedside index for severity in AP(BISAP)

The BISAP score is a simpler scoring system that can be calculated at the bedside. It includes five criteria: blood urea nitrogen (BUN) level, altered mental status, SIRS (Systemic Inflammatory Response Syndrome) criteria, age over 60 years, and pleural effusion. A BISAP score of 3 or more is associated with a higher risk of mortality and complications, making it useful for early identification of high-risk patients [14].

6.4 Modified Glasgow score

The Modified Glasgow Score is another scoring system that assesses the severity of AP based on clinical and laboratory parameters. It includes factors such as age, white blood cell count, blood glucose levels, and serum albumin. A score of 3 or more indicates a higher risk of severe disease and mortality [14].

6.5 ED-SAS score

The ED-SAS (Emergency Department – Severity Assessment Score) is a newer scoring system specifically designed for use in the emergency department. It incorporates readily available variables such as age, SpO2 levels, and the presence of SIRS criteria. The ED-SAS score has shown promise in predicting 30-day mortality in patients with acute pancreatitis, providing a rapid assessment tool for clinicians [14].

The use of mortality scores in the emergency department for patients with AP is essential for risk stratification and guiding management decisions. Each scoring system has its strengths and limitations, and the choice of which to use may depend on the clinical context and available resources. Early identification of high-risk patients can lead to timely interventions and improved outcomes.

7. Conclusion and take-home message

- AP is a life-threatening emergency.
- Prompt diagnosis and management are important to address complications.
- Severity scores can play an important role in guiding the timely management of patients coming with AP.

Acknowledgements

The author acknowledges the use of POE (AI tool) for language polishing of the manuscript.

Conflict of interest

The author declares no conflict of interest.

Acronyms and abbreviations

ED	emergency department
AP	acute pancreatitis
CBC	complete blood count
BUN	blood urea nitrogen
CT	computed tomography
MRI	magnetic resonance imaging
IV	intravenous
NPO	nil per oral
APACHE II	acute physiology and chronic health evaluation II
BISAP	bedside index for severity in AP
ED-SAS	Emergency Department – Severity Assessment Score

Author details

Nazir Najeeb Kapadia
Emergency Medicine, King Hamad University Hospital, Bahrain

*Address all correspondence to: nazirkapadia@gmail.com

References

[1] Cho JH, Kim TN, Chung HH, Kim KH. Comparison of scoring systems in predicting the severity of acute pancreatitis. World Journal of Gastroenterology. 2015;**21**:2387-2394

[2] Chen L, Lu G, Zhou Q, Zhan Q. Evaluation of the BISAP score in predicting severity and prognoses of acute pancreatitis in Chinese patients. International Surgery. 2013;**98**:6-12

[3] Szatmary P, Grammatikopoulos T, Cai W, Huang W, Mukherjee R, Halloran C, et al. Acute pancreatitis: Diagnosis and treatment. Drugs. 2022;**82**(12):1251-1276. DOI: 10.1007/s40265-022-01766-4

[4] Iannuzzi JP, King JA, Leong JH, Quan J, Windsor JW, Tanyingoh D, et al. Global incidence of acute pancreatitis is increasing over time: A systematic review and meta-analysis. Gastroenterology. 2022;**162**(1):122-134. DOI: 10.1053/j.gastro.2021.09.043

[5] Lankisch PG, Apte M, Banks PA. Acute pancreatitis. The Lancet. 2015;**386**(9998):85-96

[6] Banks PA, Bollen TL, Dervenis C, et al. Classification of acute pancreatitis—2012: Revision of the Atlanta classification and definitions by international consensus. Gut. 2013;**62**(1):102-111

[7] Juneja D, Gopal PB, Ravula M. Scoring systems in acute pancreatitis: Which one to use in intensive care units?. Journal of Critical Care. 2010;**25**:358

[8] Frossard JLSM, Masamune A. Acute pancreatitis. Lancet. 2019;**386**(9998):85-96. DOI: 10.1016/S0140-6736(19)31186-3

[9] Gapp J, Tariq A, Chandra S. Acute pancreatitis. In: StatPearls [Internet]. Treasure Island (FL): StatPearls Publishing; 2025. Available from: https://www.ncbi.nlm.nih.gov/books/NBK482468/ [Accessed: February 9, 2023]

[10] Liu Q, Ruan K, An Z, Li L, Ding C, Xu D, et al. Updated review of research on the role of the gut microbiota and microbiota-derived metabolites in acute pancreatitis progression and inflammation-targeted therapy. International Journal of Biology Sciences. 2025;**21**(3):1242-1258. DOI: 10.7150/ijbs.108858. Available from: https://www.ijbs.com/v21p1242.htm

[11] Bhat P et al., editors. Acute pancreatitis. The Washington Manual of Medical Therapeutics, 37th ed. Wolters Kluwer Health. The Washington Manual. 2023. Available from: www.unboundmedicine.com/washingtonmanual/view/Washington-Manual-of-Medical-Therapeutics/602291/all/Acute_Pancreatitis

[12] Walkowska JZN, Tubbs RS, Podgórski M, Dłubek-Ruxer J, Olewnik Ł. Diagnosis and treatment of acute pancreatitis. Diagnostics (Basel). 2022;**12**(8):1974. DOI: 10.3390/diagnostics12081974

[13] Working Group IAP/APA Acute Pancreatitis Guidelines. IAP/APA evidence-based guidelines for the management of acute pancreatitis. Pancreatology. Jul-Aug 2013;**13**(4 Suppl 2):e1-15. DOI: 10.1016/j.pan.2013.07.063. PMID: 24054878

[14] Miller JWY, Safa R, Marusca G, Bhatti S, Ahluwalia G, Dandashi J, et al. Derivation and validation of the ED-SAS score for very early prediction of mortality and morbidity with acute pancreatitis: A retrospective observational study. BMC Emergency Medicine. 2021;**21**(1):16. DOI: 10.1186/s12873-021-00410-w

Chapter 5

Bleeding in Severe Acute Pancreatitis (Pancreonecrosis)

Alexey Severtsev, Valery Vechorko, Irakly Kitiashvili, Shukhrat Dzhurakulov, Viktor Anosov, Sanal Byurchiev, Alim Huseynov and Afag Jabbarova

Abstract

The aim was to study the algorithm (outcomes) in patients with pancreonecrosis (PN)—complicated by bleedings. In 2014–2023, out of 387 patients with pancreonecrosis, 38 (9.81%) patients developed bleedings: (A) in 23 patients, it was parapancreatic bleeding; in 21 intraluminal, 6 patients had both bleedings; (B) in 37 patients – "major," in 7 – "minor"; (C) in 34 patients – primary, in 4 – postoperative. Predictors of bleeding were delayed hospitalization (specialized hospital), organ failure, infected necrosis, and systemic sepsis (bacterial, fungal). In the multivariate analysis, infected necrosis and fungal sepsis were significant factors. Patients with bleeding had much worse indices compared to those without bleeding: surgical intervention (84.2 vs. 24.1%), length of stay in the ICU (17.3 ± 4.2 vs. 8.6 ± 1.1 days), and mortality rate (63.2 vs. 20.9%). Five patients had arterial embolization, and 22 required surgical intervention, including one surgery after unsuccessful embolization. All 23 patients with intraabdominal bleeding required surgery (laparotomy, etc.); four had successful embolization. Severity index was strongly associated with bleeding that was confirmed by surgery and CT findings. Organ failure and surgery were also triggers of severe bleeding. A higher mortality rate in patients with PN is evidently associated with bleeding. Infected necrosis increases vascular wall destruction that leads to bleedings.

Keywords: erosive bleeding, splenic artery embolization, acute severe pancreatitis-pancreonecrosis, complication, systemic coagulation factors

1. Introduction

Alexander the Great died in 323 BC a few days before his 33rd birthday. He returned to Babylon after his last conquests at the Indus River in the East. To celebrate the victory, he and his generals held a large banquet where enormous amounts of food and alcohol were eaten and drunk. The next day, Alexander complained about abdominal pain, which gradually worsened, and 12 days later, he died.

For many years, poisoning was believed to be the most widely accepted reason of his death. However, according to historian Robin Lane Fox, the most common poisons at that time were strychnine and hellebore; both had a sudden effect. Therefore, Fox believes it is very unlikely that Alexander would have survived 12 days after being poisoned. It was also speculated that he might have died from malaria, as there was an outbreak of malaria in Babylon at that time. However, in 1986, Simmie Bank (Murraysburg, South Africa) suggested that that was the first reported case of alcohol-related acute pancreatitis/pancreonecrosis (PN), although it will not never be proven for certain.

PN mortality is 15–80%, even with a full range of surgical and resuscitation treatment [1–4]. Although gastrointestinal bleeding (GIB) is not identified as a specific feature of PN according to the revised Atlanta classification [1, 5], nevertheless, the consequences associated with this condition can be fatal. This is a fairly rare complication in PN, and hence, there is a lot of uncertainty around it. The overall incidence of any type of GIB in acute pancreatitis is 1–23% [6–10]. However, when this complication occurs, only it is enough to cause patients' death in 33–50% [11–13]. The greatest danger is bleeding into the peripancreatic area, which complicates the course of pancreatic necrosis and enhances the increase of mortality [6–10]. Bleeding can be developed: (1) due to the actual arrosion of the vascular wall, (2) the formation of a pseudoaneurysm, (3) microvascular ischemic complications, and (4) thrombosis of the splenic-portomesenteric veins (which in turn causes the phenomenon of subhepatic portal hypertension, with the development of GIB from varicose veins) dilated veins of the esophagus and stomach) [6, 7]. A special situation is the surgical intervention in this area ("rough" surgery, necrectomy vs. sequestrectomy) which can also lead to local bleeding [7, 11, 14, 15].

The local inflammatory response and active pancreatic enzymes in this area, which penetrate the retroperitoneum in PN, can "digest" adjacent organs, tissues, and vascular structures, including the relatively resistant arterial wall. Then, it leads to acute arrosion, rupture/weakening of the wall and the formation of a pseudoaneurysm, which can eventually rupture itself and cause bleeding [6–8, 11, 15, 16].

Furthermore, pancreatic necrosis formation itself in the area of abscess and pseudocysts can also cause similar damage to the vascular wall.

In addition, to the already mentioned errors in pancreatic sanitation, the timing of the operation and the surgical method itself have also already been identified as risk factors for the bleeding development [7, 8, 11, 15].

There are few studies on hemorrhagic complications in PN, so this research intends to determine an algorithm and assess the outcomes of PN complicated by bleeding.

2. Material and methods

From December 2014 to December 2023, 387 patients who were admitted with PN at City Clinical Hospital No. 15 (Moscow, Russia) were assessed—prospectively (54: from August 2022 to December 2023) and retrospectively (333: from December 2014 until July 2022). Insert consent form was obtained from all patients before their inclusion in the prospective group. Acute pancreatitis was diagnosed based on history, clinical examination, and imaging studies according to available National clinical guidelines (CG). The diagnosis of PN was established in accordance with the CG and the revised Atlanta classification [1, 17].

Patients were assessed based on demographic parameters, etiology of the disease, clinical manifestations, and radiological data. Patients with organ failure were provided with relevant assistance (according to CG). Dynamic evaluation was performed using hematological, biochemical, microbiological, and imaging parameters. Antibiotics were routinely used by all patients. Enteral nutrition in patients was started immediately after stabilization of their clinical condition. Patients whose condition worsened during complete conservative treatment underwent percutaneous drainage of liquid collections under X-ray (including computer tomography (CT) or ultrasound control. More extensive surgical intervention was performed for patients who had (1) progressive deterioration of their condition against the background of the most complete conservative treatment, (2) development of purulent-septic complications, and (3) life-threatening GIB. During hospitalization, patients were observed for the development of hemorrhagic complications, which were distributed according to the schemes presented below (**Figures 1** and **2**). The progress of complications and mortality associated with bleeding occurring during PN was recorded.

2.1 Assessment and distribution of acute GIB in PN

I. By localization

a. Intraluminal, clinically determined by the presence of hematemesis, melena, or fresh blood through a nasogastric tube.

b. Parapancreatic (extraluminal, intra-abdominal): there is a bleeding through drainage installed percutaneously or during surgery, or development of unexplained hemodynamic instability and/or CT findings consistent with the presence of contrast extravasation into the peripancreatic area (cyst, peritoneal cavity, or retroperitoneum). And also based on data from CT angiography and "direct" angiography.

II. By timing (Time of development of bleeding)

a. "fresh" (new): before any surgical intervention during the course of the disease (PN).

b. post-surgery: after (any) surgical intervention has been performed.

III. By severity

a. "Major" bleeding: defined as an acute decrease in hemoglobin concentration of at least 2 g/dL in a patient with obvious or proven bleeding and/or

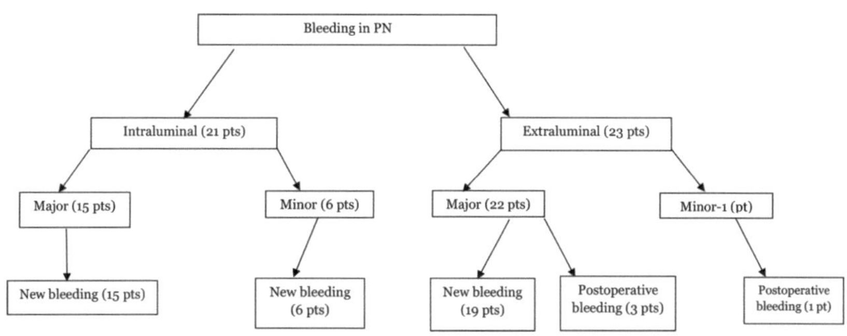

Figure 1.
Treatment of the GIB in PN, depending on the nature of the bleeding.

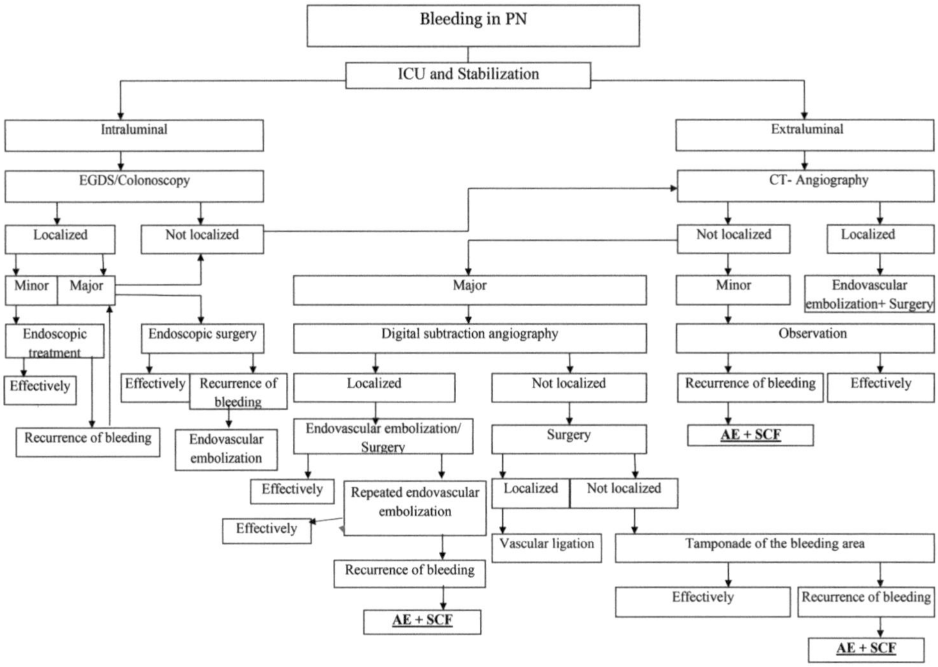

Figure 2.
General protocol for the treatment of patients with GIB with PN. ICU - intensive care unit; CT- angiography – computer angiography; AE – arterial embolization; SCF – systemic administration of coagulation factors.

hemodynamic instability of a stable patient with other conditions, and other causes of hemodynamic instability such as septic shock or abdominal compartment syndrome are excluded.

b. "Minor" ("small") bleeding: bleeding that does not fall into the category of severe ("major") bleeding.

IV. By frequency

a. one-time

b. multiple/recurrent.

V. According to anatomical sources

a. arterial

b. venous

c. capillary (parenchymal)

d. mixed

e. non-localized

Intraluminal bleeding was determined during endoscopy while patients with peripancreatic and/or postoperative bleeding as well as large intraluminal bleeding underwent computed tomography angiography (CT-angiography). Further treatment was determined based on the results of bleeding localization. For patients who were identified with bleeding and it was localized angiographically, embolization or surgery was performed depending on hemodynamic stability. When the locus was identified on a CT an`giogram, patients were assessed for severity and then an "exploratory" laparotomy was possibly performed.

All patients with severe non-localized bleeding on CT angiogram underwent "direct" angiography (DA). Patients with "minor" bleeding that was not localized on CT angiogram were monitored for the development of recurrent bleeding. In case of rebleeding, the DA was performed too (repeated).

2.2 Statistical analysis

Descriptive statistics have been applied. Data were expressed as mean ± standard deviation or median (range) depending on the situation. The Mann-Whitney U test was used to evaluate ordinal data such as CTSI. Factors recognized to be significant in univariate analysis were included in multivariate logistic regression analysis. Statistical significance was set at <0.05. Furthermore, the obtained data were presented in evaluation tables in the form of median (Me) and interquartile range (Q1; Q3).

3. Results

A total of 387 patients with PN were examined during the study period—54 prospectively and 333 retrospectively. The average age amounted to 50.12 ± 1 years (in the prospective group - 49.63 ± 1 and in the retrospective group - 50.2 ± 1). Sex ratio (M:F): 255:132 (1,93:1). Etiology: alcohol abuse in 79 (20.41%), biliary system disease in 95 (24.55%), other causes (trauma, hyperlipidemia, medications and chemicals, nutritional - other than alcohol abuse) - 40 (10.34%), the unknown reason in 173 (44.7%). The average duration between the onset of the first symptoms of the disease and hospitalization in a specialized institution was 2.4 ± 1.1 (range: 1–7) days. The average APACHE II score upon admission of patients was 10.2 ± 1.4, and the average CTSI score was 3 ± 1. At the time of admission to our hospital, 24 (6.2%) patients already had severe organ failure. However, during hospitalization, all patients who were included in the study experienced organ failure development. Infected pancreatic necrosis in the pancreatic area itself was confirmed by bacterial cultures, was detected in 131 patients out of 387 (33.9%). Among the entire group of patients, fungal (co-infection) and bacterial flora were cultured from the blood of 52 patients; only bacterial flora in 158 patients, sterile cultures were in 64, cultures were unreliable - 113. Thrombosis of the portal vein system was diagnosed in 9 (2.32%). Despite the fact that pseudoaneurysms of the peripancreatic vasculature is a logical process during a progressive destructive process in the pancreas, we were not able to reliably identify this complication during hospitalization against the background of an acute process in any case. Extensive surgical interventions (laparotomy, etc.) were required in 116 (29.97%) patients. The overall case fatality rate (from 387) was 25.1% (97). The average lengths of patient stay in the intensive care unit and hospital were 9 + 1 days and 24 + 2 days, respectively.

3.1 Source of GIB and localization

Of all 387 patients, 38 (9.81%) had GIB. Some 21 patients had intraluminal bleeding, of which 15 were "major" and 6 were "minor". Parapancreatic bleeding was observed in 23 patients, of which 22/23 (95.7%) were large and 1/23 (4.3%) were "small". CT angiogram was performed in 12 (3.1%) of all 38 patients. Among 23 patients with parapancreatic bleeding, 6 had a CT angiogram, 2 (16.67%) showed diffuse contrast extravasation, and 6 had both intraluminal and parapancreatic bleedings (21 intraluminal cases+23 parapancreatic cases = 44–6 intraluminal/parapancreatic = 38 patients).

3.2 Treatment of bleeding

3.2.1 Luminal (intraluminal) bleeding

Bleeding from an intraluminal source observed in 21 patients was stopped with endoscopic therapy (sclero, thermal coagulation, and argon plasma coagulation) (**Figures 1** and **2**; **Tables 1–4**).

False intraluminal bleeding due to rupture of the pancreatic collection, observed in 1 patient, was self-limiting (rupture of the pancreatic fluid "collection" into the lumen of the duodenum) and did not require any intervention for bleeding, and 1 patient with rupture of the colon surgical intervention required (due to sepsis) - a segmental resection of the colon was performed. In this case, there was massive intraluminal bleeding against the background of colon ischemia.

3.2.2 New ("fresh") bleeding

Nineteen patients with parapancreatic "fresh" bleeding. There was spotted compaction of structures in this area (infiltrate) on CT in 19 patients with parapancreatic "fresh" bleeding. Wait-and-see tactics and conservative treatment were applied. Two patients with postoperative minor bleeding from the drain and non-localized on CT angiogram were actively monitored, but no further active surgical management was required.

There were 6 patients who experienced "large" fresh parapancreatic bleeding development; four cases were successfully embolized; however, 1 experienced repeated bleeding development, which required "open" surgical intervention. Five cases could not have been localized by angiography, and therefore, they were operated on ("open" surgery).

3.2.3 Postoperative bleeding

No significant arterial bleeding was detected during or after surgery. Seven patients with diffuse venous (parenchymal) bleeding were treated with tight packing. In total, out of 387 patients, laparotomy was performed in 116 for the purpose of sanitation of septic lesions. At the same time, 14 had bleeding and purulent-septic focus simultaneously. Thirty-two of 38 patients with bleeding underwent laparotomy. Mortality among patients who underwent laparotomy was significantly higher (53/116 (45.69%) versus 44/271 (16.24%), $p < 0.001$) comparing with those without surgery.

Estimated indicator	**Total (n = 387)**	**While bleeding (n = 38)**	**Without bleeding (n = 349)**	**Univariate p-value**	**Multivariate p-value**	**OR (95% confidence interval)**
General indicators						
Age (in years) M ± SD/Me (Q1-Q3)	50,12 ± 16,2 48 (37–61)	52,4 ± 14,7 48 (37–61)	49,9,4 ± 16,4 48 (37–61)	0,3638	0,622	0,42 (0,28; 2,09)
Gender (M:F)	255:132	24:14	231:118	0,7351	0,837	0,88 (0,44 - 1,76)
male	255(65,89%)	24 (63,2%)	231 (66,19%)	0,7351	0,837	0,88 (0,44 - 1,76)
female	132(34,11%)	14 (36,8%)	118 (33,81%)			
Etiology						
Alcohol	79 (20,4%)	8 (21,1%)	71 (20,3%)	0,9189	0,790	1,03 (0,54 - 1,98)
Biliary	95(24,5%)	15 (39,5%)	80 (22,9%)	0,0453	0,061	1,72 (1,11 - 2,67)
Other	213 (55,0%)	15 (39,5%)	198 (56,7%)	0,0397	0,048	0,7 (0,46 - 1,04)
Resuscitation criteria						
Time interval between first symptoms and admission to hospital* (days) M ± SD/Me (Q1-Q3) 2.4 ± 1.1	2,4 ± 1,1 2 (2; 4)	3,2 ± 0,9 3 (3; 4)	2,3 ± 1,1 2 (2; 3)	0,0227	0,0405	0,25 (0,11-0,68)
Concomitant diseases	375 (96,9%)	38 (100%)	337 (96,6%)	0,7259	0,840	1,04 (1,02 - 1,06)
APACHEII*	9 (4–14)	14 (11–19)	9 (4–14)	<0,001	0,017	1,20 (1,02-2,06)
APACHEII	10,2 ± 5,8	14,8 ± 5,3	9,3 ± 4,8	<0,001	0,017	1,20 (1,02-2,06)
Number of organs in case of organ failure** M ± SD/ Me (Q1-Q3)	1,3 ± 0,6 1 (1; 2)	2,9 ± 0,5 3 (2; 4)	1,1 ± 0,2 1 (1; 2)	<0,001	0,022	1,59 (1,18 - 3,26)
Infectious lesions						
Estimated indicator	Total (n = 387)	While bleeding (n = 38)	Without bleeding (n = 349)	Univariate p-value	Multivariate p-value	OR (95% confidence interval)
Infected necrosis	131 (33,9%)	32 (84,2%)	99 (28,4%)	<0,001	<0,001	2,97 (2,39 - 3,69)
Bacterial sepsis	158(40,83%)	18 (63,2%)	140(40,11%)	<0,001	0,002	4,59 (3,21 - 6,57)

Estimated indicator	Total (n = 387)	While bleeding (n = 38)	Without bleeding (n = 349)	Univariate p-value	Multivariate p-value	OR (95% confidence interval)
Fungal sepsis + bacterial	52 (13,4%)	16 (42,11%)	36 (10,32%)	0,0001	0,009	4,08 (2,51 - 6,63)
Sterile	64 (16,5%)	3 (7,9%)	61(17,5%)	0,048	0,072	0,45 (0,15 - 1,37)
Unknown	113 (29,2%)	1 (2,6%)	112(32,1%)	0,001	0,010	0,08 (0,01 - 0,57)
Important surgical indicators						
Venous thrombosis	30 (7,8%)	8 (21,1%)	22 (6,3%)	0,0293	0,062	3,34 (1,6 - 6,98)
Need for percutaneous drainage	236 (61%)	36 (94,7%)	200 (57,3%)	<0,001	0,032	1,65 (1,47 - 1,86)
Need for surgical intervention	116 (30%)	32 (84,2%)	84 (24,1%)	<0,001	<0,001	3,5 (2,78 - 4,41)
Important general medical indicators						
Mortality	97 (25,1%)	24 (63,2%)	73 (20,9%)	<0,001	0,007	3,02 (2,2 - 4,15)
ICU Stay	9,0 + 4,3	17,3 + 4,2	8,6 + 1,1	<0,001	0,031	1,29 (1,06 - 4,33)
ICU Stay*	5 (3; 11,5)	11,5 (7; 23,5)	5 (3; 10)	<0,001	0,031	1,29 (1,06 - 4,33)
Total length of hospitalization	26,8 + 4,0	41,2 + 3,7	26,3 + 1,6	<0,001	0,018	1,7 (1,09 - 2,45)
Total length of hospitalization*	18 (13; 30)	33,5 (17; 60)	18 (12; 26)	<0,001	0,018	1,7 (1,09 - 2,45)

**Admission to an expert institution.*
***At the time of hospitalization.*
APACHE, acute physiology and chronic health evaluation; CTA - CT angiography; PCD, percutaneous drainage (percutaneous drainage); ICU, intensive care unit (intensive care unit/ resuscitation unit).

Table 1.
General comparative data between patients with and without bleeding.

Assessment parameter	Intraluminal bleeding (n = 21)	Intra-abdominal bleeding (n = 23)	p-value
Age	53.3 ± 15,2 50 (45; 63)	49.9 ± 13,2 50 (45; 60)	0,4414
Gender M:F	18:3	13:10	0,0283
male	18 (85,7%)	13 (56,5%)	0,0283
female	3 (14,3%)	10 (43,5%)	
Interval between attack and bleeding*	3,0 ± 0,6	3,1 ± 0,5	0,764
APACHE II*	14,9 ± 5,7 14(11; 20)	144 ± 4,72 14 (11; 18)	0,728
CTSI	2.9 ± 0,9 3,0 (2; 4)	3,1 ± 0,9 3,0 (2; 4)	0,537
Average number of organs – their failure**	2,9 ± 0,2	3,0 ± 0,2	0,686
Thrombosis of the portal vein system	5 (23,8%)	5 (21,7%)	0,871
Infected pancreatic necrosis (pancreas itself)	15 (71,4%)	23 (100%)	0,1317
Sepsis	14 (66,7%)	15 (65,2%)	0,9197
Need for surgery	15 (71,4%)	23 (100%)	0,1317
Mortality	14 (66.67%)	15 (65,2%)	0,9197
Duration in hospital*	21,0 ± 34,8 21(14; 60)	47,6 ± 33,2 39 (18; 75)	0,356
Stay in ICU*	16,8 ± 15,8 11(8; 23)	19,0 ± 19,7 11,5(7; 28)	0,707

**From the immediate moment of an attack of pancreatitis.*
***Upon admission.*
APACHE, acute physiology and chronic health evaluation; CTSI, CT severity index; ICU, intensive care.

Table 2.
Assessment of patients with intraluminal and parapancreatic (intra-abdominal).

Indicator	"Major" bleeding (n = 31)	"Minor" bleeding (n = 7)	p-value
Age (in years)	51,9 ± 12,2 50 (37; 68)	53,3 ± 19,2 50 (28; 71)	0,793
Gender (M:F)	22 (71,0%) : 9 (29,0%)	3 (42,9%): 4 (57,1%)	0,1568
Time (in days) between the attack of PN and the development of bleeding*	26 ± 4,6	10 ± 2,9	0,016
APACHE II*	14,7 ± 4,8 15 (11; 18)	15,6 ± 6,5 13 (10,5; 21)	0,244
CTSI	3,2 ± 0,98 3 (1; 4)	3,1 ± 0,6 3 (2; 3)	0,315
Average number of organs in a state of organ failure**	2,9 ± 0,2	3	0,627

Indicator	"Major" bleeding (n = 31)	"Minor" bleeding (n = 7)	p-value
Thrombosis of the portal vein system	8 (25,81%)	0 (7,7%)	0,5845
Infected pancreatic necrosis (pancreas itself)	24 (77,42%)	3 (42,86%)	0,0686
Sepsis	21 (67,41%)	3 (42,86%)	0,2177
Need for surgery	22(70,97%)	3 (42,86%)	0,1568
Mortality	22 (70,97%)	2 (28,57%)	0,0357
Length of hospital stay*	48,3 ± 31,2 39 (21; 69)	29,4 ± 32,9,2 17 (11; 32)	0,009
Stay in ICU*	20,1 ± 18,8 13 (8; 31)	11,3 ± 7,5 11 (7; 16)	<0,001

**Primary attack of pancreatitis.*
***At the time of admission.*
APACHE, acute physiology and chronic health evaluation; CTSI, CT severity index; ICU, intensive care.

Table 3.
Comparison of "large" and "small" bleeding.

Indicator	New ("fresh") bleeding (n = 34)	Postoperative bleeding (n = 4)	p-value
Age (in years)	52,09	52,75	0,745
Gender (M:F)	24:10	2:2	0,849
Male	24 (70,6%)	2 (50%)	0,849
Female	10 (29,4%)	2 (50%)	
Time (in days) between the attack of PN and the development of bleeding*	19 ± 6,2	45 ± 11,7	<0,001
APACHE II	15,1 ± 1,6	12,9 ± 1,1	0,728
CTSI	4,0 ± 0,9	3,1 ± 0,4	0,008
Average number of organs in a state of organ failure**	3,2 ± 0,4	3	0,637
Thrombosis of the portal vein system	6 (17,65%)	1 (25%)	0,847
Infected pancreatic necrosis	26 (76,47%)	3 (75%)	0,8077
Sepsis	23 (67,65%)	1 (25%)	0,5796
Mortality	23 (67,65%)	2 (50%)	0,5796
Length of hospital stay*	38,3 ± 9,5	57,4 ± 8,2	0,131
Stay in ICU*	17,22 ± 3,8	10,1 ± 3,5	0,415

**Primary attack of pancreatitis.*
***At the time of admission.*
APACHE, acute physiology and chronic health evaluation; CTSI, severity index; ICU, intensive care.

Table 4.
Comparison of new ("fresh") and postoperative bleeding.

3.3 Predictors of bleeding and complications

According to univariate analysis, predictors of bleeding and complications were a delay in admission to a specialized expert medical institution, a higher APACHE II score, a greater number of "labels" for organ failure at admission, the presence of infected necrosis, and the development of systemic sepsis during the course of the disease (**Table 1**). In multivariate analysis, the presence of infected necrosis and the presence of fungal sepsis were significant factors for bleeding.

Intraluminal and parapancreatic bleeding. Patients with peripancreatic bleeding had more severe PN and a higher need for surgical intervention (**Table 2**).

"Major" and "Minor" bleeding: patients with major bleeding had a lower average number of organ failure "marks" and a higher need for surgical intervention (**Table 3**).

New ("fresh") bleeding versus postoperative bleeding: Both groups were comparable in severity and need for intervention (**Table 4**).

4. Discussion

Despite centuries of studies, the problem of the complicated course of PN remains unresolved. Furthermore, despite extensive experience of the authors of this article [18, 19], we can now state that the solution to the problems associated with the treatment of this pathology remains as it was 40 years ago.

Our study carried out an analysis of GIB diseases in PN that had occurred in City Clinical Hospital No. 15 of Moscow for the period from 2014 to 2023. Based on data analysis, a treatment algorithm was proposed (including an extremely difficult situation with parapancreatic non-localized bleeding). Given the rarity of such complications, it is extremely difficult to evaluate the available data. However, the need for any option (invasive, including surgical or minimally invasive) intervention can already be determined based on the proposed algorithm. Although bleeding associated with PN should be most often treated surgically, we observe a group of patients with non-localized bleeding that could be controlled without "open" surgery (embolization one of the main pancreatic artery + SCF). This is due to the fact that the possibilities of intervention in such cases are very limited due to the nature and type of bleeding, the lack (primarily) of their clear topic, as well as the general, extremely severe, general condition. Another important group of patients includes those with a rupture (breakthrough) of the pancreatic collection (infected/uninfected) into a hollow organ. As a rule, there was observed minor intraluminal bleeding followed by clinical improvement (most often spontaneous). These patients needed to have subsequent intervention if it was due to the development of infectious complications resulting from contamination of the pancreatic collection or the development of gastrointestinal fistulas (especially those associated with the colon).

The development of GIB in PN is a poor prognostic sign, as it sharply increases mortality. Approximately one third to half of patients who experienced progress bleeding die after this complication [6, 7, 10, 15]. Reports on the incidence of bleeding associated with PN greatly vary due to the relative rarity of this complication and various manifestations, due to the fact that in most of the cases, it develops during the recovery stage of the patient [6–11, 14, 15]. As mentioned earlier, according to other researchers, the greatest danger is pseudoaneurysms. In our work, we did not diagnose this complication. But it does not mean that they did not exist. A number of special studies attach great importance to this complication. The most significant work on pseudoaneurysms associated with pancreatitis, including both acute and chronic, was carried out on the basis of 46 intensive care units [15]. In general, data on bleeding in PN are as follows: Wei et al. [10] - 15% frequency, Tang et al. [20] - 11.5%, and Gupta V et al. [5] - 13%. In our work, this figure was 9.81% (in 38 out of 387 patients).

The development of bleeding is certainly associated with the severity of the disease [8–10, 15, 20, 21]. We observed a higher average number of "marks" of organ failure in patients with bleeding that has developed (both at the stage of admission and the ongoing development of this process during the hospital stay). Other studies have also identified higher rates of process severity and organ failure associated with the development of bleeding in PN. A relatively recent study (2018) has reported 7.7 and 19.2% bleeding rates, respectively, based on the APACHE II score [20]. In our work, similar figures were 9.3 and 14.8%, respectively.

The work of Labarca et al. [15] has noted the importance of age and etiology as risk factors in multivariate analysis. Another fairly large study showed that sepsis developing BEFORE undergoing surgery for PN is a risk factor in multivariate analysis [10]. Shen et al. [22] observed a higher incidence of bleeding in the presence of pancreatic necrosis. In the presence of infected necrosis, the bleeding rate is 29.5% [15]. According to multivariate analysis [5], infected necrosis and the presence of sepsis were risk factors associated with the occurrence of bleeding. The relevant results we obtained look even more dramatic. Thus, during infected pancreatic necrosis, the probability of bleeding increases to 82.4% (vs. 28.4%). Moreover, the addition of fungal flora to the bacterial component further increases the likelihood a developing of this complication (from 10.32 to 42.11%).

The incidence of venous thrombosis of the portal vein system in this study accounted to 2.32%, and it was not an independent factor predicting the risk of bleeding. According to the literature, the frequency of this indicator ranges from 2 to 23% [7, 14, 23].

The incidence of GIB was higher among patients who had a delay in admission to an expert medical center or when transferred from hospitals that did not specialize in the treatment of such patients. The importance of this factor was also noted by other authors [9]. Bleeding is usually a late complication during the development and dynamics of PN [7]. A study was performed that showed a poor overall outcome in patients admitted to a specialized institution after a week of onset of the disease/PN [2]. The treatment of these patients is difficult due to the presence of a peripancreatic inflammatory process, ongoing sepsis, poor general status due to the duration of the disease, and the inability to accurately localize the source of bleeding. Detection of pseudoaneurysms by angiography is considered a prognostically favorable situation, since this allows successful embolization [24]. However, even with the availability of CT angiography and "direct" angiography, we were unable to identify a single observation in the acute period. Probably, in the course of subsequent work with these patients, more careful attention should be paid to this factor. According to the literature, the most common location of pseudoaneurysm is the splenic artery [6, 7, 9, 10, 12, 13, 25]. A study [5] reported pseudoaneurysms as the cause of bleeding in one third of cases. A number of studies have reported the incidence of bleeding due to the presence of pseudoaneurysm to be 10% [14] and 18% [9].

The effectiveness of treatment for non-localized bleeding remains to be further elucidated in future studies. A recent review from 2017 has reported that capillary and venous bleeding was present in 20% of cases [6, 7]. In a study by Gupta et al., bleeding could not be accurately localized in 30% of patients. The cause is usually slow, diffuse venous, or capillary bleeding, which is difficult to accurately diagnose and localize.

Patients with "major" non-localized bleeding have very limited surgical options and high mortality. In our study, we tried to take these data into account and, based on them, developed a method for treating venous and parenchymal bleeding using angioembolization in combination with the introduction of SCF (**Figure 2**) [26]. Endovascular blockade of arterial blood flow in the splenic artery (as the main artery supplying the body and tail of the pancreas) slows down, but does not completely stop, the total blood flow in the distal parts of the pancreas. This occurs even when the source of bleeding is not localized during angiography. Thus, arterial blood flow slows down, but does not stop, in the small arterial vessels of the superior mesenteric artery basin, the gastroduodenal artery basin, the splenic vein system, and the vessels of the pancreas parenchyma itself. It should be noted that endovascular embolization of the splenic artery, even at the level of its origin from the celiac trunk, rarely causes serious complications [27]. At the same time, maintaining an alternative arterial blood supply to the gland (in this case from the superior mesenteric artery system) ensures relevant medications' access to the target organ. Using coagulation factors (primarily YII, during a defect in any vessel with damaged endothelium) against the backdrop of SLOW blood flow in the pancreas ensures to successfully stop NON-PROFUSE (NON-ARTERIAL) bleeding, which cannot be stopped during an open surgery.

5. Conclusions

In conclusion, there is the COMPLETE (even for non-localized bleeding) algorithm based on the nature, location, time, frequency, and source and severity of bleeding. The actions for treatment planning in a severe group of patients with PN become clear. The work done allows us to identify "weak points" in the treatment of a serious complication (GIB in PN) and determine further directions of research in its treatment.

Conflict of interest

Each author declares that he/she has no commercial associations (e.g., consultancies, stock ownership, equity interest, patent/licensing arrangement, etc.) that might pose a conflict of interest in connection with the submitted article.

Author details

Alexey Severtsev[1,2*], Valery Vechorko[1,2], Irakly Kitiashvili[2], Shukhrat Dzhurakulov[1,2], Viktor Anosov[1,2], Sanal Byurchiev[1], Alim Huseynov[2] and Afag Jabbarova[1]

1 N.I. Pirogov Russian National Research Medical University, Moscow, Russia

2 O.M. Philatov Moscow City Hospital, Moscow, Russia

*Address all correspondence to: sev-alex@mail.ru

References

[1] Working Group IAP/APA Acute Pancreatitis Guidelines. Pancreatology. 2013;**13**(4 Suppl. 2):e1-e15. DOI: 10.1016/j.pan.2013.07.063

[2] Mallick B, Dhaka N, Sharma V, Malik S, Sinha SK, et al. Impact of timing of presentation of acute pancreatitis to a tertiary care centre on the outcome. Pancreatology. 2019;**19**:143-148. DOI: 10.1016/j.pan.2018.10.005

[3] Manrai M, Kochhar R, Gupta V, Yadav TD, Dhaka N, Kalra N, et al. Outcome of acute pancreatic and peripancreatic collections occurring in patients with acute pancreatitis. Annals of Surgery. 2018;**267**:357-363. DOI: 10.1097/sla.0000000000002854

[4] Топузов ЭЭ, Балашов ВК, Цатинян БГ, Аршба ЭА, et al. Хирургическое лечение острого панкреатита: возможности чрескожного дренирования. Хирургия. Журнал им. Н.И. Пирогова. 2017;**8**:91-94 [Topuzov E.E., Balashov V.K., Tsatinyan B.G., Arshba E.A. et al. Surgical treatment of acute pancreatitis: possibilities of percutaneous therapy. Pirogov Rus J of Surg. 2017;8:91-94. In Russian]. DOI: 10.17116/hirurgia2017891-94

[5] Gupta V, Krishna P, Kochhar R, et al. Hemorrhage complicating the course of severe acute pancreatitis. Annals of Hepato-Biliary-Pancreatic Surgery. 2020;**24**:292-300. DOI: 10.14701/ahbps.2020.24.3.292

[6] Andersson E, Ansari D, Andersson R. Major haemorrhagic complications of acute pancreatitis. The British Journal of Surgery. 2010;**97**:1379-1384. DOI: 10.1002/bjs.7113

[7] Evans RP, Mourad MM, Pall G, Fisher SG, Bramhall SR. Pancreatitis: Preventing catastrophic haemorrhage. World Journal of Gastroenterology. 2017;**23**:5460-5468. DOI: 10.3748/wjg.v23. i30.5460

[8] Flati G, Andrén-Sandberg A, La Pinta M, Porowska B, Carboni M. Potentially fatal bleeding in acute pancreatitis: Pathophysiology, prevention, and treatment. Pancreas. 2003;**26**:8-14. DOI: 10.1097/00006676-200301000-00002

[9] Sharma PK, Madan K, Garg PK. Hemorrhage in acute pancreatitis: Should gastrointestinal bleeding be considered an organ failure? Pancreas. 2008;**36**:141-145. DOI: 10.1097/mpa.0b013e318158466e

[10] Wei AL, Guo Q, Wang MJ, Hu WM, Zhang ZD. Early complications after interventions in patients with acute pancreatitis. World Journal of Gastroenterology. 2016;**22**:2828-2836. DOI: 10.3748/wjg.v22.i9.2828

[11] Ammori BJ, Madan M, Alexander DJ. Haemorrhagic complications of pancreatitis: Presentation, diagnosis and management. Annals of the Royal College of Surgeons of England. 1998;**80**:316-325

[12] Bergert H, Hinterseher I, Kersting S, Leonhardt J, Bloomenthal A, Saeger HD. Management and outcome of hemorrhage due to arterial pseudoaneurysms in pancreatitis. Surgery. 2005;**137**:323-328. DOI: 10.1016/j.surg.2004.10.009

[13] Mendelson RM, Anderson J, Marshall M, Ramsay D. Vascular complications of pancreatitis. ANZ

Journal of Surgery. 2005;**75**:1073-1079. DOI: 10.1111/j.1445-2197.2005.03607.x

[14] Balthazar EJ, Fisher LA. Hemorrhagic complications of pancreatitis: Radiologic evaluation with emphasis on CT imaging. Pancreatology. 2001;**1**:306-313. DOI: 10.1159/000055829

[15] Labarca E, Zubia F, Maraví-Poma E, Martinez F, EPAMI Group. Early predictors of abdominal hemorrhage among critically ill patients with pancreatitis: A prospective cohort study. Pancreas. 2018;**47**:1027-1032. DOI: 10.1097/mpa.0000000000001135

[16] Репин ИГ, Савостьянов КА, Мизин СП, Столяров АА, Репин ДИ. Ложная аневризма селезеночной артерии как причина желудочно-кишечного кровотечения. Хирургия. Журнал им. Н.И. Пирогова. 2017;**5**:87-90. [Repin I.G., Savostiyanov K.A., Mizin S.P., Stolyarov A.A., Repin D.I. Acute bleeding from upper gastrointestinal tract due to splenic artery pseudoaneurysm in a cavity of pancreatic pseudocyst. Pirogov Rus J of Surg. 2017;5:87-90. In Russian]. DOI: 10.17116/hirurgia2017587-90

[17] Banks PA, Bollen TL, Dervenis C, Gooszen HG, Johnson CD, Sarr MG, et al. Classification of acute pancreatitis – 2012: Revision of the Atlanta classification and definitions by international consensus. Gut. 2013;**62**:102-111. DOI: 10.1136/gutjnl-2012-302779

[18] Брехов ЕИ, Литвин ГД, Кирпичев АГ, Северцев АН. Применение лазера при комбинированных операциях у больных раком желудка. Хирургия. Журнал им. Н.И. Пирогова. 1987;**7**:70-74 [Brekhov E.I., Litvin G.D., Kirpichev A.G., Severtsev A.N. The use of laser in combined operations in patients with gastric cancer. Pirogov Rus J of Surg. 1987;7:70-74. In Russian]

[19] Брехов ЕИ, Северцев АН, Чегин АГ, Кулешов ИЮ. Динамическая оментопанкреатостомия в лечении острого деструктивного панкреатита. Хирургия. Журнал им. Н.И. Пирогова. 1991;**2**:127-133 [Brekhov E.I., Severtsev A.N. , Chegin V.M., Kuleshov I. Yu. Dynamic omentopancreatostomy in the treatment of acute destructive pancreatitis. Pirogov Rus J of Surg. 1991;2:127-133. In Russian]

[20] Tang MY, Chen TW, Bollen TL, Wang YX, Xue HD, Jin ZY, et al. MR imaging of hemorrhage associated with acute pancreatitis. Pancreatology. 2018;**18**:363-369. DOI: 10.1016/j.pan.2018.03.004

[21] Balthazar EJ. Complications of acute pancreatitis: Clinical and CT evaluation. Radiologic Clinics of North America. 2002;**40**:1211-1227. DOI: 10.1016/s0033-8389(02)00043-x

[22] Shen X, Sun J, Zhang J, Ke L, Tong Z, Li G, et al. Risk factors and outcome for massive intra-abdominal bleeding among patients with infected necrotizing pancreatitis. Medicine (Baltimore). 2015;**94**:e1172. DOI: 10.1097/md.0000000000001172

[23] Law NM, Freeman ML. Emergency complications of acute and chronic pancreatitis. Gastroenterology Clinics of North America. 2003;**32**:1169-1194. DOI: 10.1016/s0889-8553(03)00089-x

[24] Gupta V, Irrinki S, Sakaray YR, Moond V, Yadav TD, Kochhar R, et al. Treatment strategies for bleeding from gastroduodenal artery pseudoaneurysms complicating the course of chronic pancreatitis-a case series of 10 patients. Indian Journal of Gastroenterology. 2018;**37**:457-463. DOI: 10.1007/s12664-018-0897-y

[25] Udd M, Leppäniemi AK, Bidel S, Keto P, Roth WD, Haapiainen RK.

Treatment of bleeding pseudoaneurysms in patients with chronic pancreatitis. World Journal of Surgery. 2007;**31**:504-510. DOI: 10.1007/s00268-006-0209-z

[26] Северцев АН, Вечорко ВИ, Репин ИГ, Аносов ВД, et al. Первый опыт использования эмболизации и системного введения факторов свертывания в комплексном лечении рецидивного аррозивного кровотечения при панкреонекрозе. Кремлевская медицина. Клинический вестник. 2024;**1**:133-136. [Severtsev A.N., Vechorko V.I., Repin I.G., Anosov V.D., et al. The first experience of using embolization and systemic administration of coagulation factors in the complex treatment of recurrent erosive bleeding in pancreatic necrosis. Kremlin Medicine J. 2024;1:133-136. In Russian]. DOI: 10.48612/cgma/pggk-1h1v-rtev

[27] Yamaguchi T, Toshihito T, Komemushi A, Suwa K, et al. Acute necrotizing pancreatitis as a fatal complication following DC bead transcatheter arterial chemoembolization for hepatocellular carcinoma: A case report and review of the literature. Molecular and Clinical Oncology. 2018;**9**:403-407. DOI: 10.3892/mco.2018.1690

Chapter 6

Pancreatic Cancer and Pancreatitis

Ahmet Ziya Bayhan

Abstract

Pancreatic cancer is still fatal despite effective treatment. Due to the special anatomy of the pancreas, symptoms do not occur in the early period and metastases occur frequently. The majority of pancreatic cancers have adenocarcinoma histology. Cystic neoplasm and neuroendocrine tumors are primary malignancies with a more indolent course. There is a complicated relationship between pancreatitis and pancreatic cancers. The risk factors, and clinical and radiological appearances of the two entities share common features. Moreover, with the progress in genetic science, it has been revealed that common genetic factors may play a role in the development of pancreatitis and pancreatic cancers. In this section, common pancreatic malignancies will be defined and their relationship with pancreatitis will be examined.

Keywords: pancreatitis, pancreatic cancer, autoimmune pancreatitis, abdominal pain, chronic pancreatitis

1. Introduction

According to GLOBOCAN in 2022, an estimated 510,992 people were diagnosed with pancreatic cancer and 467,409 people died from the disease in the world [1].

Primary pancreatic malignant neoplasm is divided into two main groups: exocrine pancreatic neoplasm and neuroendocrine tumors of the pancreas. Cystic neoplasms of the pancreas are considered a separate entity and basically define the premalignant period of exocrine pancreatic neoplasm. Pancreatic cystic neoplasms share many genetic and environmental risk factors with exocrine gland pancreatic cancers. Pancreatic ductal adenocarcinoma (PDAC) constitutes up to 95% of exocrine gland malignant neoplasm. For this reason, pancreatic cancer and PDAC are often used synonymously. Acinar cell-derived malignancies, squamous cell cancer, and undifferentiated carcinomas are very rare histological types.

The relationship between pancreatitis and pancreatic cancer is complicated. The role of acute pancreatitis in the development of pancreatic cancer is not clearly defined. Chronic pancreatitis is a better defined risk factor for the development of pancreatic cancer [2]. Some genetic risk factors are common cause both pancreatitis and pancreatic cancer. Moreover, conversely, pancreatic cancer can cause an attack of acute pancreatitis due to mechanical obstruction. Cystic neoplasms can also cause pancreatitis with similar mechanism.

Apart from the etiological similarity pancreatitis is also included in the differential diagnosis of pancreatic cancer.

2. Cystic neoplasms of the pancreas

With the increase in the use of radiological imaging, pancreatic cysts are detected more frequently incidentally. More than 50% of these are pancreatic cystic neoplasms, while the remainder are clinically insignificant cysts (small pseudocysts, retention cysts, etc.).

Cystic neoplasms are diverse tumors that range from harmless benign cysts to invasive, potentially lethal, cancers. Approximately 5 to 15% of all pancreatic cysts are neoplastic; these constitute less than 5% of all pancreatic neoplasms [3].

Pancreatic cystic neoplasm are classified into four main groups (**Table 1**) [4].

2.1 Serous cystadenoma

Serous cystadenomas account for approximately 25% of all pancreatic cystic neoplasms; histologically, they are composed of glycogen-rich cuboidal cells. The pathophysiology of pancreatic serous cystadenomas is poorly understood. Often, pancreatic serous cystadenomas are detected incidentally by abdominal ultrasonography or cross-sectional imaging studies performed for another condition. Serous cystadenoma shows low viscosity, low amylase level (unlike psödokist), and low carcinoembryonic antigen (CEA) levels. Malignancy potential is low. The female: male ratio is 2:1. It is often diagnosed in the seventh decade of life. Large cyst can cause pain and may lead to extrahepatic cholestasis or pancreatitis through mechanical obstruction. Somatic von-Hippel Lindau (VHL) mutation is common [5] and surgery provides almost complete cure.

2.2 Mucinous cystic neoplasm (MCN)

The cystic spaces are filled with thick, tenacious mucin, and the cysts are lined by a columnar mucinous. The female: male ratio is 2:1. One-third shows malignant transformation, located in the body or tail of pancreas. The most common and early genetic alteration occurring in MCN is the KRAS gene.

Serous neoplasm
Serous cystadenoma
Serous cystadenocarcinoma
Mucinous cystic neoplasm
Mucinous cystic neoplasm with low-grade dysplasia
Mucinous cystic neoplasm with high-grade dysplasia
Intraductal papillary mucinous neoplasm
Intraductal papillary mucinous neoplasm with low-grade dysplasia
Intraductal papillary mucinous neoplasm with high grade dysplasia
Solid pseudopapillary neoplasm

Table 1.
Pancreatic cystic neoplasm classification.

2.3 İntraductal papillary mucinous neoplasm (IPMN)

İt is often seen in men and located in the head of the pancreas. PMNs arise in the main pancreatic ducts, or one of its major branch ducts, and lack the cellular stroma seen in mucinous cystic neoplasms [6]. Therefore, it may present with obstructive symptoms and mechanical pancreatitis Recurrent attacks of acute pancreatitis are common due to mucin plugs. Up to two-thirds of IPMNs harbor oncogenic mutations of GNAS on chromosome 20q13, which encode the alpha subunit of a stimulatory G-protein [7].

2.4 Solid pseudopapillary neoplasm

Unlike other cystic neoplasms, it is diagnosed in early age. Diagnosis is common in the second and third decades. The female: male ratio is 2:1. İt is frequently detected incidentally and may cause obstructive symptoms. Cross-sectional imaging reveals large, solitary, well-circumscribed lesions that can have a completely cystic, mixed cystic and solid, or purely solid appearance [8]. Surgery is curative [9].

3. Pancreatic cancer and acute pancreatitis

Acute pancreatitis is an inflammatory disease of the pancreas that develops suddenly. Previous experimental studies have suggested that acute pancreatitis can cause pancreatic cancer, whereas epidemiological studies have reported conflicting results. However, the association between acute pancreatitis and pancreatic cancer remains controversial. Otherwise, a retrospective analysis revealed a relationship between recurrent attacks of acute pancreatitis and the incidence of pancreatic cancer development [10]. The possible mechanism appears to be neutrophil infiltration, inflammation, and formation of free oxygen radicals [11]. Many patients have common risk factor for developing both acute pancreatitis and pancreatic cancer, such as diabetes, alcoholism, and obesity. Therefore, it seems difficult to reveal the direct effect of development of acute pancreatitis on the occurrence of pancreatic cancer in clinical studies.

Pancreatic cancer often presents with symptoms such as weight loss, jaundice, and pain. However, there are also pancreatic cancer patients who rarely present with acute pancreatitis [12]. Obstructive pancreatitis due to pancreatic cancer was considered. In this case, wait for pancreatitis-related inflammation to regress may be necessary to reduce postsurgical complication. Radiological imaging with CT or MRI the backbone of differential diagnosis.

Drug-associated pancreatitis constitutes a rare group of disease [13]. 5-FU is a drug reported in relation to drug-associated pancreatitis and is the one of the most commonly used chemotherapy drugs in the treatment of pancreatic cancer.

4. Autoimmune pancreatitis (AIP) in the differential diagnosis of pancreatic cancer

Autoimmune pancreatitis (AIP) is a distinct form of chronic pancreatitis that is characterized by striking infiltration of the pancreas by lymphocytes and plasma cells, many of which are positive for IgG4, accompanied by a "swirling" fibrosis and venulitis (aka lymphoplasmacytic sclerosing pancreatitis) [14].

Autoimmune pancreatitis is not a clearly established risk factor for the development of pancreatic cancer and it has not been clearly demonstrated as a risk factor in case series [15]. On the other hand, there are patient series in which 1–2% of patients diagnosed with AIP by biopsy are accompanied by pancreatic cancer [16].

For instance, Kamisawa et al. found that codon-12 mutation of K-ras was significantly more frequent in the pancreato-biliary regions of patients with autoimmune pancreatitis (AIP) than in those affected with chronic alcoholic pancreatitis [17]. K-ras mutation is the most frequently detected genetic mutation in PDAC. More recently, Kinugawa et al. also described some methylation abnormalities of tumor suppressor genes in AIP patients. Promoter region hypermethylation with consequent gene silencing was reported for several genes in pancreatic cancer [18]. TPFI2 is a tumor suppressor gene. TPFI2 has previously been associated with pancreatic cancer [19] and has been seen with increased frequency in AIP, however genetic mutation similarities have been shown the clinical relationship has not been clearly established.

AIP can present with clinical and radiologic characteristics of pancreatic cancer, such as jaundice, weight loss, elevated CA 19-9 level, and the presence of diffuse pancreatic enlargement, a pancreatic ductal stricture (**Figure 1**), or a focal pancreatic mass [20]. Therefore, it is included in the differential diagnosis of pancreatic cancer. Diffusely enlarged pancreas, late-phase enhancement on MRI, increased Ig4 level in serum, and normal or near-normal CA 19.9 are helpful in diagnosis. Biopsy is required definitive diagnosis. Response to steroid is often dramatic. However, as stated before, the association of pancreatic cancer should be taken into consideration. If steroid is used without a biopsy due to an emergency, radiological and clinical follow-up should continue.

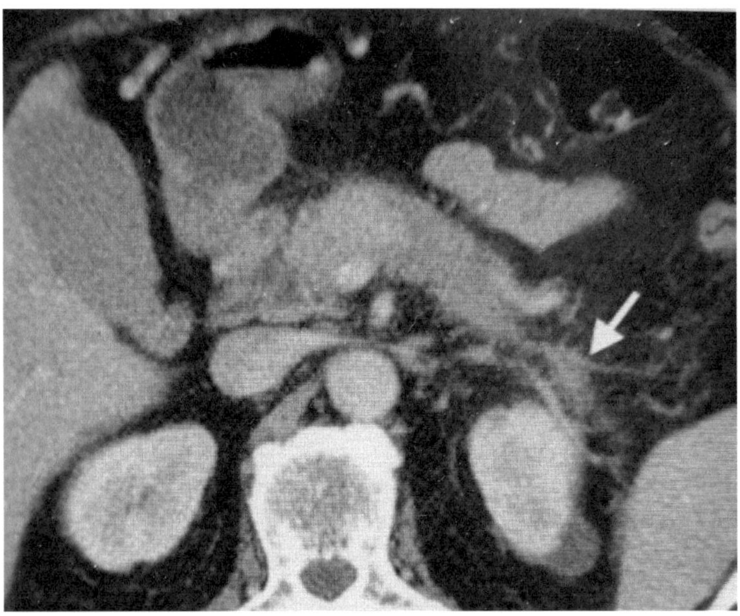

Figure 1.
Tomography image of autoimmune pancreatitis.

5. Pancreatic cancer and chronic pancreatitis

Like all cancers, pancreatic cancer arises as a consequence of inherited and acquired mutations in cancer-associated genes. There is a progressive accumulation of genetic changes in pancreatic epithelium as it proceeds from non-neoplastic to noninvasive precursor lesions, and to invasive carcinoma [21]. The main risk factors for pancreatic cancer are modifiable and include tobacco smoking, obesity, physical inactivity, and high-calorie/fat diets; these lifestyle-related risk factors clearly contributed to the increase of the disease incidence in the last three decades, especially in the developed countries, where diagnostic improvements and increased life expectancy have played a role as well [22].

Most of the PDAC cases are sporadic, but about 5–10% report a hereditary predisposition [23]. The recent sequencing of the pancreatic cancer genome has confirmed that four genes are most commonly affected by somatic mutations in this neoplasm: KRAS, CDKN2A/p16, SMAD4, and TP53. KRAS is the most frequently altered oncogene in pancreatic cancer; it is activated by a point mutation in greater than 90% of cases. These mutations impair the intrinsic GTPase activity of the KRAS protein so that it is constitutively active. In turn, KRAS activates a number of intracellular signaling pathways that promote carcinogenesis. CDKN2A/p16, SMAD4, and TP53 mutations result in tumor suppressor gene inactivation [24]. Ultimately, it results in escape from apoptosis and uncontrolled proliferation. ATM, BRCA 1, and BRCA 2 are genes involved in cell repair pathways and are associated with familiar pancreatic cancer [25, 26].

Chronic pancreatitis is a disease characterized by recurrent parenchymal inflammation and subsequent fibrosis. It may be caused by mechanical ductal obstruction, repeated toxin exposure (alcohol, etc.), autoimmune pancreatitis, or some genetic mutations. The final result is exocrine and endocrine pancreatic insufficiency. Also, chronic pancreatitis has been demonstrated as a risk factor for the development of pancreatic cancer [27].

Like pancreatic cancer, many genes have been identified for the development of chronic pancreatitis. PRSS1 (Katyonik tripsinojen) and SPİNK1 (tripsin inhibitör gen) are two genes that regulate trypsin activation. Activation of trypsin converts other zymogens into their active forms. Mutation in these regions has been associated with hereditary pancreatitis, resulting in chronic pancreatitis. Chronic pancreatitis that begins in childhood, such as hereditary pancreatitis secondary to PRSS1 mutations, confers a 40 to 55% lifetime risk for pancreatic cancer [28, 29]. CFTR gene mutation also causes the development of chronic pancreatitis as a component of cystic fibrosis [30]. These mutations cause chronic pancreatitis but do not appear to be direct factor in the development of malignancy. Although malignancy is thought to be due to repeated physical damage and inflammation, common genetic disorders for chronic pancreatitis and pancreatic cancer are also being identified.

Chronic pancreatitis may be asymptomatic or present only with steatorrhea. However, it can sometimes mimic symptoms of pancreatic cancer, such as pain, increased bilirubin, and weight loss. CT, MRI-MRCP, or EUS are often help to exclude pancreatic cancer (**Figure 2**). However, sometimes a local mass imaging may be present in chronic pancreatitis. CA 19.9 has low sensitivity and specificity. Considering the increased frequency of pancreatic cancer in chronic pancreatitis, a biopsy should be performed if necessary. There is no globally accepted practice for screening for malignancy in patients with chronic pancreatitis.

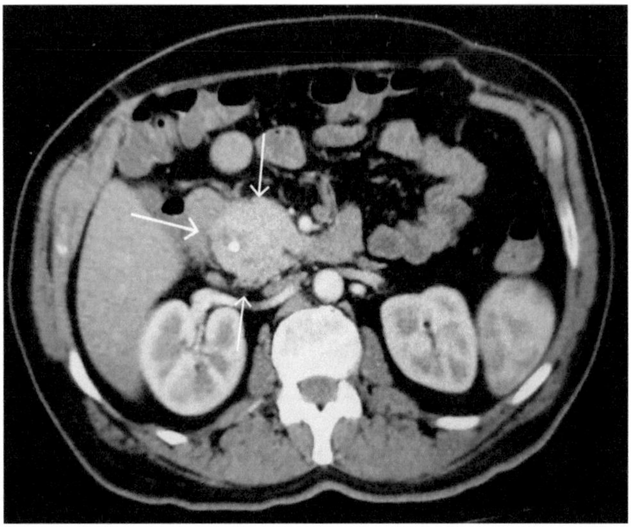

Figure 2.
Tomography image of chronic pancreatitis.

6. Pancreatic neuroendocrine tumors

They constitute 1% of pancreatic cancers and approximately 80% are non-functional [31]. Well-differentiated grade 3 neuroendocrine tumors (NETs) were introduced as a new category in the 2017 WHO classification update of pancreatic neuroendocrine neoplasia (**Table 2**) [32].

Nonfuntionaş tumors generally do not cause symptoms and are detected incidentally. As a result, they often present later in the course of the disease with symptoms of local compression or metastatic disease [33]. On the other hand, functional tumors generally become symptomatic earlier due to the peptides they secrete. İnsulinoma with hypoglycemia attacks; gastrinoma with peptic ulcer; glucagonoma diabetes and necrolytic migratory erythema; and VIPoma may present with secretory diarrhea and hypokalemia. These tumors may also present with metastasis. Pancreatic neuroendocrine carcinomas lead to an aggressive clinic with a poor prognosis. These tumors are often diagnosed as metastasis.

Pancreatic neuroendocrine tumors can theoretically cause pancreatitis. However, there are very few clinically reported cases [34].

Grade	Ki67 İndex (%)	Mitotik İndex
Well-differentiated pancreatic neuroendocrine tumors		
Grade 1	<3	<2
Grade 2	3–20	2–20
Grade 3	>20	>20
Poor differentiated pancreatic neuroendocrine tumors		
Neuroendocrine carcinoma (Grade 3)	>20	>20

The mitotic index is based on the evaluation of (0.2 mm^2 each) in areas of higher density.

Table 2.
Pancreatic neuroendocrine neoplasm, basic histologic WHO classification.

7. Metastatik pancreatic tumors

Metastasis to the pancreatic gland is extremely rare. Lymphoma, renal cell carcinoma, colon, and esophagus cancer metastases have been reported rarely [35, 36]. Although it is theoretically possible for this tumor to cause pancreatitis, it has not been reported clinically.

Duodenum, distal biliary tract, and ampulla tumors can also cause pancreatitis through obstruction. But these tumors are beyond the scope of this section of the book.

Lymphoma is clinically characterized by absence of jaundice and distinct constitutional (weight loss, fever, and night sweats) symptoms. It is important to consider in the differential diagnosis of autoimmune pancreatitis and PDA. Elevated levels of LDH and beta-2 microglobulin and widespread lymph node positivity are primarily favor lymphoma [37].

8. Conclusion

Recurrent acute pancreatitis and chronic pancreatitis constitute risk factor for the development of pancreatic cancer. Additionally, pancreatic cancer may rarely present with an attack of pancreatitis.

Conflict of interest

The authors declare no conflict of interest.

Thanks

Thanks to Dr. Öznur Yağmurkaya and Dr. Ebru Kahraman for figure.

Author details

Ahmet Ziya Bayhan
Adana City Education and Research Hospital, Adana, Turkey

*Address all correspondence to: bayhanahmetziya@gmail.com

References

[1] WHO. Global cancer observatory. Available from: https://gco.iarc.who.int/en

[2] Malka D, Hammel P, Maire F, et al. Risk of pancreatic adenocarcinoma in chronic pancreatitis. Gut. 2002;**51**:849-852

[3] Horvath KD, Chabot JA. An aggressive resectional approach to cystic neoplasms of the pancreas. American Journal of Surgery. 1999;**178**:269-274

[4] Gill AJ, Klimstra DS, Lam AK, et al. Tumours of the pancreas. In: WHO Classification of Tumours. 5th ed. Lyon: IARC Press; 2019. p. 296

[5] Springer S et al. A combination of molecular markers and clinical features improve the classification of pancreatic cysts. Gastroenterology. 2015;**149**(6):1501-1510

[6] Xiao S-Y. Intraductal Papillary Mucinous Neoplasm of the Pancreas: An Update Scientifica (Cairo). 2012;**28**:893632

[7] Ohtsuka T et al. Clinical assessment of the GNA mutation status in patients with intraductal papillary mucinous neoplasm of pankreas. Surgery Today. 2019;**49**(11):887-893

[8] De Robertis R et al. Solid Pseudopapillary neoplasms of the pancreas: Clinicopathologic and radiologic features according to size. American Journal of Roentgenology. 2019;**213**(5):1073-1080

[9] Lanke G et al. Clinical update on the management of pseuopapillary tumor of pancreas. World Journal of Gastrointestinal Endoscopy. 2018;**10**(9):145-155

[10] Jeong SH et al. Risk of pancreatic cancer after acute pancreatitis: A retrospective analysis of the Korean National Sample Cohort. Journal of Korean Medical Science. 2024;**39**(4):e21

[11] Jeon CY et al. Bidirectional relationship between acute pancreatitis and pancreatic cancer. Current Opinion in Gastroenterology. 2024;**40**(5):431-438

[12] Jiang R et al. Progress in the diagnosis and treatment of pancreatic cancer with acute pancreatitis as the initial symptom. Zhounghua Wai Ke Za Zhi. 2024;**62**(10):971-975

[13] Badalov N et al. Drug induced acute pancreatitis: An evidence-based review. Clinical Gastroenterology and Hepatology. 2007;**5**:648

[14] Matsubayashi H. Diagnosis of autoimmune pancreatitis. World Journal of Gastroenterology. 2014;**20**(44):16559-16569

[15] Buijs et al. The long-term impact of autoimmune pancreatitis on pancreatic function, quality of life, and life expectancy. Pancreas. 2015;**44**:1065-1071

[16] Shimosegawa T et al. International consensus diagnostic criteria for autoimmune pancreatitis. Pancreas. April 2011;**40**(3):352-358

[17] Kamisawa T, Tsuruta K, Okamoto A, Horiguchi S, Hayashi Y, Yun X, et al. Frequent and significant K-ras mutation in the pancreas, the bile duct, and the gallbladder in autoimmune pancreatitis. Pancreas. 2009;**38**:890-895. DOI: 10.1097/MPA.0b013e3181b65a1c

[18] Kinugawa Y, Uehara T, Sano K, Matsuda K, Maruyama Y, Kobayashi Y, et al. Methylation of tumor suppressor genes in autoimmune pancreatitis. Pancreas. 2017;**46**:614-618. DOI: 10.1097/MPA.0000000000000804

[19] Sato N, Parker AR, Fukushima N, Miyagi Y, Iacobuzio-Donahue CA, Eshleman JR, et al. Epigenetic inactivation of TFPI-2 as a common mechanism associated with growth and invasion of pancreatic ductal adenocarcinoma. Oncogene. 2005;**24**:850-858. DOI: 10.1038/sj.onc.1208050

[20] Kajiwara M, Kojima M, Konishi M, et al. Autoimmune pancreatitis with multifocal lesions. Journal of Hepato-Biliary-Pancreatic Surgery. 2008;**15**:449-452

[21] Brosens LAA et al. Pancreatic adenocarcinoma pathology: Changing "landscape". Journal of Gastrointestinal Oncology. Aug 2015;**6**(4):358-374

[22] Khalaf N, El-Serag HB, Abrams HR, Thrift AP. Burden of pancreatic cancer: From epidemiology to practice. Clinical Gastroenterology and Hepatology. 2021;**19**:876-884. DOI: 10.1016/j.cgh.2020.02.054], 10.1016/j.cgh.2020.02.054]

[23] Pilarski R. The role of BRCA testing in hereditary pancreatic and prostate cancer families. American Society of Clinical Oncology Educational Book. 2019;**39**:79-86

[24] Kumar V et al. Robbins Basic Pathology. 10th ed. Philadelphia, PA: Elsevier-Health Sciences Division; 2017. 687 p

[25] Roberts NJ et al. ATM mutations in patients with hereditary pancreatic cancer Nicolas. Journal of Cancer Discovery. 2012;**2**(1):41-46

[26] Vietri MT et al. Pancreatic cancer with mutation in BRCA ½, MLH1 and APC genes: Phenotype correlation and detection of a novel germline BRCA2 mutation. Genes. 2022;**13**:321. DOI: 10.3390/genes13020321

[27] Munigala S, Kanwal F, Xian H, et al. Increased risk of pancreatic adenocarcinoma after acute pancreatitis. Clinical Gastroenterology and Hepatology. 2014;**12**:1143-1150 e1141

[28] Kumar V et al. Robbins Basic Pathology. 10th ed. Philadelphia, PA: Elsevier-Health Sciences Division; 2017. 685 p

[29] Girodon E et al. Clinical interpretation of PRSS1 variants in patients with pancreatitis. Clinic and Research in Hepatology and Gastroenterology. 2021;**45**:101497

[30] Kumar V et al. Robbins Basic Pathology. 10th ed. Philadelphia, PA: Elsevier-Health Sciences Division; 2017. 683 p

[31] Yao JC, Eisner MP, Leary C, et al. Population-based study of islet cell carcinoma. Annals of Surgical Oncology. 2007;**14**:3492-3500

[32] Coriat R, Walter T, Terris B, et al. Gastroenteropancreatic well differentiated grade 3 neuroendocrine tumors: Review and position statement. The Oncologist. 2016;**21**:1191-1199

[33] Vagefi PA et al. Evolving patterns in the detection and outcomes of pancreatic neuroendocrine neoplasms: The Massachusetts General Hospital experience from 1977 to 2005. Archives of Surgery. 2007;**142**(4):347

[34] De Cesare A et al. Acute pancreatitis secondary ton on-functioning pancreatic neuroendocrine tumor:Uncommon

clinical presentation. Clinical case and review of literature. Annali Italiani di Chirurgia. 2021;**10**:S2239253X21034939

[35] Eghlimi H et al. A rare case of colorectal cancer metastasis to the pancreas: A case report. Journal of Surgical Case Reports. 2024;**2024**(3):rjae173

[36] Denda Y et al. Simultaneous presentation and resection of esophageal cancer and metastasis to the pancreas: Alpha case report and literature review. Molecular and Clinical Oncology. 2023;**20**(1):2

[37] Rock J et al. The spectrum of hematologic malignancies involving the pancreas: Potential clinical mimics of pancreatic adenocarcinoma. American Journal of Clinical Pathology. 2012;**137**(3):41422

Chapter 7

Microbiota Involvement in Acute and Chronic Pancreatitis

Sandica Bucurica

Abstract

The microbiota plays a significant role in the development, progression, and severity of both acute and chronic pancreatitis through mechanisms involving immune modulation, microbial translocation, and gut permeability. The intricate relationship between gut microbiota and pancreatitis reveals distinct mechanisms through which acute and chronic forms of the disease manifest. In acute pancreatitis, microbial dysbiosis leads to significant alterations in gut flora, characterized by reduced diversity and an overrepresentation of pathogenic bacteria. This dysbiosis is associated with compromised gut barrier integrity and increased bacterial translocation, resulting in heightened systemic inflammation mediated by lipopolysaccharides and Toll-like receptor activation. In contrast, chronic pancreatitis is marked by persistent microbial imbalances driven by ongoing inflammation and malnutrition, further exacerbating the disease state. The interactions between gut microbiota and pancreatic function demonstrate a bidirectional relationship, where dysbiosis contributes to pancreatic injury and is also a consequence of impaired exocrine function. Overall, advancing our knowledge of the gut-pancreas axis will enhance our understanding of disease pathology and inform more effective treatment strategies for individuals affected by pancreatic disorders.

Keywords: acute pancreatitis, chronic pancreatitis, gut-microbiota, gut-pancreas axis, oral microbiota

1. Introduction

The gastrointestinal and oral microbiota play a significant role in health and disease, influencing immune function, inflammation, and systemic homeostasis. Recent research has identified the connection between gut microbiota and pancreatic health, finding the imbalance in microbial communities as a contributing factor in the pathogenesis of pancreatic diseases. This chapter explores how microbiota may influence pancreatitis onset, progression, and severity, addressing recent findings that uncover the microbiota's roles in inflammation, immune modulation, and potential therapeutic interventions.

Although pancreatic diseases encompass a vast range of conditions, acute and chronic pancreatitis are the most prevalent alongside pancreatic cancer, with increasing rates despite medical advancements [1–5] Acute pancreatitis (AP) is characterized by a critical tissue inflammation that can lead to severe systemic complications.

In contrast, chronic pancreatitis (CP) involves prolonged inflammation and fibrosis, often resulting in exocrine and endocrine insufficiencies [6, 7].

The etiopathogenetic factors involved in pancreatic disease are various, and microbiota imbalances are one of them [8, 9]. The human microbiota consists of a vast and complex community of microorganisms that play essential roles in maintaining health by aiding digestion, synthesizing vitamins, and modulating immune responses. Gut microbiota, including species from the phyla Firmicutes, Bacteroidetes, Proteobacteria, and Actinobacteria, influences human health, from immune function to metabolic regulation. Recent research has shown that these microbial communities are not limited to the gut but populate other organs also, including the pancreas [10, 11].

2. The gut-microbiota and gut-pancreas axis

2.1 Gut microbiota balance

The gut microbiota represents an extensive and complex ecosystem, with over 3500 microbial species identified. While most of these species belong to the bacterial domain, a minority (17 species) fall under the Archaea domain, with *Methanobrevibacter smithii* being a predominant archaeal member [12]. This biosystem includes fungi, viruses, and phages in addition to bacteria. The major bacterial phyla in the gut are *Bacteroidetes*, *Firmicutes*, *Proteobacteria*, *Actinobacteria*, *Fusobacteria*, and *Verrucomicrobia*. *Firmicutes* and *Bacteroidetes* are the dominant groups, while the other phyla constitute approximately 10% of the gut microbiota [13]. Fungal species such as *Candida*, *Saccharomyces*, *Malassezia*, and *Cladosporium* also contribute to this microbiome ecosystem [14–16]. The proper and balanced state of the gut microbiota population characterizes the eubiosis status. For instance, the balance between Firmicutes and Bacteroidetes has a role in maintaining gut health, and shifts in their ratio have been linked to dysbiosis [15, 17]. Consequently, dysbiosis represents an imbalanced state in one's gut microbiota by disrupting the symbiotic relationship between the microbiota and the host, leading to a heightened risk of systemic diseases or inflammatory conditions [13].

Multiple factors are involved in microbiota changes that affect the host's health. The intestinal barrier represents one of these factors and plays an important role in host defense. The gastrointestinal tract, with its vast luminal surface, interacts directly with dietary particles and microbial components, making it the body's primary defense interface.

The intestinal barrier comprises several key elements: the mucus layer, commensal microbes, antimicrobial peptides, secretory immunoglobulin A (IgA), a monolayer of specialized epithelial cells, and immune cells within the lamina propria [18]. Each component works harmoniously to protect the host from potential pathogens and prevent the translocation of harmful substances from the gut lumen into circulation. This barrier integrity is critical in preventing endotoxemia [19]. The barrier itself can be disrupted at both molecular and physical levels. Under normal conditions, tight junctions between epithelial cells maintain low permeability, preventing the passage of pathogens and large molecules. However, when these tight junctions are weakened or "loosened," the result is increased gut permeability, often termed "leaky gut" [20]. This condition allows pathogen-associated molecular patterns (PAMPs) to cross the barrier and enter the bloodstream, where they can trigger inflammatory responses [21, 22].

Zonulin, a protein that modulates the permeability of tight junctions, is central to regulating gut barrier integrity. Elevated levels of zonulin are a hallmark of dysbiosis and increased gut permeability. This allows microbial products and toxins to enter the bloodstream, thereby promoting systemic inflammation and endotoxemia [20, 23]. In conditions where gut dysbiosis is prevalent, zonulin release increases, leading to a compromised barrier and setting the stage for various metabolic and inflammatory diseases [20].

The interaction between the gut microbiota and the intestinal barrier begins at birth and evolves throughout life. Gut microbes influence mucus production and quality by stimulating epithelial cells in the intestine and colon, reinforcing the barrier against pathogens [24, 25]. Besides physical barrier enhancement, the microbiota regulates immune responses by balancing pro- and anti-inflammatory signals. For example, certain bacteria stimulate the production of short-chain fatty acids (SCFAs), which support regulatory T-cell (Treg) differentiation, foster immune tolerance, and reduce inflammation in the gut [26].

Moreover, the gut microbiota also plays an essential role in the developing process of the enteric nervous system and in shaping the immune system's response to intestinal antigens. These microorganisms influence the gut-brain axis, a bidirectional communication network between the gut and the central nervous system (CNS). By producing neuroactive compounds like SCFAs, neurotransmitters, and bioactive peptides, the microbiota contributes to gut-brain signaling that can impact brain function, mood, and stress responses [27].

Another level of defense provided by the intestinal barrier is the chemical defense. The gut barrier is protected by a chemical defense layer that includes antimicrobial proteins, bile acids, and enzymes. Antimicrobial proteins prevent barrier erosion by inhibiting bacterial overgrowth, while bile acids support gut epithelial growth, regeneration, and mucus production. The stomach has a low pH, which further aids in limiting bacterial colonization in the upper GI tract and protecting the small intestine from pathogen invasion [28, 29].

The gut microbiota maintains a symbiotic relationship with the host's immune system. In a state of eubiosis (a balanced microbial population), the gut microbiota promotes overall health by aiding in immune modulation, pathogen defense, and the metabolic processing of nutrients. Beyond digestion, the microbiota synthesizes bioactive compounds, such as secondary bile acids, SCFAs, and neurotransmitters, which participate in gut-liver and gut-brain axis signaling. These compounds regulate distant organs and systemic physiological processes, highlighting the microbiota's role in metabolic health, immune homeostasis, and nervous system function. SCFAs, for instance, influence the hypothalamic-pituitary-adrenal (HPA) axis, modulating stress responses and indirectly affecting CNS function [30, 31].

In sum, the gut microbiota's intricate relationship with the host underscores its essential role in health. Disruption of this balanced ecosystem through dysbiosis can lead to compromised intestinal integrity, systemic inflammation, and a predisposition to various metabolic and inflammatory diseases.

2.2 The gut-pancreas axis and molecular pathways

Among the multiple gut-organ axes described, such as the gut-brain axis, gut-liver axis, or gut-skin axis, the gut-pancreas axis is represented by the bidirectional relationship between the gut and the pancreas, mediated by gut microbiota, immune cells, and metabolites. Disruption in this axis due to dysbiosis has been implicated in pancreatic diseases, marked by alterations in gut microbiota composition, increased gut permeability, bacterial translocation, and systemic inflammation—all factors contributing to pancreatic pathology [32].

Since the exocrine pancreas is the primary producer of digestive enzymes, such as amylases, proteases, and lipases secreted by acinar cells into the small intestine, acute and chronic pancreatitis are associated with various exocrine pancreatic dysfunction. Besides the breakdown of ingested food into the primary absorbable forms, pancreatic enzymatic digestion provides essential nutrients for the gut microbiota [33].

The gut-pancreas axis comprises a multilevel interaction mechanism, including microbial metabolites, increased intestinal permeability, and immune system modulation [34].

Dysbiosis may increase intestinal permeability ("leaky gut"), allowing bacterial antigens and endotoxins to enter the bloodstream and exacerbate pancreatic inflammation. Increased lipopolysaccharides (LPS) levels from gut bacteria are associated with higher inflammation markers in pancreatitis [35, 36]. On the other hand, microbial metabolites, such as short-chain fatty acids (SCFAs) and other signaling molecules, influence pancreatic health by modulating immune responses and inflammatory signaling pathways. Moreover, SCFA production impacts the gut barrier's integrity [36, 37].

The immune system plays a central role in maintaining pancreatic health and regulating inflammation. Gut microbiota communicates directly with the immune system through various signaling mechanisms, impacting inflammatory responses that influence pancreatic diseases like pancreatitis and pancreatic cancer. Microbial components interact with pattern recognition receptors (PRRs) such as Toll-like receptors (TLRs) and Nod-like receptors (NLRs) on immune cells, triggering cytokine release and influencing immune cell differentiation. In states of dysbiosis, these signaling pathways can become overactivated, leading to chronic inflammation that contributes to disease progression [38].

Toll-like receptors (TLRs) are a class of PRRs that detect microbial-associated molecular patterns (MAMPs) and initiate immune responses. In the pancreas, TLRs are expressed on immune cells like macrophages and dendritic cells and on pancreatic acinar and ductal cells, which can respond to microbial signals originating from the gut. Under healthy conditions, the microbiota interacts with TLRs at controlled levels, promoting immune tolerance and maintaining gut barrier integrity. However, increased exposure to microbial products, such as lipopolysaccharides (LPS) from Gram-negative bacteria during dysbiosis can lead to heightened TLR activation [36, 39].

TLR4, the receptor for LPS, is especially relevant in acute pancreatitis. Studies have shown that increased circulating LPS levels in AP patients activate TLR4 signaling, triggering a cascade of pro-inflammatory cytokine production, including TNF-α, IL-1β, and IL-6, contributing to systemic inflammatory responses [40, 41]. This inflammation can lead to further pancreatic tissue damage, exacerbate gut permeability, and allow more microbial translocation, creating a vicious cycle of immune activation and inflammation [41].

In chronic pancreatitis, persistent TLR activation contributes to fibrosis and immune cell infiltration in pancreatic tissue. Studies suggest that TLR4 and TLR2 (receptor for peptidoglycans from Gram-positive bacteria) are upregulated in CP, leading to sustained inflammatory signaling and increased production of fibrogenic cytokines like transforming growth factor-beta (TGF-β) [41]. These findings underscore the role of TLR-mediated immune activation in maintaining chronic inflammation, which can lead to irreversible pancreatic damage over time [42].

Another pathway involved in gut microbiota interference with the pancreatic inflammatory process is through Nod-like receptors (NLRs) and inflammasome activation. NLRs are another group of PRRs that detect intracellular microbial components. Upon activation, NLRs assemble into inflammasomes, protein complexes that trigger the release of pro-inflammatory cytokines, including IL-1β and IL-18. NLRs play a significant role in regulating inflammation within the pancreas, particularly through the NLRP3 inflammasome, which is highly expressed in pancreatic immune cells and acinar cells [43].

In acute pancreatitis, NLRP3 inflammasome activation has been shown to exacerbate pancreatic inflammation. Dysbiosis-induced bacterial translocation into systemic circulation can activate NLRP3 in pancreatic tissue, which promotes the release of IL-1β, a potent mediator of inflammation [44, 45]. Elevated IL-1β levels contribute to acinar cell injury, edema, and the infiltration of immune cells into pancreatic tissue, all of which worsen AP severity. Furthermore, studies have found that inhibiting NLRP3 activity can reduce inflammatory damage in experimental models of AP, highlighting its role in the immune response to dysbiosis [44, 45].

NLRP3 activation also contributes to chronic pancreatitis's persistent inflammation and fibrosis [46]. Chronically activated NLRP3 inflammasomes result in prolonged IL-1β production, promoting a feedback loop of inflammation and tissue remodeling that leads to fibrotic changes. This process has been associated with alterations in the gut microbiota, where increased pathogenic bacterial populations promote NLRP3 activation *via* bacterial products that reach the pancreas [47].

Both TLR and NLR activation release cytokines, which are critical in orchestrating the immune response. Cytokines such as IL-6, IL-1β, and TNF-α are elevated in patients with pancreatic diseases, particularly during acute inflammatory episodes in AP. In chronic inflammation, such as in CP and pancreatic cancer, cytokine signaling sustains a low-grade, systemic inflammatory response that facilitates disease progression and immune suppression [47].

In pancreatitis, the cytokine response to dysbiosis involves both pro-inflammatory and anti-inflammatory signals. TNF-α and IL-6 are initially beneficial in containing infection and clearing damaged tissue. However, persistent cytokine release due to continued microbial exposure results in systemic inflammatory response syndrome (SIRS), which is common in severe AP and a major cause of AP-associated mortality [48]. In addition, cytokines like IL-10, which typically downregulate inflammation, are often dysregulated in chronic pancreatic diseases, resulting in insufficient immune control and chronic inflammation [42].

The protective mechanisms intervene by activation of regulatory T cells and anti-inflammatory signals. The pancreatic acinar cells produce most of the Regs, which belong to the C-type lectin family and provide protective action of the host against bacteria [49]. Of the increased REG2, 3β, and 3ϒ, the last one has the role of multifunctional antimicrobial peptide and action mainly on Gram-positive bacteria. Alongside the counteract of Reg 3β, which acts against Gram-negative bacteria, both could retain microorganisms in luminal intestinal space and minimize microbial translocation through a leaky gut [32].

Regulatory T cells (Tregs) are a subset of T cells that maintain immune homeostasis and prevent excessive inflammation by suppressing pro-inflammatory responses. The gut microbiota influences Treg populations primarily by producing short-chain fatty acids (SCFAs), which enhance Treg differentiation and function. However, in pancreatic diseases, dysbiosis can reduce SCFA-producing bacteria, leading to impaired Treg function and uncontrolled inflammation (**Figure 1**) [50].

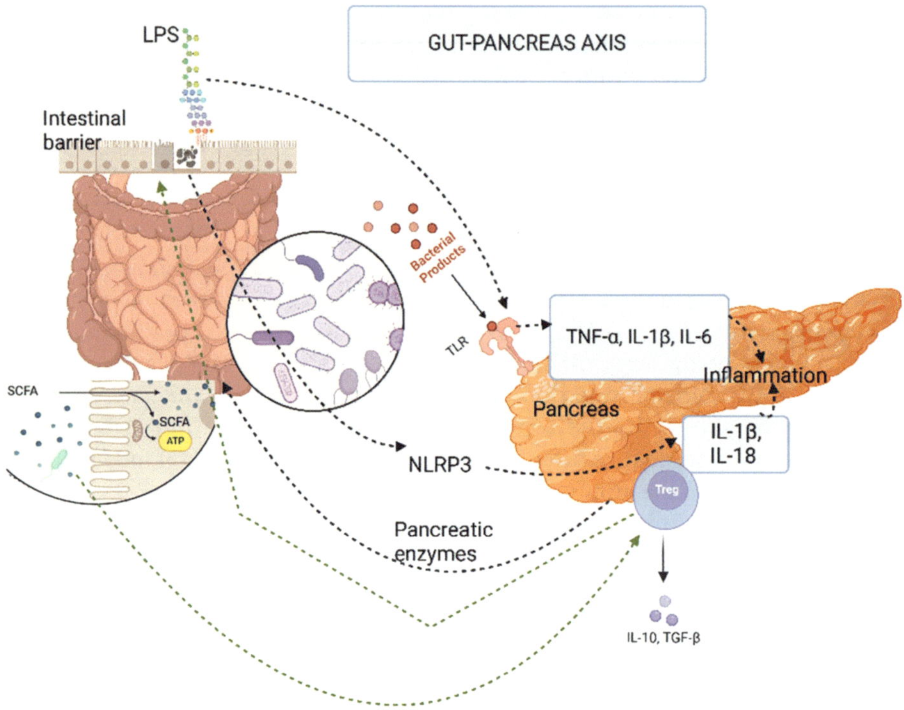

Figure 1.
Gut-pancreas axis. Pancreatic enzymes (amylases, proteases, and lipases) provide essential nutrients for the gut microbiota. The integrity of the intestinal barrier is essential in maintaining the eubiosis state. When the integrity is lost, bacterial antigens and endotoxins enter the bloodstream and activate the immune system. The activation of the immune system is intermediated by bacterial LPS, which activates TLR4 and promotes a cascade of pro-inflammatory cytokine production, including TNF-α, IL-1β, and IL-6, contributing to systemic inflammatory responses. The other inflammatory pathway is through NLRs and inflammasome activation, resulting in IL-1β and IL-18 release. Activating Treg represents the protective pancreatic response and releases TGF-β and IL-10, with roles in maintaining immune homeostasis. The gut microbiota influences Treg populations primarily by producing SCFAs, which enhance Treg differentiation and function. Abbreviations: TLR—Toll-like receptor, LPS—lipopolysaccharides, NLRP3—NOD-, LRR- and pyrin domain-containing protein 3, TNF-α—tumor necrosis factor-α, IL—1β-interleukin-1β, IL-6—interleukin 6, Treg—Regulatory T cells, SCFAs—short-chain fatty acids, IL-10—interleukin-10, TGF-β—transforming growth factor-β. (Created in BioRender).

Studies in both AP and CP have shown that reduced Treg activity correlates with increased pancreatic inflammation and disease severity. In the context of pancreatic cancer, Tregs are paradoxically involved in immune suppression within the tumor microenvironment. Tumor-associated Tregs suppress anti-tumor immune responses, facilitating cancer progression. Dysbiosis in cancer patients promotes Treg recruitment to the tumor site, contributing to an immunosuppressive environment that allows cancer cells to evade immune surveillance [51, 52].

Therapeutically, efforts to enhance Treg function through microbiota modulation, such as probiotic supplementation or fecal microbiota transplantation (FMT), have shown promise in reducing inflammation in pancreatic diseases. Probiotics that promote SCFA production have been found to increase Treg levels, potentially restoring immune balance and preventing excessive inflammation in pancreatitis [53].

3. Gut microbiota and pancreatitis

Although both diseases represent an inflammatory impairment of the pancreas, acute and chronic pancreatitis display different pathways and patterns of gut microbiota imbalance. In acute pancreatitis, bacterial translocation and immune activation are described through increased gut permeability and LPS and TLR activation; meanwhile, in chronic pancreatitis, the studies found microbial dysbiosis associated with persistent inflammation. Also, the nutritional impairment related to chronic pancreatitis promotes microbiota changes and different immune modulation.

3.1 Gut microbiota and acute pancreatitis

The gut microbiota dysbiosis in acute pancreatitis is often characterized by decreased diversity in beneficial bacteria, such as *Faecalibacterium* and *Bifidobacterium*, and an increase in pathogenic bacteria from the *Proteobacteria* phylum, including *Escherichia coli* and *Klebsiella* [50]. This shift in microbiota composition disrupts gut barrier integrity, enabling bacterial translocation into the systemic circulation and triggering an inflammatory cascade.

Dysbiosis is a common feature in AP patients, with studies showing distinct microbial signatures compared to healthy individuals. Specifically, AP is associated with reduced levels of *Bacteroidetes* and *Firmicutes* and an overrepresentation of *Proteobacteria* and *Fusobacteria*, especially in severe cases. These microbial shifts disrupt gut barrier function, enabling the translocation of bacterial products like lipopolysaccharides (LPS) into the systemic circulation, which can trigger a heightened inflammatory response in the pancreas. This study by Wang et al. showed a variability of microbial gut species with the grade of pancreatitis severity [54]. *Synergistota*, *Patescibacteria*, *Desulfobacterota,* and *Fusobacteriota* were predominant in the peak phase of AP compared with the remission stage. *Fusobacteriota* was related to the evolution of chronic inflammation or carcinogenesis. *Desulfobacterota* and *Synersistota* were associated with an acute inflammatory response by damaging the intestinal barrier and LPS luminal discharge [54]. The same study found that a decreased level of *Verrucomicrobiota* was related to a more severe stage of acute pancreatitis. Moreover, *Akkermansia muciniphila*, a component of the *Verrucomicrobiota* family, has proven protective activity by enhancing the defensive immune response by stimulating dendritic cells and increasing Treg cell expression [54]. Another affected population was *Proteobacteria*, which maintain a proper intestinal immune response. The Wang et al. study concluded that the more microbiota is influenced and imbalanced, the more severe course of AP will follow [54].

Two Mendelian randomization studies found causal or positive associations between acute pancreatitis and changes in the amount of *Eubacterium*, *Coprococcus*, *Clostridiaceae*, *Lachnospiraceae*, *Proteobacteria*, and *Bacteroidales* [55, 56]. These studies also found that the *Firmicutes* phylum, genus *Flavonifractor*, *Methanobrevibacter*, *Prevotella*, *Ruminiclostridium*, and *Ruminococcaceae* were protective factors against acute pancreatitis [55, 56].

Further published literature described the same changes in gut microbiota and their effects on damaging the intestinal barrier and bacterial translocation. Even more, it related acute pancreatitis with inflammatory bowel diseases, stating that these patients are at higher risk of developing necrotizing forms [32]. In normal conditions, pancreatic enzymes maintain beneficial populations of microorganisms in the intestinal lumen. Pancreatic lipase favors the thriving of protective species such as *Akkermansia muciniphila* and *Lactobacillus reuteri*, which strengthens the intestinal barrier and suppresses mucosal inflammation [32]. The impaired exocrine secretion of lipase, which occurs in acute pancreatitis, disables fat and protein absorption, impedes the national status of the host and the host's microbiota, and balances the intestinal barrier [57]. In addition, increased populations of *Escherichia coli* and *Enterococcus* were found in acute pancreatitis [58].

LPS, as bacterial endotoxin from Gram-negative bacteria in the *Proteobacteria* phylum, is one of AP's most potent inflammation triggers. Elevated LPS levels in AP patients correlate with disease severity due to their activation of immune cells through TLR4, leading to systemic inflammation and tissue damage [11]. Gut bacteria and their metabolites interact with Toll-like receptors, specifically TLR4, which play a critical role in immune activation. In AP, dysbiotic microbiota can overstimulate these receptors, increasing pro-inflammatory cytokines and activating the NF-κB pathway, which amplifies pancreatic inflammation [41, 59].

The pathogenic bacteria, including *Enterococcus*, *Escherichia coli*, and *Klebsiella*, are often abundant in AP patients. These bacteria can translocate across the gut barrier, particularly in necrotic pancreatitis, where infections complicate the disease course. These bacteria are associated with increased morbidity and mortality in AP patients, underscoring the need for effective infection control and microbial modulation strategies [11, 60].

Microbial metabolites, such as SCFAs and secondary bile acids, play essential roles in maintaining gut and pancreatic health. *Verrucomicrobiota* produces SCFAs, consequently stimulating the production of the beneficial and protective propionic acid and butyric acid [54]. In AP, dysbiosis reduces SCFA production, removing an essential anti-inflammatory mechanism. Conversely, dysbiosis increases the production of pro-inflammatory metabolites, which can exacerbate the disease's inflammatory cascade.

3.2 Gut microbiota and chronic pancreatitis

The data showed a drastically decreased microbial variety, with a predominance of facultative microbial pathogens in chronic pancreatitis cases with chronic pancreatitis compared to healthy individuals [61]. Moreover, the gut microbiota in CP has a significantly different composition from that found in a healthy gut [62].

The relationship between gut microbiota and pancreatic exocrine insufficiency is bidirectional since microbiota dysbiosis disrupts the regulatory pathways in the gut-pancreas axis, and impaired exocrine pancreatic function exerts a significant alteration of intestinal microbial state [63]. The first study on pancreatic exocrine insufficiency and gut microbiota-associated changes showed that in conjunction with a reduction in pancreatic elastase, dysbiotic changes included a significant increase in *Prevotella*, a bacterium that promotes chronic inflammation [63]. The interrelationship between microbial components in the gut and pancreatic function is demonstrated by the *Prevotella* species' production of hydrogen sulfate, a compound known to trigger pancreatic injury *via* apoptosis, potentially worsening the decline in exocrine pancreatic function [63]. The LPS production pathway is also involved in the complex interrelationship between dysbiosis and chronic pancreatitis. *Escherichia-Shigella's* production of LPS promotes the inflammatory process, activates TLR 4, and leads to pancreatic fibrosis through TGF-beta 1 activation of pancreatic stellate cells [36]. Type 3c diabetes is the endocrine insufficiency associated with exocrine insufficiency;

another consequence of the pancreatic fibrotic process had a gut microbiota characterized by a decline of the *Faecalibacterium prausnitzii* population [64].

Metabolite studies showed that gut dysbiosis contributes to malnutrition, reduced SCFA production, and vitamin deficiencies that worsen CP symptoms and disease progression [34].

The decreased *Faecalibacterium prausnitzii* and *Ruminococcus bromine* enables endotoxemia. Moreover, the chronic consumption of alcohol, which may be present in patients with CP, favors the overgrowth of potential pathogens such as *Klebsiella*, *Enterococcus*, and *Pseudomonas* [65].

Frost et al. found a significantly larger Enterococcus, Streptococcus, and *Escherichia Shigella* population in patients with chronic pancreatitis and without any relationship with exocrine pancreatic insufficiency. On the contrary, the beneficial SCFAs-producing species, such as *Faecalibacterium*, were decreased, and in previously antibiotic-treated patients, *Enterococcus* was specifically overgrowth [61]. Other studies described a predominant growth of *Escherichia-Shigella*, *Enterococcus*, *Klebsiella*, and *Streptococcus* in chronic pancreatitis patients compared to in healthy individuals, with overall changes characterized by increased Proteobacteria and decreased Bacteroidetes and Actinobacteria phylum [62, 66]. The overgrowth of these in chronic pancreatitis cases unfavored the development of *Faecalibacaterium*, *Bifidobacterium*, *Coprococcus*, *Paraprevotella*, *Fusicatenibacter*, and *Roseburia*, different from healthy gut microbiota [66].

4. Oral microbiota and acute and chronic pancreatitis

The oral microbiota, comprising bacteria, fungi, and viruses residing in the oral cavity, plays an increasingly recognized role in systemic diseases, including pancreatic diseases such as acute and chronic pancreatitis and pancreatic cancer. Dysbiosis, or an imbalance in the oral microbiota, can lead to bacterial translocation to distal organs and drive inflammation, thereby influencing disease outcomes in the pancreas [67].

Research suggests that bacteria from the oral cavity can translocate to the gastrointestinal (GI) tract and ultimately reach the pancreas, particularly during episodes of dysbiosis or oral infections like periodontitis. *Porphyromonas gingivalis* and *Fusobacterium nucleatum*, two common pathogens associated with periodontitis, have been implicated in contributing to inflammation that can exacerbate conditions like pancreatitis [62]. *Porphyromonas gingivalis* can influence pancreatic disease by activating toll-like receptors (TLR)-2 and TLR-4, key molecules in innate immune response and pro-inflammatory signaling [68]. In acute pancreatitis (AP) patients, the diversity and abundance of oral microorganisms increased, with a decline in beneficial bacteria like *Streptococcus*, *Neisseria*, and *Gemella* and a rise in *Prevotella*, *Veillonella*, *Granulicatella*, *Actinomyces*, and *Peptostreptococcus*. As disease severity progressed, beneficial bacteria (*Neisseria*, *Haemophilus*, and *Gemella*) decreased further in moderately severe and severe AP (MSAP and SAP) compared to in mild AP (MAP). The analysis identified *Prevotella*, *Peptostreptococcus*, *Actinomyces*, and *Porphyromonas* as key microbial markers for AP, suggesting that oral microbiome changes could not only distinguish AP patients from healthy individuals but also serve as potential early indicators of disease severity [69].

In acute pancreatitis (AP), an inflammatory cascade in response to digestive enzymes and bacterial translocation may result in systemic inflammatory response syndrome (SIRS). The presence of oral pathogens in the pancreas, possibly translocated via the bloodstream or GI tract, can worsen inflammation, leading to severe cases of AP [69]. Chronic exposure to inflammatory mediators due to continuous oral bacteria translocation may promote chronic pancreatitis (CP) by facilitating fibrosis and repeated tissue injury. CP therefore is likely exacerbated by these ongoing inflammatory signals derived from persistent oral pathogens [70].

In the study of Farrel et al., *Streptococcus mitis* and *Granulicatella adiacens* became evident in distinguishing chronic pancreatitis patients from healthy individuals [70].

Additionally, oral pathogens may indirectly influence pancreatitis through endotoxins and virulence factors. For example, *P. gingivalis* produces gingipains, which are proteolytic enzymes that stimulate cytokine production and immune cell activation. These immune responses may subsequently travel systemically, creating a pro-inflammatory environment that worsens the pathophysiology of CP [71].

The studies are still equivocal regarding the potential microbiota-targeted therapies as interventions in acute and chronic pancreatitis. Administration of a symbiotic blend of *Lactobacillus casei*, *L. rhamnosus*, *L. acidophilus*, *Bifidobacterium bifidum*, and fructooligosaccharides showed improvements in bowel habits and laboratory markers in patients with chronic pancreatitis [72]. This suggests that symbiotics may enhance nutritional status in CP patients. Although promising, further research is needed. Additionally, fecal microbiota transplantation (FMT) could theoretically benefit CP patients with persistent pancreatic exocrine insufficiency (PEI), but no studies currently address FMT in CP [36].

The use of probiotics in treating pancreatitis remains debated. Some studies have shown that *Lactobacillus plantarum*, delivered *via* enteral feeding or nasojejunal tube, may reduce sepsis in pancreatitis, while *Bifidobacterium* has been associated with decreased gastrointestinal dysfunction. However, other research found that a combination of *Lactobacillus* and *Bifidobacterium* did not prevent infectious complications in pancreatitis patients, possibly due to factors such as nutrient excess and delayed treatment administration. This highlights the need for further investigation into optimal probiotic strategies for pancreatitis management [32].

5. Conclusion

The intricate relationship between gut microbiota and pancreatitis reveals distinct mechanisms through which acute and chronic forms of the disease manifest. In acute pancreatitis, microbial dysbiosis leads to significant alterations in gut flora, characterized by reduced diversity and an overrepresentation of pathogenic bacteria. This dysbiosis is associated with compromised gut barrier integrity and increased bacterial translocation, resulting in heightened systemic inflammation mediated by lipopolysaccharides and Toll-like receptor activation. In contrast, chronic pancreatitis is marked by persistent microbial imbalances, driven by ongoing inflammation and malnutrition, which further exacerbate the disease state. The interactions between gut microbiota and pancreatic function demonstrate a bidirectional relationship, where dysbiosis not only contributes to pancreatic injury but also is a consequence of impaired exocrine function.

Acknowledgements

The author acknowledges the use of Grammarly for the corrections and rearrangement of the manuscript.

Author details

Sandica Bucurica
University of Medicine and Pharmacy Carol Davila, Bucharest, Romania

*Address all correspondence to: sandica.bucurica@umfcd.ro

References

[1] Cai Q-Y et al. Incidence, prevalence, and comorbidities of chronic pancreatitis: A 7-year population-based study. World Journal of Gastroenterology. 2023;**29**(30):4671-4684. DOI: 10.3748/wjg.v29.i30.4671

[2] Ouyang G et al. The global, regional, and national burden of pancreatitis in 195 countries and territories, 1990-2017: A systematic analysis for the Global Burden of Disease Study 2017. BMC Medicine. 2020;**18**(1):388. DOI: 10.1186/s12916-020-01859-5

[3] Spagnolo DM et al. Acute and chronic pancreatitis disease prevalence, classification, and comorbidities: A cohort study of the UK BioBank. Clinical and Translational Gastroenterology. 2022;**13**(1):e00455. DOI: 10.14309/ctg.0000000000000455

[4] Li C, Jiang M, Pan C, Li J, Xu L. The global, regional, and national burden of acute pancreatitis in 204 countries and territories, 1990-2019. BMC Gastroenterology. 2021;**21**(1):332. DOI: 10.1186/s12876-021-01906-2

[5] Partyka O et al. Overview of pancreatic cancer epidemiology in Europe and recommendations for screening in high-risk populations. Cancers. 2023;**15**(14):3634. DOI: 10.3390/cancers15143634

[6] Hewitt DB et al. A phase 3 randomized clinical trial of chemotherapy with or without algenpantucel-L (hyperacute-pancreas) immunotherapy in subjects with borderline resectable or locally advanced unresectable pancreatic cancer. Annals of Surgery. 2022;**275**(1):45-53. DOI: 10.1097/SLA.0000000000004669

[7] Ma Y, Chen S, Dai G. Exploring prognostic factors for survival in patients with advanced pancreatic cancer undergoing PD-1 inhibitor immunotherapy. Human Vaccines & Immunotherapeutics. 2024;**20**(1):2376429. DOI: 10.1080/21645515.2024.2376429

[8] Li P, Zhang H, Dai M. Current status and prospect of gut and oral microbiome in pancreatic cancer: Clinical and translational perspectives. Cancer Letters. 2024;**604**:217274. DOI: 10.1016/j.canlet.2024.217274

[9] Zhu Y et al. Microbiota and metabolite alterations in pancreatic head and body/tail cancer patients. Cancer Science. 2024;**115**(8):2738-2750. DOI: 10.1111/cas.16238

[10] Pushalkar S et al. The pancreatic cancer microbiome promotes oncogenesis by induction of innate and adaptive immune suppression. Cancer Discovery. 2018;**8**(4):403-416. DOI: 10.1158/2159-8290.CD-17-1134

[11] Zhou R, Wu Q, Yang Z, Cai Y, Wang D, Wu D. The role of the gut microbiome in the development of acute pancreatitis. International Journal of Molecular Sciences. 2024;**25**(2):1159. DOI: 10.3390/ijms25021159

[12] Leviatan S, Shoer S, Rothschild D, Gorodetski M, Segal E. An expanded reference map of the human gut microbiome reveals hundreds of previously unknown species. Nature Communications. 2022;**13**(1):3863. DOI: 10.1038/s41467-022-31502-1

[13] Hou K et al. Microbiota in health and diseases. Signal Transduction and Targeted Therapy. 2022;**7**(1):135. DOI: 10.1038/s41392-022-00974-4

[14] De Filippo C et al. Impact of diet in shaping gut microbiota revealed by a comparative study in children from Europe and rural Africa. Proceedings. National Academy of Sciences. United States of America. 2010;**107**(33):14691-14696. DOI: 10.1073/pnas.1005963107

[15] Magne F et al. The firmicutes/bacteroidetes ratio: A relevant marker of gut dysbiosis in obese patients? Nutrients. 2020;**12**(5):1474. DOI: 10.3390/nu12051474

[16] Sokol H et al. Fungal microbiota dysbiosis in IBD. Gut. 2017;**66**(6):1039-1048. DOI: 10.1136/gutjnl-2015-310746

[17] Stojanov S, Berlec A, Štrukelj B. The influence of probiotics on the firmicutes/bacteroidetes ratio in the treatment of obesity and inflammatory bowel disease. Microorganisms. 2020;**8**(11):1715. DOI: 10.3390/microorganisms8111715

[18] Vancamelbeke M, Vermeire S. The intestinal barrier: A fundamental role in health and disease. Expert Review of Gastroenterology & Hepatology. 2017;**11**(9):821-834. DOI: 10.1080/17474124.2017.1343143

[19] Rosendo-Silva D, Viana S, Carvalho E, Reis F, Matafome P. Are gut dysbiosis, barrier disruption, and endotoxemia related to adipose tissue dysfunction in metabolic disorders? Overview of the mechanisms involved. Internal and Emergency Medicine. 2023;**18**(5):1287-1302. DOI: 10.1007/s11739-023-03262-3

[20] Fasano A. All disease begins in the (leaky) gut: Role of zonulin-mediated gut permeability in the pathogenesis of some chronic inflammatory diseases. F1000Res. 2020;**9**:69. DOI: 10.12688/f1000research.20510.1

[21] Mouries J et al. Microbiota-driven gut vascular barrier disruption is a prerequisite for non-alcoholic steatohepatitis development. Journal of Hepatology. 2019;**71**(6):1216-1228. DOI: 10.1016/j.jhep.2019.08.005

[22] Assimakopoulos SF, Triantos C, Maroulis I, Gogos C. The role of the gut barrier function in health and disease. Gastroenterology Research. 2018;**11**(4):261-263. DOI: 10.14740/gr1053w

[23] Tripathi A et al. The gut-liver axis and the intersection with the microbiome. Nature Reviews. Gastroenterology & Hepatology. 2018;**15**(7):7. DOI: 10.1038/s41575-018-0011-z

[24] Santilli A, Stefanopoulos S, Cresci GAM. The gut barrier and chronic diseases. Current Opinion in Clinical Nutrition and Metabolic Care. 2022;**25**(3):178-185. DOI: 10.1097/MCO.0000000000000820

[25] Rogers AP, Mileto SJ, Lyras D. Impact of enteric bacterial infections at and beyond the epithelial barrier. Nature Reviews. Microbiology. 2023;**21**(4):260-274. DOI: 10.1038/s41579-022-00794-x

[26] Liu X-F et al. Regulation of short-chain fatty acids in the immune system. Frontiers in Immunology. 2023;**14**:1186892. DOI: 10.3389/fimmu.2023.1186892

[27] Cryan JF et al. The microbiota-gut-brain axis. Physiological Reviews. 2019;**99**(4):1877-2013. DOI: 10.1152/physrev.00018.2018

[28] Liu L, Yin M, Gao J, Yu C, Lin J, Wu A, et al. Intestinal Barrier Function in the Pathogenesis of Nonalcoholic Fatty Liver Disease. Journal of Clinical and Translational Hepatology. 2023;**11**(2):452-458. DOI: 10.14218/JCTH.2022.00089

[29] Donaldson GP, Lee SM, Mazmanian SK. Gut biogeography

of the bacterial microbiota. Nature Reviews. Microbiology. 2016;**14**(1):20-32. DOI: 10.1038/nrmicro3552

[30] Ding J-H et al. Role of gut microbiota via the gut-liver-brain axis in digestive diseases. World Journal of Gastroenterology. 2020;**26**(40):40. DOI: 10.3748/wjg.v26.i40.6141

[31] Butler MI, Cryan JF, Dinan TG. Man and the microbiome: A new theory of everything? Annual Review of Clinical Psychology. 2019;**15**(1):1. DOI: 10.1146/annurev-clinpsy-050718-095432

[32] Zhang Z, Tanaka I, Pan Z, Ernst PB, Kiyono H, Kurashima Y. Intestinal homeostasis and inflammation: Gut microbiota at the crossroads of pancreas-intestinal barrier axis. European Journal of Immunology. 2022;**52**(7):1035-1046. DOI: 10.1002/eji.202149532

[33] Lange R et al. Examination of duodenal and colonic microbiome changes in mouse models of acute and chronic pancreatitis. Scientific Reports. 2024;**14**(1):24754. DOI: 10.1038/s41598-024-75564-1

[34] Pan L, Yin N, Duan M, Mei Q, Zeng Y. The role of gut microbiome and its metabolites in pancreatitis. mSystems. 2024;**9**(10):e00665-24. DOI: 10.1128/msystems.00665-24

[35] Xia L et al. Impaired autophagy increases susceptibility to endotoxin-induced chronic pancreatitis. Cell Death & Disease. 2020;**11**(10):889. DOI: 10.1038/s41419-020-03050-3

[36] Schepis T et al. Microbiota in pancreatic diseases: A review of the literature. Journal of Clinical Medicine. 2021;**10**(24):5920. DOI: 10.3390/jcm10245920

[37] Du Y et al. The role of short chain fatty acids in inflammation and body health. International Journal of Molecular Sciences. 2024;**25**(13):7379. DOI: 10.3390/ijms25137379

[38] Yoo JY, Groer M, Dutra SVO, Sarkar A, McSkimming DI. Gut microbiota and immune system interactions. Microorganisms. 2020;**8**(10):1587. DOI: 10.3390/microorganisms8101587

[39] Tang J, Xu L, Zeng Y, Gong F. Effect of gut microbiota on LPS-induced acute lung injury by regulating the TLR4/NF-kB signaling pathway. International Immunopharmacology. 2021;**91**:107272. DOI: 10.1016/j.intimp.2020.107272

[40] Kamada N, Seo S-U, Chen GY, Núñez G. Role of the gut microbiota in immunity and inflammatory disease. Nature Reviews. Immunology. 2013;**13**(5):321-335. DOI: 10.1038/nri3430

[41] Mattke J et al. Toll-like receptor 4 in pancreatic damage and immune infiltration in acute pancreatitis. Frontiers in Immunology. 2024;**15**:1362727. DOI: 10.3389/fimmu.2024.1362727

[42] Glaubitz J et al. Immune response mechanisms in acute and chronic pancreatitis: Strategies for therapeutic intervention. Frontiers in Immunology. 2023;**14**:1279539. DOI: 10.3389/fimmu.2023.1279539

[43] Hoque R et al. TLR9 and the NLRP3 inflammasome link acinar cell death with inflammation in acute pancreatitis. Gastroenterology. 2011;**141**(1):358-369. DOI: 10.1053/j.gastro.2011.03.041

[44] Ferrero-Andrés A, Panisello-Roselló A, Roselló-Catafau J, Folch-Puy E. NLRP3 inflammasome-mediated inflammation in acute pancreatitis. International Journal of

Molecular Sciences. 2020;**21**(15):5386. DOI: 10.3390/ijms21155386

[45] Qiang R, Li Y, Dai X, Lv W. NLRP3 inflammasome in digestive diseases: From mechanism to therapy. Frontiers in Immunology. 2022;**13**:978190. DOI: 10.3389/fimmu.2022.978190

[46] Kanak MA, Shahbazov R, Yoshimatsu G, Levy MF, Lawrence MC, Naziruddin B. A small molecule inhibitor of NFκB blocks ER stress and the NLRP3 inflammasome and prevents progression of pancreatitis. Journal of Gastroenterology. 2017;**52**(3):352-365. DOI: 10.1007/s00535-016-1238-5

[47] Liu T et al. The trigger for pancreatic disease: NLRP3 inflammasome. Cell Death Discovery. 2023;**9**(1):246. DOI: 10.1038/s41420-023-01550-7

[48] Kınacı E, Sevinc MM, Demir A, Erdogan E, Ahlatci FA, Idiz UO. Changes in cytokines and chemokines in an acute pancreatitis model. Ulusal Travma ve Acil Cerrahi Dergisi. 2024;**30**(4):229-235. DOI: 10.14744/tjtes.2024.18049

[49] Shin JH, Seeley RJ. Reg3 proteins as gut hormones? Endocrinology. 2019;**160**(6):1506-1514. DOI: 10.1210/en.2019-00073

[50] Tan J, Taitz J, Sun SM, Langford L, Ni D, Macia L. Your regulatory T cells are what you eat: How diet and gut microbiota affect regulatory T cell development. Frontiers in Nutrition. 2022;**9**:878382. DOI: 10.3389/fnut.2022.878382

[51] Wheatley RC, Valle JW, McNamara MG. The microbiome as a potential diagnostic biomarker for pancreatic ductal adenocarcinoma (PDAC). Hepatobiliary Surgery and Nutrition. 2022;**11**(5):752-754. DOI: 10.21037/hbsn-22-380

[52] Riquelme E et al. Tumor microbiome diversity and composition influence pancreatic cancer outcomes. Cell. 2019;**178**(4):795-806.e12. DOI: 10.1016/j.cell.2019.07.008

[53] Rau S, Gregg A, Yaceczko S, Limketkai B. Prebiotics and probiotics for gastrointestinal disorders. Nutrients. 2024;**16**(6):778. DOI: 10.3390/nu16060778

[54] Wang Z et al. Intestinal microflora and metabolites affect the progression of acute pancreatitis (AP). Gut Pathogens. 2024;**16**(1):64. DOI: 10.1186/s13099-024-00652-6

[55] Nan BB, Jin L, Wang T, Long CB, Zhao H, Wang C, et al. Correlation between gut microbiota and pancreatitis: A bidirectional Mendelian randomization. European Journal of Gastroenterology & Hepatology. 31 Oct 2024. DOI: 10.1097/MEG.0000000000002861

[56] Zhou F, Liu Y, Shi Y, Wu N, Xie Y, Zhou X. Association between gut microbiota and acute pancreatitis: A bidirectional Mendelian randomization study. Journal of Gastroenterology and Hepatology. 2024;**39**(9):1895-1902. DOI: 10.1111/jgh.16658

[57] Nishiyama H et al. Supplementation of pancreatic digestive enzymes alters the composition of intestinal microbiota in mice. Biochemical and Biophysical Research Communications. 2018;**495**(1):273-279. DOI: 10.1016/j.bbrc.2017.10.130

[58] Zhu Y et al. Gut microbiota dysbiosis worsens the severity of acute pancreatitis in patients and mice. Journal of Gastroenterology. 2019;**54**(4):347-358. DOI: 10.1007/s00535-018-1529-0

[59] Singh P, Garg PK. Pathophysiological mechanisms in acute pancreatitis:

Current understanding. Indian Journal of Gastroenterology. 2016;**35**(3):153-166. DOI: 10.1007/s12664-016-0647-y

[60] Gu R et al. Angiotensin-(1-7) improves intestinal microbiota disturbances and modulates fecal metabolic aberrations in acute pancreatitis. The FASEB Journal. 2024;**38**(20):e70134. DOI: 10.1096/fj.202401565RR

[61] Frost F et al. The gut microbiome in patients with chronic pancreatitis is characterized by significant dysbiosis and overgrowth by opportunistic pathogens. Clinical and Translational Gastroenterology. 2020;**11**(9):e00232. DOI: 10.14309/ctg.0000000000000232

[62] Vilà-Quintana L et al. Metagenomic study reveals phage–bacterial interactome dynamics in gut and oral microbiota in pancreatic diseases. International Journal of Molecular Sciences. 2024;**25**(20):10988. DOI: 10.3390/ijms252010988

[63] Frost F et al. Impaired exocrine pancreatic function associates with changes in intestinal microbiota composition and diversity. Gastroenterology. 2019;**156**(4):1010-1015. DOI: 10.1053/j.gastro.2018.10.047

[64] Jandhyala SM et al. Altered intestinal microbiota in patients with chronic pancreatitis: Implications in diabetes and metabolic abnormalities. Scientific Reports. 2017;**7**(1):43640. DOI: 10.1038/srep43640

[65] Ciocan D et al. Characterization of intestinal microbiota in alcoholic patients with and without alcoholic hepatitis or chronic alcoholic pancreatitis. Scientific Reports. 2018;**8**(1):4822. DOI: 10.1038/s41598-018-23146-3

[66] Hong J et al. Gut microbiome changes associated with chronic pancreatitis and pancreatic cancer: A systematic review and meta-analysis. International Journal of Surgery. 2024;**110**(9):5781-5794. DOI: 10.1097/JS9.0000000000001724

[67] Memba R et al. The potential role of gut microbiota in pancreatic disease: A systematic review. Pancreatology. 2017;**17**(6):867-874. DOI: 10.1016/j.pan.2017.09.002

[68] Gallimidi AB et al. Periodontal pathogens *Porphyromonas gingivalis* and *Fusobacterium nucleatum* promote tumor progression in an oral-specific chemical carcinogenesis model. Oncotarget. 2015;**6**(26):22613-22623. DOI: 10.18632/oncotarget.4209

[69] Liu Y et al. Alterations of oral microbiota are associated with the development and severity of acute pancreatitis. Journal of Oral Microbiology. 2023;**15**(1):2264619. DOI: 10.1080/20002297.2023.2264619

[70] Farrell JJ et al. Variations of oral microbiota are associated with pancreatic diseases including pancreatic cancer. Gut. 2012;**61**(4):582-588. DOI: 10.1136/gutjnl-2011-300784

[71] de Jongh CA, de Vries TJ, Bikker FJ, Gibbs S, Krom BP. Mechanisms of *Porphyromonas gingivalis* to translocate over the oral mucosa and other tissue barriers. Journal of Oral Microbiology. 2023;**15**(1):2205291. DOI: 10.1080/20002297.2023.2205291

[72] Dos Santos PQ, Guedes JC, De Jesus RP, Santos RRD, Fiaconne RL. Effects of using symbiotics in the clinical nutritional evolution of patients with chronic pancreatitis: Study prospective, randomized, controlled, double blind. Clinical Nutrition ESPEN. 2017;**18**:9-15. DOI: 10.1016/j.clnesp.2017.01.005

Chapter 8

Role of EUS in Diagnosis and Therapy of Chronic Pancreatitis

Naren S. Nallapeta and Srushti Sahukar

Abstract

Endoscopic ultrasound (EUS) plays a crucial role in the diagnosis and management of chronic pancreatitis. This chapter explores the utility of EUS in detecting early parenchymal and ductal changes, its superiority over other imaging modalities, and its therapeutic applications. EUS provides high-resolution imaging of the pancreas, allowing for the visualization of subtle abnormalities such as hyperechoic foci, stranding, and lobularity. The Rosemont criteria, which standardize EUS findings for chronic pancreatitis diagnosis, are discussed in detail. The chapter also highlights EUS effectiveness in detecting small (<2 cm) and isoattenuating pancreatic tumors, outperforming computerized tomography (CT) and magnetic resonance imaging (MRI) in this aspect. The ability to perform fine-needle aspiration cytology (FNAC) under EUS guidance further enhances its diagnostic capabilities for neoplasia. In pain management, EUS-guided celiac plexus neurolysis (EUS-CPN) is presented as an effective intervention. The chapter describes various approaches to EUS-CPN, including central, bilateral, and direct techniques, along with their respective advantages and limitations. Other EUS-guided pain relief interventions, such as splanchnic nerve neurolysis and celiac ganglia block, are also discussed. The effectiveness of EUS-CPN in providing significant pain relief for patients with chronic pancreatitis is emphasized, noting that pain control typically lasts between one to 6 months.

Keywords: endoscopic ultrasound, chronic pancreatitis, Rosemont criteria, celiac plexus neurolysis, pancreatic neoplasia

1. Introduction

Chronic pancreatitis is a disorder of autodigestion and damage to acinar cells that precedes the fibrotic response of the pancreatic stellate cells that surround the acini. While there are no set number of episodes of acute pancreatitis or a set duration of chronic alcoholism that cause the onset of chronic pancreatitis, recurrent and frequent episodes of acute pancreatitis inevitably cause early initiation of the pathological processes involved in chronic pancreatitis, begetting morphological changes that are often permanent. See **Figure 1** for an overview of relevant histology for pancreatic tissue.

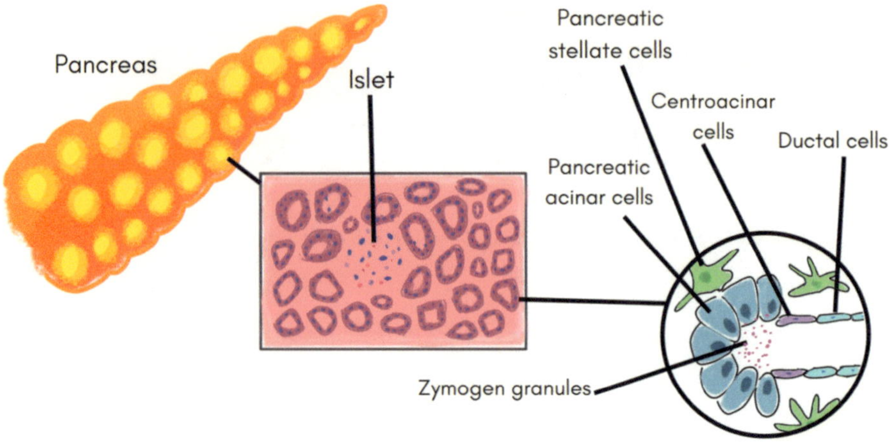

Figure 1.
The disease-free pancreas on endoscopic ultrasound.

While endoscopic ultrasound (EUS), endoscopic retrograde cholangiopancreatography (ERCP), magnetic resonance imaging (MRI), and computerized tomography (CT) have comparable diagnostic accuracy, EUS and ERCP are outperformers. In this chapter, we delve into the role of endoscopic ultrasound in diagnosis and management of chronic pancreatitis.

Endoscopic ultrasound, like ultrasound, uses high-frequency sound waves that create images in shades of light and dark depending on tissue density and composition. On endoscopic ultrasound, a normal pancreas with no obvious risk factors for chronic pancreatitis appears homogeneous with smooth margins and has a finely reticular or granulated appearance. It is especially good at detecting both ductal and parenchymal changes in the early stages of the disease. Even subtle parenchymal changes like hyperechoic foci, stranding, small cystic changes, and lobularity are discernable. Endoscopic ultrasound is especially better than transabdominal ultrasound when it comes to detecting cystic lesions and calcifications. The closer proximity eliminates interference from bowel gas and provides a more accurate assessment with higher resolution for subtle variations in echogenicity. The pancreatic duct is seen as a thin, tubular structure running through the center of the pancreas and appears anechoic and dark due to pancreatic juice contained within it. The average diameter of the pancreatic duct lumen is 1.7 mm (ranging from 1 to 3 mm), and it gets progressively narrow from the head to the body and tail.

2. Tissue changes with chronic pancreatitis, their appearances on endoscopic ultrasound imaging, and the Rosemont criteria

One of the most prominent features of chronic pancreatitis in EUS is the hyperechoic foci, representing calcifications. Chronic pancreatic inflammation alters the composition of pancreatic juice and its flow. This leads to the formation of protein plugs that contain precipitates of calcium carbonate. These act as nucleation sites for the plug to grow further and eventually form a stone. This can obstruct flow, increase ductal pressure, and cause further damage to the organ. These calcifications, when dense, are associated with *posterior acoustic shadowing*. Calcifications are highly echogenic and therefore bright on ultrasound, and they reflect most of the sound waves back to the transducer. This leaves fewer sound waves to penetrate deeper structures, resulting in a dark area or shadow behind the calcification on the EUS image, known as posterior acoustic shadowing. The absence of posterior acoustic shadowing is indicative of calcifications that are smaller or less dense and thus allow for ultrasound waves to pass through. Fibrosis from chronic inflammation also contributes to shadowing behind fibrotic areas as they cause some degree of ultrasound wave scattering.

The clusters of acinar cells are organized into lobules. The lobularity of normal pancreas is very subtle as compared with the exaggerated lobularity seen in chronic pancreatitis. In fact, the lobularity is so subtle, fine, and uniform in the disease-free pancreas that it is often not picked up. In contrast, when the disease process sets in, the fibrosis and scarring cause the lobules to become larger and more distorted, creating a coarse, irregular pattern on EUS. Depending on the extent of inflammation, fibrosis, and calcification, the lobularity can be more widespread, termed *contiguous lobularity*. Here, the lobular changes in pancreatic parenchyma cover a continuous region, suggesting advanced and more diffuse pancreatic pathology. Contiguous lobularity and honeycombing refer to similar but slightly different patterns of structural change within the pancreatic tissue. With contiguous lobularity, the pancreas exhibits a uniform and consistent lobular pattern. With honeycombing, fibrosis is extensive and the normal pancreatic tissue is significantly disrupted. *Non-contiguous* lobularity, on the other hand, is more focal and localized, leading to a more scattered lobularity with normal pancreatic tissue interspersed, indicating early stages of chronic pancreatitis.

Ongoing inflammation can also cause cysts and stranding to form in the pancreatic tissue. Cysts are fluid-filled sacs and therefore will not generate a shadow as the sound waves can pass through the fluid. Stranding is another phenomenon that occurs in chronic inflammation – the fibrotic response causes normal pancreatic tissue to be replaced by scar tissue that appears as bright, linear structures that disrupt the otherwise smooth texture of pancreas.

The pancreatic duct itself can undergo several changes when enduring chronic inflammation. The duct walls can undergo calcification and fibrosis, causing the duct wall to appear hyperechoic [1]. Scarring can disrupt the smooth appearance of duct wall [1]. Focal thickening can cause irregular narrowing and dilatation and cause the duct to kink and have a jagged appearance. Recurrent inflammation can cause fibrosis, which in turn can cause strictures [1]. This can cause stasis of pancreatic secretions. This allows for protein to accumulate and form a plug. Calcium then precipitates and forms stones. Loosely, and to put it simply, early stones are more proteinaceous and less calcified, while mature stones are composed mainly of calcium carbonate. The composition of the pancreatic juice itself also changes over time, becoming more lithogenic.

While CT and MRI are widely used, they have limitations in detecting early-stage changes. EUS stands out for its ability to identify subtle parenchymal and ductal alterations in the pancreas, particularly in early chronic pancreatitis. EUS can visualize fine details such as hyperechoic foci, stranding, small cystic changes, and lobularity, which are often missed by CT. The high-resolution imaging provided by EUS, due to its close proximity to the pancreas, allows for the detection of calcifications, ductal irregularities, and early fibrotic changes. This makes EUS particularly valuable for the diagnosis of chronic pancreatitis in its initial stages before more obvious structural changes become apparent in other imaging modalities.

The *Rosemont* criteria very clearly outline and define the rules for diagnosing chronic pancreatitis on the basis of EUS detection of the pathological changes described.

Rosemont criteria and features (**Table 1**) [1].

Diagnosis (**Table 2**).

Major criteria A	Parenchymal features: • Hyperechoic foci with shadowing: echogenic focus ≥2 mm in length and width that generates a shadow Ductal features: • Main pancreatic duct calculi: echogenic structures within the main pancreatic duct that cause acoustic shadowing
Major criterion B	Parenchymal features: • Honeycomb pattern of lobularity
Minor criteria	Parenchymal features • Lobularity without honeycombing • Hyperechoic foci without shadowing • Cysts • Strands Ductal features: • Irregular pancreatic duct contour • Hyperechoic duct wall • Dilated main pancreatic duct • Dilated side ducts

Table 1.
Rosemont criteria and features [1–3].

Consistent with chronic pancreatitis	• One major A feature + three or more minor features • One major A feature + one major B feature • Two major A features
Suggestive of chronic pancreatitis	• One major A feature + three minor features • One major B feature ± three minor features • Five or more minor features
Indeterminate for chronic pancreatitis	• Three to four minor features, no major features • Major B feature alone • Major B + up to three minor features
Normal	• Less than two minor features, no major features

Table 2.
Diagnosis of chronic pancreatitis based on Rosemont criteria [1].

3. Role of endoscopic ultrasound in neoplasia

Onset of neoplastic changes in the setting of chronic pancreatitis varies from patient to patient, and hinges on factors like the cause of pancreatitis, genetic predispositions, and lifestyle factors such as smoking and alcohol use. The general timeline, though, is 10–20 years after the onset of pancreatitis. Early-stage pancreatic masses are especially challenging because of smaller size, isoattenuation, and absence of ductal abnormalities. Endoscopic ultrasound is particularly valuable for the diagnosis of malignancy both as an imaging modality and as a guide for biopsy. While the sensitivity of CT for the detection of larger tumors (>2 cm) approaches 100%, smaller (<2 cm) and isoattenuating tumors are easily missed. Isoattenuating tumors are often indistinct from normal pancreatic tissue, and up to 11% of pancreatic adenocarcinomas are isoattenuating. These tumors tend to blend in with normal pancreatic tissue. While MRI and magnetic resonance cholangiopancreatography (MRCP) are more sensitive than CT in detecting masses, they may still miss very small tumors and those in difficult-to-image locations. Tumors in the tail and deeper in location like ones closer to the spleen and left kidney are considered difficult to image.

Endoscopic ultrasound is far superior to CT and MRI when it comes to detecting tumors smaller than 2 cm. EUS directly visualizes the pancreas in high resolution. The close proximity of the ultrasound probe allows for clearer, more detailed imaging of pancreatic tissue, enabling it to pick up on subtle abnormalities like small masses, early fibrosis, and mild disruptions in pancreatic architecture.

A major advantage of EUS is the ability to perform fine-needle aspiration cytology (FNAC), which is crucial for tissue sampling and cytological and histological analysis. CT-guided biopsy does the job too but is less preferred due to lower accuracy when sampling smaller lesions, and higher risk of complications like bleeding, acute pancreatitis, infection, abscess formation, accidental injury to surrounding structures, and, although rare, tumor seeding that might advance the stage.

4. Pain management in chronic pancreatitis

Pain management in chronic pancreatitis almost always involves a multimodal approach. Alcohol abstinence is of supreme importance. Dietary changes are essential – small, low-fat meals are encouraged. This reduces stimulus for pancreatic enzyme production and decreases pain associated with eating. Pancreatic enzyme supplementation is a useful adjunct as it helps digestion and reduces the need for the pancreas to secrete enzymes. Acetaminophen or non-steroidal anti-inflammatory drugs (NSAIDs) are the first-line pharmacotherapy for moderate pain, and tramadol and stronger opioids [4]. Adjuvant pain medications like tricyclic antidepressants (amitriptyline and nortriptyline) and gabapentinoids (gabapentin and pregabalin) may also be prescribed. Some surgical options to note are pancreatic resection, pancreatectomy, and pancreaticojejunostomy.

5. Pain pathway

Our focus is on endoscopic intervention, particularly Endoscopic ultrasound-guided celiac plexus neurolysis, which is commonly abbreviated as EUS-CPN. The celiac plexus block (CPB) is a similar procedure but uses anesthetic medications like bupivacaine instead of neurolytic.

Before proceeding to these modalities, it is essential to first understand the course of the pain pathway between the pancreas and the central nervous system. The greater splanchnic nerves (T5-T9) are sympathetic nerves that carry pain fibers from

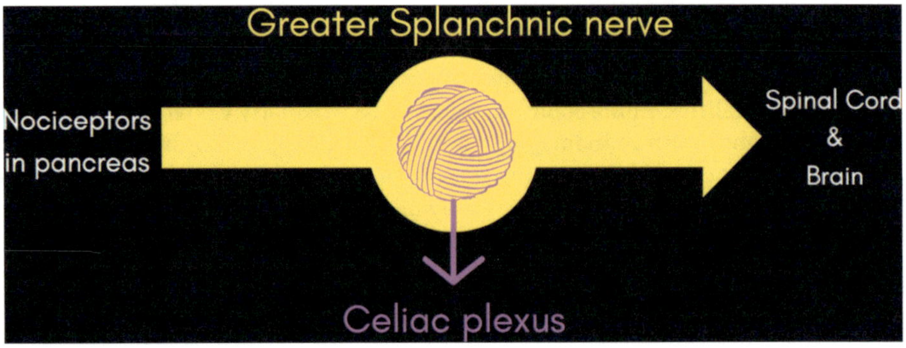

Figure 2.
Formation of celiac plexus.

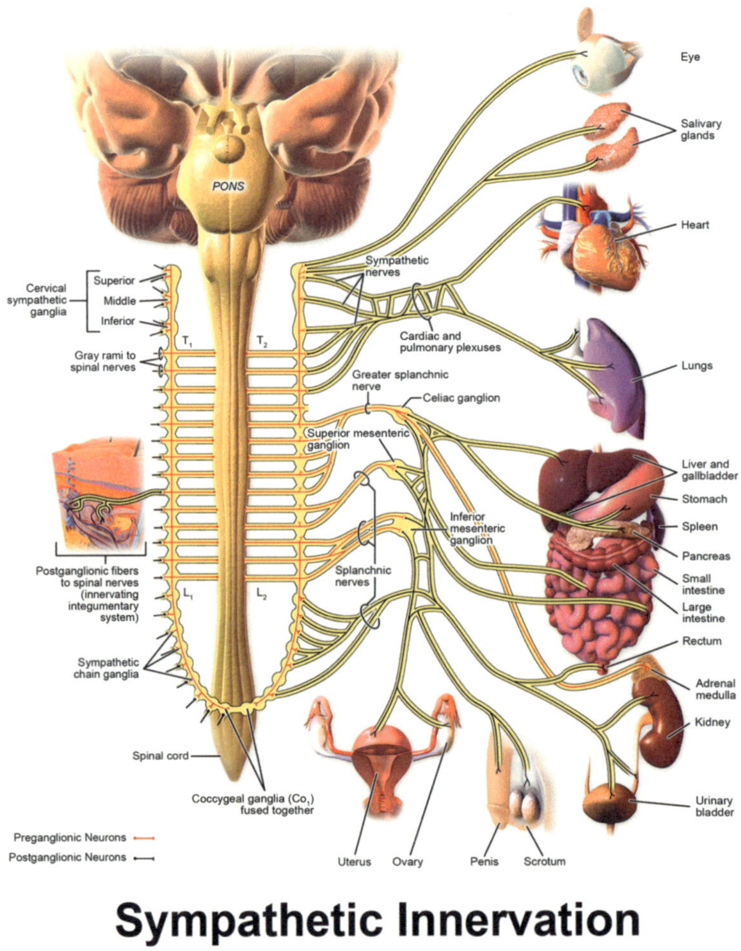

Figure 3.
Celiac plexus formation.

the pancreas and other abdominal structures [2, 5]. The visceral afferent fibers in the greater splanchnic nerve carry pain sensation from the nociceptors in the pancreas through the celiac plexus, which acts as a relay station [2, 5]. It is important to note that there are no synapses in the celiac plexus. It simply acts as a conduit for the fibers to pass through on their way to the spinal cord. It carries signals from the stomach, liver, and other upper abdominal organs as well [5]. Please refer to **Figures 2** and **3** for diagrammatic depictions of the pain pathway specific to the pancreas.

6. Endoscopic ultrasound-guided celiac plexus neurolysis

EUS-CPN uses neurolytic like ethanol (50–100%) and phenol (5–10% in glycerol) to chemically destroy nerve fibers by dehydrating the nerve cell, coagulating nerve cell proteins, and dissolving lipid membranes. Ethanol is preferred because of its profound and longer-lasting neurolytic effect, more predictable spread, and high efficacy. It permanently destroys the sympathetic pain fibers and therefore is the preferred choice, especially in cancer pain. CPB provides a more temporary relief of symptoms as opposed to neurolysis [4]. CPB may often precede CPN as a way to confirm the location of the celiac plexus and reduce discomfort during the procedure [4]. Doppler ultrasound is additionally used to minimize risks of vascular injury and bleeding and significantly enhances safety by enabling careful navigation around vascular structures [6].

There are several approaches, the central approach being the most straightforward and safe one [6, 7]. Here, the aorta is visualized through the posterior wall of the upper gastric body with the echoendoscope. The celiac artery is identified and a needle is passed through the stomach wall until it reaches the point where the celiac artery originates from the aorta. The neurolytic agent is injected just above the celiac artery until an echogenic cloud is visualized.

The bilateral technique is superior to the central approach in terms of pain relief because two injections are administered, one each for the right and left celiac plexuses on either side of the aorta [6, 8]. This is done by rotating the echoendoscope and injecting at the left and right lateral bases of the superior mesenteric artery. The direct approach is another technique wherein each of the celiac ganglia is visualized and targeted directly, hence the name. This approach is more time-consuming and

Approach	Target area	Key features	Advantages	Disadvantages
Central	Anterior to aorta at the origin of the celiac trunk	Single injection into the central area of the plexus	Easier, faster, good pain relief for most patients	May provide less coverage of the entire plexus
Bilateral	Left and right sides of the aorta near celiac trunk	Two injections, one on each side of the aorta	Better coverage of the celiac plexus	Longer procedure, slightly higher risk of complications
Direct	Individual celiac ganglia	Precise targeting of specific celiac ganglia	Targeted, potentially better pain relief	More technically demanding, not always feasible

Table 3.
Summary of the main approaches in EUS-CPN [2, 3, 6, 7].

technically difficult. But it reduces the risk of neurolytic agent diffusion to areas outside the intended target, potentially minimizing side effects (**Table 3**).

7. Other approaches

EUS-guided pain relief interventions are not limited to the aforementioned modalities. Splanchnic nerve neurolysis is another one wherein a neurolytic agent is injected into the nerve bundle bilaterally. This is technically more challenging and has a higher risk of complications due to damage to adjacent structures (kidney and spinal cord), but it may provide a longer-lasting effect compared to traditional celiac plexus neurolysis. The retrocrural approach also targets the splanchnic nerves and can be combined with the celiac ganglia block. The celiac ganglia block (CGB) is similar to the direct approach but focuses specifically on blocking rather than neurolysis of the celiac ganglia. It involves the injection of a local anesthetic (with or without steroids) into the celiac ganglia to block pain transmission without destroying the nerve tissue. Steroids are added if inflammation is suspected to contribute to the pain. Less commonly, when a posterior approach is not feasible, the anterior approach may be opted for after localizing the celiac plexus. This too is a technically challenging procedure and has a higher risk of complications.

Summary of additional approaches (**Table 4**):

8. Pain control outcomes

Within days of the procedure, a significant number of patients report a reduction in pain [3]. The control lasts anywhere between 1 and 6 months [3]. The resurgence of pain is due to the regeneration of nerve fibers, as neurolysis causes only temporary destruction of nerve fibers. Repeat intervention may be necessary for continued pain control, and the use of adjunct therapies after neurolysis is not uncommon.

Approach	Target Area	Key Features	Advantages	Disadvantages
Splanchnic Nerve Neurolysis (EUS-SN)	Splanchnic nerves (T11–T12 level)	Bilateral injections targeting nerves outside plexus	Potentially more effective, longer-lasting relief	Technically more challenging, higher complication risk
Celiac Ganglia Block (EUS-CGB)	Specific celiac ganglia	Temporary block with local anesthetic	Diagnostic, temporary relief	Short-term requires repeat treatments
Celiac Plexus Block (EUS-CPB)	Celiac plexus	Temporary block with anesthetics (and sometimes steroids)	Diagnostic tool, lower risk than neurolysis	Short-lived effect may need neurolysis later
Retrocrural Approach	Splanchnic nerves (retrocrural space)	Targets nerves behind the diaphragm	Effective for hard-to-treat pain	Technically challenging, higher risk of complications
Anterior Transgastric Approach [5]	Celiac plexus	Through anterior gastric wall instead of posterior	Useful when posterior approach is not feasible	More complex, higher risk of complications

Table 4.
Summary of additional approaches in EUS-CPN [6, 7].

In conditions like pancreatic cancer, the spread of cancer can cause the involvement of new nerves not targeted by neurolysis. Alternatively, tumors can stimulate new nerve pathways to develop.

9. Conclusions

Endoscopic ultrasound has summoned an exciting era of more precise imaging, better pain control, and advances in medicine. It helps detect early structural changes in the pancreas and provides a means for tissue biopsy, ruling out malignancy in high-risk patients. Our ability to grade the severity with Rosemont criteria is useful in staging the disease and offering treatment options to patients. On the therapeutic front, EUS-guided celiac plexus neurolysis offers significant relief from the often debilitating pain associated with chronic pancreatitis, improving the quality of life in patients with refractory symptoms.

Author details

Naren S. Nallapeta[1*] and Srushti Sahukar[2]

1 Strand GI Associates, Myrtle Beach, SC, USA

2 Department of Medicine, The State University of New York at Syracuse, NY, USA

*Address all correspondence to: naren.nallapeta@gmail.com

References

[1] Catalano MF, Sahai A, Levy M, Romagnuolo J, Wiersema M, Brugge W, et al. EUS based criteria for the diagnosis of chronic pancreatitis: The Rosemont classification. Gastrointestinal Endoscopy. 2009;**69**(7):1251-1261

[2] Ohno E, Kawashima H, Ishikawa T, Lida T, Suzuki H, Uetsuki K, et al. Current status of tissue harmonic imaging in endoscopic ultrasonography (EUS) and EUS-elastography in pancreaticobiliary disease. Digestive Endoscopy. 2019;**31**(S1):55-61

[3] Koulouris AI, Alexandre L, Hart AR, Clark A. Endoscopic ultrasound-guided celiac plexus neurolysis for pancreatic cancer-related pain: A review. Journal of Clinical Medicine; **10**(21):5083

[4] Sakamoto H, Kitano M, Komaki T, Imai H, Kamata K. Masatoshi Kudo Endoscopic ultrasound-guided neurolysis in pancreatic cancer. Pancreatology. 2011;**11**(Suppl 2):52-58

[5] Gardner TB, Taylor DJ, Gordon SR. Reported findings on endoscopic ultrasound examinations for chronic pancreatitis: Toward establishing an endoscopic ultrasound quality benchmark. Pancreas. 2014;**43**(1):37-40

[6] Yamashita Y, Kato J, Ueda K, Nakamura Y, Kawaii Y, Abe H, et al. Endoscopic ultrasound-guided celiac plexus neurolysis for pancreatic cancer-related pain: A review. Journal of Clinical Medicine. 2021;**10**(21):5083

[7] Fusaroli P, Jenssen C, Hocke M, Burmester E, Havre RF, Ignee A, et al. EFSUMB guidelines on interventional ultrasound (INVUS), part V: EUS-guided therapeutic interventions. Ultraschall in der Medizin. 2020;**41**(3):252-275

[8] Fan L, Dong J, Tang Y, Huang H, Liu H, Song L, et al. Bilateral vs. unilateral endoscopic ultrasound-guided celiac plexus neurolysis for abdominal pain management in patients with pancreatic malignancy: A systematic review and meta-analysis. Support Care Cancer. 2018;**26**(2):353-359

Chapter 9

Emerging Innovations in the Management of Acute Pancreatitis

Elena Ramírez-Maldonado, Sandra López Gordo and Rosa Jorba

Abstract

Recent advances in acute pancreatitis (AP) management have revolutionised care, improving outcomes and patient experiences. Early oral refeeding in mild AP accelerates recovery and allows for the safe implementation of outpatient protocols, minimising hospital stays and enhancing quality of life. In severe AP, early enteral nutrition and step-up approaches for managing pancreatic necrosis have become standard, while emerging tools like biomarkers, proteomics, genetics, and radiomics are refining diagnostic precision. Artificial intelligence (AI) has further transformed the field by enabling accurate diagnosis, predicting disease severity, and personalising treatment plans through the analysis of clinical data and imaging. These AI-driven innovations enhance decision-making and optimise patient outcomes. Collectively, these developments, spanning early refeeding, outpatient care, and cutting-edge technologies are shaping a more efficient, personalised, and patient-centred approach to AP management, offering hope for better prognoses and improved quality of care in both mild and severe cases.

Keywords: acute pancreatitis, innovations, early refeeding, ambulatorisation, new biomarkers, step-up approach, artificial intelligence, machine learning

1. Introduction

The pancreas, once regarded as an enigmatic and elusive organ, was largely unexamined until the nineteenth century, with most insights derived through autopsies and retrospective diagnoses. Its retroperitoneal location and indistinct morphology made it difficult to differentiate from surrounding tissues, limiting early detection and intervention for pancreatic diseases [1]. However, significant technological and medical advancements have since transformed our understanding of the pancreas, enabling more effective diagnosis and treatment of conditions such as acute pancreatitis (AP) [1].

Acute pancreatitis, characterised by sudden pancreatic inflammation, continues to present a broad clinical spectrum, ranging from mild, self-limiting cases to severe, life-threatening forms with substantial risks of organ failure and mortality. Since its initial description by Fitz and Senn in the late nineteenth century, the optimal management of AP has been a subject of considerable debate, particularly regarding the balance between medical and surgical approaches and the timing of interventions [1].

Historically, the concept of "pancreatic rest" dominated the therapeutic landscape, contributing to prolonged hospitalisations and increased complication rates. However, as the global incidence of AP rises, there is a pressing need to adopt evidence-based strategies that reflect the latest research and technological advancements [2]. Over the past two decades, significant progress has been made in refining diagnostic techniques, advancing nutritional support, optimising antibiotic use, and managing gallstone-related AP. Despite these advancements, integrating innovative practices into routine care has been slow, and adherence to clinical guidelines remains inconsistent [2].

By leveraging cutting-edge technologies, including proteomics, radiomics, and artificial intelligence (AI), clinicians now have the tools to enhance risk stratification, predict complications, and personalise treatment. Bridging the persistent gap between scientific evidence and clinical practice is essential to improving outcomes, minimising healthcare costs, and reducing mortality in patients with AP [2].

This chapter explores significant innovations in the management of AP, focusing on advancements that hold the greatest promise for transforming current clinical practice and improving patient care.

2. Innovations in imaging: Greater precision and less invasiveness

Refinement in imaging techniques has played a pivotal role in optimising AP management. In recent decades, advances in computed tomography (CT) and magnetic resonance imaging (MRI) have enabled increasingly detailed evaluations of pancreatic anatomy and its potential complications. Multiphasic dynamic CT and functional MRI provide high-resolution images of the pancreas and surrounding structures, facilitating early detection of necrosis, fluid collections, and other local abnormalities [3–5].

Endoscopic ultrasound (EUS) has also gained prominence, offering a meticulous visualisation of the pancreatic parenchyma and ducts. It is a less invasive, safer alternative, particularly for patients with more severe conditions or high surgical risk. In cases of recurrent idiopathic AP, EUS can identify an underlying cause in most patients [3–5].

These imaging advancements have enabled a more accurate, safer, and more efficient approach to AP management and monitoring of complications without invasive procedures. However, routine abdominal CT use is not justified for most AP cases, as diagnosis is typically straightforward, and most cases are mild and uncomplicated. Current guidelines recommend performing a CT scan upon admission only when the diagnosis is unclear or if the patient does not improve clinically. Both CT and MRI are unreliable for determining severity in the early stages of AP; local changes, such as pancreatic necrosis, are typically identified after 48–72 hours [3–5].

CT and MRI provide similar quality in AP evaluation. CT offers lower cost, quicker acquisition times, and is less problematic for patients with claustrophobia. MRI is better suited for patients with iodinated contrast allergies or renal insufficiency and is more effective in detecting choledocholithiasis [3–5].

In the context of severe AP (SAP), clinical guidelines recommend a contrast-enhanced CT scan 7–10 days after the initial study. Follow-up CT scans are advised only if the patient's clinical status deteriorates, fails to improve, or if invasive interventions become necessary [3–5].

The integration of segmentation, radiomics, and AI is transforming the diagnosis and management of AP. These tools improve risk stratification, optimise treatment plans, and reduce variability in radiological interpretation. By combining radiomics with clinical and proteomic data, AI enhances personalised medicine, offering tailored approaches for patients at higher risk of severe outcomes. This multidisciplinary approach marks a significant advancement in precision diagnostics and therapeutic planning for AP [6, 7].

3. Early nutrition and metabolic management: Challenging established paradigms

Nutritional management in AP has undergone significant changes over the last decade. Traditionally, patients were subjected to prolonged fasting under the assumption that providing 'pancreatic rest' would avoid stimulating the organ's enzymatic activity [2]. Recent evidence supports that early enteral nutrition is both safe and beneficial, even in severe cases [2–5, 8–11].

3.1 Mild acute pancreatitis

In cases of mild AP (MAP), an immediate oral refeeding approach has been introduced, allowing patients to start a low-fat solid diet directly from the emergency department. This strategy eliminates the need for prolonged fasting and a gradual reintroduction of diet [2–5, 8–11].

Systematic reviews and meta-analyses [8–11], which thoroughly evaluate studies on the timing (**Table 1**) and type (**Table 2**) of diet for early refeeding, emphasise that initiating an immediate, low-fat solid diet reduces hospital stay [12–24], a recommendation also highlighted in recent clinical guidelines [5]. While standardising criteria and increasing patient sample sizes are essential to strengthen research, the evidence is clear: early oral feeding in patients with MAP is safe and beneficial. A 2021 study concluded that this immediate diet approach

Studies	Oral refeeding condition	LOS p-value
Eckerwald, 2007 [12]	Immediately	<0.05
Teich, 2010 [13]	No abdominal pain, decreased laboratory levels	NS
Li, 2013 [14]	Subjective feeling of hunger	<0.001
Lariño-Noia, 2014 [15]	Subjective feeling of hunger	<0.001
Khan, 2017 [16]	First 12h	<0.001
Karabulut, 2019 [17]	Immediately	<0.001
Lozada, 2020 [18]	Immediately	0.042
Horibe, 2020 [19]	Immediately	<0.001
Ramírez-Maldonado, 2021 [20]	Immediately	<0.001

LOS: Length of Stay, NS: no significantly differences.

Table 1.
Analysis oral refeeding time.

Studies	Type of diet	LOS p-value
Jacoboson, 2007 [21]	Low fat solid diet	NS
Sathiaraj, 2008 [22]	Solid diet	<0.001
Moraes, 2010 [23]	Solid diet	NS
Rajkumar, 2013 [24]	Solid diet	<0.001
Lozada, 2020 [18]	Soft diet	0.001
Horibe, 2020 [19]	Low fat solid diet	<0.001
Ramírez-Maldonado, 2021 [20]	Low fat solid diet	<0.001

LOS: Length of Stay, NS: no significantly differences.

Table 2.
Analysis oral refeeding type.

promotes faster recovery, enhances pain relief, shortens hospital stays, and lowers healthcare costs, offering significant benefits for both patients and healthcare systems [20].

3.2 Severe acute pancreatitis

Over the past few decades, the nutritional management of SAP has evolved substantially, overturning long-standing clinical paradigms. Patients with SAP now benefit from early enteral nutrition (EEN), ideally within the first 48 hours. EEN offers multiple advantages over parenteral nutrition [2–5, 25–27]:

- Reduced infectious complications: EEN preserves intestinal mucosal integrity, prevents bacterial translocation, and decreases the risk of systemic infections and infected necrosis.

- Decreased systemic inflammation: Moderate gastrointestinal tract stimulation modulates the inflammatory response, helping prevent progression to multiple organ dysfunction syndrome.

- Improved mortality rates: Recent studies and meta-analyses demonstrate that EEN is associated with lower mortality in SAP patients compared to parenteral nutrition.

- Cost-effectiveness: EEN is more affordable and widely available, easing the economic burden on both patients and healthcare systems [2–5, 8, 25–27].

For patients unable to eat orally due to vomiting, ileus, or intolerance, nasoenteral tube placement has become standard practice. Both gastric and jejunal feeding routes can be administered safely and effectively [2–5, 25–28]. Advances in enteral formulas and supplementation with immunomodulatory nutrients, such as omega-3 fatty acids, arginine, and nucleotides, have shown promise in improving outcomes. Omega-3 fatty acids possess anti-inflammatory properties, arginine supports immune function, and nucleotides aid tissue regeneration and repair. Future strategies, such as personalised EEN tailored to specific inflammatory markers and energy metabolism, are being explored [28]. Monitoring the intestinal microbiota and modulating it with probiotics is gaining importance as a complementary measure in managing SAP [28–30].

4. Outpatient treatment in selected cases: Moving towards more flexible management

Acute pancreatitis ranks among the leading causes of hospitalisation for gastrointestinal conditions worldwide, posing significant clinical and economic challenges. SAP consumes substantial healthcare resources and incurs higher costs due to the need for intensive care and specialised treatments. However, approximately 70% of hospitalisations are attributed to MAP [1–5].

Despite the absence of complications, MAP often requires hospitalisation. In some cases, hospital stays are prolonged by the outdated practice of extended fasting aimed at 'resting the pancreas'. This fasting approach, frequently unnecessary, increases the risk of complications, elevates costs, and places additional strain on healthcare resources [20].

Adopting more efficient strategies for managing MAP, such as early initiation of feeding and outpatient care, offers a promising solution to reduce costs and improve healthcare system sustainability. At the same time, these strategies must ensure that high standards of patient safety and care quality are maintained [31–36].

In recent years, outpatient management of MAP has gained acceptance. While hospitalisation was once the standard, recent studies have demonstrated that selected MAP patients can be safely managed outside the hospital setting, sits as home care or outpatient management, under specific conditions. This approach has proven effective in maintaining treatment safety and efficacy without increasing the risk of complications. Moreover, it reduces hospital stays and associated costs while enhancing the patient experience by allowing recovery in a more comfortable setting [31–36].

To support this transition, both completed and ongoing studies (**Table 3**) have developed rigorous protocols and selection criteria to identify suitable candidates for outpatient management [31–38]. These completed studies demonstrate that, with appropriate clinical oversight and regular follow-up, low-risk patients can achieve favourable outcomes [31–36]. In the future, telemedicine models and remote monitoring systems are expected to provide continuous, real-time supervision, enhancing patient safety and presenting a promising alternative to traditional hospitalisation.

Studies	Selection criteria
Ince, 2014 [31]	• No comorbidities with hospitalization • No dilated pancreatic duct or pancreatic calcifications • Imrie score ≤5 and HAP score ≤2 within first 24 h • No alcohol etiology • No OF within first 24 h • No clinical signs of non-biliary sepsis • Presentation <48h of symptoms onset • Hematocrit ≤44% • No coagulopathy, INR < 1.4 and/or platelet <50.000/mm^3

Studies	Selection criteria
Serra, 2017 [32]	• No active comorbidities • No OF, no local or systemic complications • No fever • CRP < 150 mg/dl • Bilirrubin below the upper normal limit • BUN $\leq$ 5 mg/dl in two consecutive samples by an interval of 24 h • Tolerance of oral intake • Good pain control • Family support
Kothari, 2017 [33]	• No OF, no local or systemic complications • No HR > 130 bpm and/or RR > 25 rpm > 2 h • No severe hypotension (SBP < 80 mmHg) • Oxygin saturation > 90% • Temperature < 102°F (38.9°C) • <10% immature WBC (bands) • Glucose < 400 mg/dl • No evidence of end-organ damage • No altered consciousness • No ischemic changes on electrocardiogram • No concern for cholangitis or choledocholitiasis • No previous pancreatic surgery, pancreatic malignant, chronic pancreatic • No history of severe cardiac and renal failure • No any condition requiring admission • Tolerating a LFSD and oral pain medication • Reduction in 2 points on VAS • Improved nausea/presence of hunger • Stable vital signs • Stable laboratory data
Kumar, 2018 [34]	• Ranson's score $\leq$ 3 within 48 h of presentation to the hospital • No OF • Absence of sepsis on clinical or laboratory criteria • Requiring ERCP for gallstone pancreatitis • No patients who self-discharged or were transferred to another hospital • No chronic pancreatic • Pain score < 5 • Temperature < 38°C • WBC < 18,000 • Diet tolerance • No severity on imaging

Studies	Selection criteria
Ahmed, 2021 [35]	• No history of severe cardiac and renal failure • No previous pancreatic surgery, pancreatic malignant, chronic pancreatic • No any condition requiring admission • No OF, no local or systemic complications • No HR > 130 bpm and/or RR > 25 rpm for 2 h • No severe hypotension • Oxygin saturation >90% • Temperature < 102°F (38.9°C) • No altered consciousness • <10% immature WBC • Glucose <400 mg/dl • No ischemic changes on electrocardiogram • No concern for cholangitis or choledocholitiasis • No evidence of end-organ damage • Tolerating a LFSD and oral pain medication • Improved nausea/presence of hunger • Reduction in 2 points on VAS • Stable vital signs • Stable laboratory data
Anderson, 2023 [36]	• No OF, no local or systemic complications • No HR > 130 bpm and/or RR > 25 rpm for >2 h • No severe hypotension (SBP > 80 mmHg) • Oxygin saturation > 90% • Temperature < 102°F (38.9°C) • <10% immature WBC • Glucose < 400 mg/dl • No evidence of end-organ damage • No altered consciousness • No ischemic changes on electrocardiogram • No concern for cholangitis or choledocholitiasis • No previous pancreatic surgery, pancreatic malignant, chronic pancreatic • No history of severe cardiac and renal failure • No any condition requiring admission • Tolerating a LFSD and oral pain medication • Improved nausea/presence of hunger • Pain control • Stable vital signs • Stable laboratory data

Studies	Selection criteria
Ongoing studies about early discharge	
Busquets, 2022 [37]	• No cognitive capacity and without any previous diagnose of psychiatric disease • No previous pancreatic surgery, pancreatic malignant, chronic pancreatic • Comorbidities that required previous hospitalization (myocardial infarction, liver cirrhosis, chronic kidney disease, chronic lung disease • BMI $\leq$ 35 kg/m^2 • No evidence of SIRS in the emergency room • BISAP $\leq$ 2 at the time of randomization • CRP levels < 150 mg/dl • Marked increase in the WBC • Absence of coagulopathy (INR < 1.4) • Hematocrit < 44% • Creatinine < 170 umol/L • Hyperbilirrubinemia >3×ULN • Absence organ failure • No local or systemic complications • No concern for cholangitis or choledocholitiasis • Patients with good pain response to 12-h supportive care in the ER • VAS < 4 • Adequate oral feeding tolerability • Hospital home care criteria
Ramírez-Maldonado, 2023 [38]	• ASA < 3 • No cognitive impairment • No previous pancreatic surgery, pancreatic malignant, chronic pancreatic • SIRS $\leq$ 2 criteria • BISAP $\leq$ 2 score • No OF, no local or systemic complications • No concern for cholangitis or choledocholitiasis • Diet tolerance $\geq$ 50% • Absence of nausea/vomiting • Pain controlled with analgesics

ASA: American Society of Anesthesiologists; BISAP: Bedside Index of Severity of Acute Pancreatitis; BMI: Body Mass Index; ER: Emergency Room; CRP: C-Reactive Protein; ERCP: Endoscopic Retrograde Cholangiopancreatography; HR: Heart Rate; INR: International Normalized Ratio; LFSD: Low Fat Solid Diet; MAP: Mild Acute Pancreatitis; OF: Organ Failure; RR: Respiratory Rate; SAP: Severe Acute Pancreatitis; SBP: Systolic Blood Pressure; SIRS: Systemic Inflammatory Response Syndrome; VAS: Visual Analogue Scale; WBC: White Blood Cells.

Table 3.
Studies about early discharge.

5. Minimally invasive interventions: Effective alternatives to open surgery

Before proceeding, it is essential to emphasise that successful treatment of SAP relies heavily on close interdisciplinary collaboration amongst gastroenterologists, intensivists, radiologists, and surgeons. Establishing committees or holding multidisciplinary meetings can be essential to achieving this goal.

Historically, local complications of SAP, such as pancreatic necrosis or fluid collections, often required open surgery, which carried significant risks of infection, morbidity, and mortality. The introduction of stepwise and minimally invasive management has revolutionised the treatment of SAP [39]. The "Step-up approach" [39] begins with draining infected or necrotic tissue and progresses to minimally invasive techniques, such as laparoscopic cystogastrostomy and video-assisted retroperitoneal debridement (VARD). Additionally, transluminal drainage, using percutaneous and EUS-guided techniques, has proven to be effective in clinical practice, offering a safer approach, reducing complications and mortality, and optimising resource utilisation [3–5, 8, 39–44].

A recent meta-analysis of 10 studies on necrotising AP, despite small sample sizes, identified the step-up approach as the preferred strategy. Delayed surgery (DS), delayed step-up surgery (DSU), and delayed endoscopic step-up (DEU) were associated with low mortality and fewer major complications. Secondary analyses emphasised the benefits of DEU and DSU in reducing organ failure, fistulas, pancreatic insufficiencies, and hospital stays. Delaying interventions for at least four weeks is recommended to optimise outcomes [44].

6. Biomarkers, proteomics, genetics, and personalised medicine: Towards a more specific approach in acute pancreatitis

The traditional diagnosis of AP relies on clinical, biochemical (amylase, lipase), and imaging parameters [3–5]. However, these methods have limitations in accurately predicting disease progression and the risk of complications. Biomarkers offer a more nuanced understanding, allowing earlier intervention, risk stratification, and personalised therapeutic strategies [30].

Current research focuses on identifying new biomarkers, including proteins, inflammatory molecules, and microRNAs, with the following goals.

6.1 Early diagnostic and prediction of severity

Biomarkers play a critical role in identifying patients at risk of developing SAP or complications such as pancreatic necrosis and organ failure. Early detection can significantly reduce morbidity and mortality by facilitating timely interventions. Key biomarkers include:

- *C-Reactive Protein (CRP)*: Elevated CRP levels within the first 48 hours of admission correlate with severe AP [3–5, 30, 45–47].

- *Procalcitonin (PCT)*: PCT is a valuable marker for predicting pancreatic infections and systemic inflammatory response syndrome (SIRS). Higher levels are linked to the development of infected pancreatic necrosis [3–5, 30, 45–47].

- *Interleukin-6 (IL-6)*: IL-6 is a promising early indicator of severe inflammation and correlates with systemic complications, making it a potential predictor of organ failure [30, 45–47].

6.2 Predicting organ failure and complications

Significant challenges in managing AP are identifying patients at risk for multi-organ failure and other systemic complications. Biomarkers offer a non-invasive method to monitor disease progression and predict adverse outcomes. Essential biomarkers include:

- *Blood urea nitrogen (BUN)*: BUN is a valuable biomarker in AP, reflecting early renal dysfunction and intravascular volume depletion. Elevated BUN levels on admission or rising within the first 24 hours are associated with increased severity and mortality. Monitoring BUN helps guide fluid resuscitation and assess prognosis in acute pancreatitis patients [3–5, 30, 45–47].

- *Lactate dehydrogenase (LDH)*: Elevated LDH levels indicate pancreatic cell injury and are associated with necrotising pancreatitis [30, 45–47].

- *Urinary trypsinogen activation peptide (uTAP)*: This biomarker reflects premature trypsinogen activation and can predict the severity of AP at an early-stage [45–47].

6.3 Guiding therapeutic interventions

Biomarkers also support the customisation of therapeutic approaches by identifying patients who may benefit from specific interventions, such as EEN, aggressive fluid resuscitation, or minimally invasive procedures. Important biomarkers include:

- *Lymphocyte-to-monocyte ratio (LMR)*: A low LMR is associated with poor prognosis and higher rates of pancreatic necrosis, suggesting the need for closer monitoring and aggressive management [46].

- *MicroRNAs (miRNAs)*: miRNAs, such as miR-551 and miR-216, are emerging as potential biomarkers for differentiating MAP from SAP, guiding decisions on the intensity of care required [30, 45–47].

By incorporating these biomarkers, clinicians can minimise unnecessary therapeutic exposures, reduce risks, and enable more precise risk stratification and targeted treatment strategies.

6.4 Proteomics

Proteomics has emerged as a transformative tool for understanding the pathophysiology of AP and advancing towards a more personalised treatment approaches. By analysing protein expression profiles and their interaction networks, researchers aim to identify key biomarkers that improve disease stratification, treatment optimisation, and enhance prognosis predictions [48].

Historically, conventional statistical methods, such as parametric tests and regression models, were used to identify biomarkers. However, these methods often fall short in handling the vast and complex datasets generated by proteomic studies. Machine learning (ML) algorithms have revolutionised omics data analysis, facilitating the management of large datasets and the creation of multibiomarker panels.

These panels capture complex patterns associated with AP, significantly enhancing diagnostic and prognostic accuracy [48].

Recent advancements, such as single-cell proteomics and mass spectrometry imaging (MSI), have further expanded the ability to study proteins at the tissue level. These technologies provide detailed insights into the spatial distribution of biomarkers in the pancreas and other affected organs, offering a deeper understanding and its progression [48].

6.5 Genetics and proteomics

The discovery of pancreatic digestive genes encoding trypsinogen (PRSS1 and PRSS2) marked a significant step in understanding the genetic basis of AP [8]. Since then, further genetic variants have been classified based on their pathogenic mechanisms into three primary pathways [8]:

- *Trypsin-dependent pathway*: Includes PRSS1, PRSS2, Kazal-type 1 trypsin inhibitor (SPINK1), and chymotrypsin (CTRC) genes. Dysregulation in this pathway can lead to uncontrolled trypsin activation, a known trigger for pancreatic injury.

- *Ductal physiological pathway*: Comprises the cystic fibrosis transmembrane conductance regulator (CFTR), claudin 2 (CLDN2), calcium-sensing receptor (CASR), and calcium channel genes (TRPV6). Variants in these genes disrupt ductal bicarbonate secretion and ion transport, contributing to impaired pancreatic duct function.

- *Misfolding-dependent pathway*: This includes distinct variants of PRSS1, carboxypeptidase A1 (CPA1), and rare variants of carboxyl ester lipase (CEL). Protein misfolding within the endoplasmic reticulum can result in cellular stress, contributing to pancreatitis onset.

Genetics complements proteomics by identifying individual predispositions to severe or recurrent forms of AP. Specific genetic polymorphisms have been associated with increased susceptibility to complications, while whole-genome studies allow the identification of genes involved in inflammatory responses and metabolic dysfunction [8, 48].

On the other hand, proteomics provides a dynamic view of the inflammatory and metabolic processes during AP. The integration of proteomic, genomic, and metabolic biomarkers represents a crucial step towards personalised medicine in AP [48]. While genetic studies reveal inherited susceptibilities and pathways prone to dysfunction, proteomics captures the evolving biological landscape during active disease. This complementary approach enhances risk stratification, aids in early diagnosis, and guides tailored therapeutic interventions, ultimately improving patient outcomes and reducing complications [8, 48].

6.6 Challenges and future directions

Despite advancements, challenges remain, as universal biomarkers do not yet exist due to clinical heterogeneity, sample processing difficulties, and limitations in translational applicability. However, the future points towards the creation of multimolecular panels that integrate proteomic, genetic, and clinical information, facilitating more precise and personalised stratification of AP [8, 48].

Proteomics and biomarkers are transforming the approach to AP, providing tools that go beyond conventional diagnostics. As technology advances, the combination of genomics, proteomics, and ML will enable a more accurate, personalised, and effective approach to managing AP, ultimately improving clinical outcomes and the quality of life for patients [8, 48].

7. Artificial intelligence in acute pancreatitis: A new era in diagnosis and management

The advent of AI and its subset ML represents a revolutionary step in the field of AP. These technologies enable the analysis of complex, nonlinear datasets, uncovering subtle relationships that conventional tools cannot detect. Through AI, healthcare systems can achieve more precise diagnostics, enhanced prognostication, and personalised treatment approaches, ultimately improving patient outcomes.

7.1 Artificial intelligence, radiomics, and machine learning: A brief overview

AI refers to the simulation of human intelligence by machines to perform tasks such as decision-making, problem-solving, and pattern recognition. AI encompasses various subfields, including ML and Deep Learning (DL). ML, a subset of AI, relies on statistical algorithms to learn from structured, high-quality data and make predictions, often requiring advanced computing power for model training. DL, a specialised branch of ML, leverages neural networks to process and learn directly from raw, complex datasets, such as medical images, identifying intricate patterns without manual feature engineering. DL models are capable of learning complex features and representations from raw data by themselves, without the need for manual feature engineering, enabling them to continuously improve with more data [49, 50].

Radiomics is an advanced AI-driven application in medical imaging that focuses on extracting a wealth of high-dimensional, quantitative features from medical images, such as CT, MRI, and PET scans. These features, often imperceptible to the human eye, capture complex patterns, textures, shapes, and intensities within the images, providing a deeper layer of analysis. By converting imaging data into a rich set of measurable variables, radiomics enables precise predictions about disease characterisation, prognosis, and treatment response [6].

7.2 AI in diagnosis of acute pancreatitis

Traditionally, AP diagnosis relies on clinical criteria, elevated enzyme levels (amylase/lipase), and imaging studies in case of diagnostic uncertainty. However, AI-powered diagnostic models have proven superior in identifying AP severity and distinguishing between different pancreatic conditions.

- Imaging enhancement: AI algorithms improve radiologist workflows through segmentation and detection of pancreatic changes in CT and MRI scans. Some authors demonstrated that a DL classifier achieved high accuracy in recognising AP and identifying critical lesions like necrosis or abscess formation [6].

- Radiomic analysis: Advanced radiomic features extracted from CT images enable differentiation between AP, chronic pancreatitis, and functional abdominal pain with accuracies exceeding 80% [7].

AI also optimises imaging protocols by reducing the need for repeated scans and providing real-time analysis, particularly in emergency settings where timely intervention is critical.

7.3 AI in severity prediction, complications and mortality

Accurate prognosis and early identification of complications in AP are crucial for improving outcomes, especially in severe cases. AI models have emerged as powerful tools, leveraging multimodal data, including clinical parameters, laboratory values, and imaging features, to provide superior predictive accuracy compared to traditional scoring systems like Bedside Index of Severity of Acute Pancreatitis (BISAP), Ranson, and Acute Physiology and Chronic Health Disease Classification System II (APACHE II). ML algorithms allow the real-time stratification of high-risk patients and early intervention, minimising complications such as acute kidney injury (AKI), acute respiratory distress syndrome (ARDS), pancreatic necrosis, and persistent organ failure [50].

7.3.1 Severity prediction

ML algorithms significantly outperform conventional tools in predicting SAP within the critical early phase. The following examples illustrate some of these advanced algorithms and their applications

- *EASY-APP model*: Incorporating clinical parameters available at admission, achieved an area under the curve (AUC) of 0.81 for predicting SAP. Its ability to identify early symptoms makes it highly valuable for the early stratification of SAP risk and the timely identification of high-risk patients at admission [51].

- *PANCREATIA model*: Like EASY-APP predicts SAP but focuses solely on baseline clinical variables without requiring lab or imaging data. While EASY-APP integrates additional findings to achieve an AUC of 0.81 for SAP prediction, PANCREATIA delivers comparable AUCs of 0.849 for mortality and 0.783 for persistent organ failure using only early-stage data. This makes PANCREATIA ideal for resource-limited settings, offering rapid triage for referrals, timely interventions, and optimised patient management [52].

- *PrismSAP*: By integrating radiomics features from CT scans, deep learning insights from 2D imaging, and clinical data from electronic health records (EHRs), PrismSAP achieved superior performance compared to traditional scoring systems such as BISAP and Ranson with an impressive AUC of 0.916 [6].

7.3.2 Complications prediction

Acute pancreatitis can lead to a range of severe complications, including AKI, ARDS, pancreatic necrosis, sepsis, and even mortality. Predicting these outcomes early is critical for timely intervention and improving patient outcomes. ML and AI models have revolutionised this process by leveraging clinical, laboratory, and imaging data to assess the risk of these complications with high accuracy [53–55].

7.3.2.1 Acute kidney injury (AKI)

AKI is a life-threatening complication that can occur early in SAP. AI algorithms, such as Gradient Boosting Machines (GBM) and Random Forest Models, utilise biomarkers (e.g., blood urea nitrogen, procalcitonin) and vital signs for prediction.

- GBM models have achieved AUCs between 0.814 and 0.867 in AKI prediction, outperforming traditional regression models [54].
- Random Forest models yielded an AUC of 0.809, while Support Vector Machines (SVM) performed comparably with an AUC of 0.810 [54].

7.3.2.2 Acute respiratory distress syndrome (ARDS)

This condition contributes significantly to early mortality in SAP, accounting for nearly 60% of deaths within the first week of disease onset. Early identification and intervention are crucial to improving outcomes, underscoring the importance of predictive tools and models. ML models, such as the Bayesian Classifier (BC), Artificial Neural Networks (ANN), and Support Vector Machines (SVM), have demonstrated substantial promise in predicting ARDS by integrating clinical and laboratory parameters like BISAP scores, procalcitonin, prothrombin time, serum calcium, and PaO2. Amongst these, the BC model achieved the highest AUC of 0.891, outperforming the ANN model, which had an AUC of 0.853. These tools enhance clinicians' ability to identify high-risk patients early, facilitating timely interventions and reducing mortality rates associated with SAP-related ARDS [56, 57].

7.3.2.3 Pancreatic necrosis

Pancreatic necrosis is a critical complication of SAP, marked by the death of pancreatic tissue due to inflammation and ischaemia. This condition is associated with a high-risk of secondary infections, organ failure, and mortality. Early prediction is vital for guiding timely interventions. NECRO-APP, an AI-driven model, has been specifically developed for predicting pancreatic necrosis, achieving AUC of 0.757 with XGBoostClassifier. By integrating clinical data and radiomics features extracted from CT scans, NECRO-APP provides a detailed assessment of necrosis risk, enabling clinicians to identify high-risk patients with precision. Furthermore, DL models trained on non-contrast CT scans using the Computed Tomography Severity Index (CTSI) as a reference has achieved even higher accuracy, with AUC values reaching 0.980. These AI tools leverage subtle imaging features, such as textural heterogeneity and intensity changes, to enhance diagnostic and prognostic capabilities, surpassing traditional scoring systems. The integration of AI in necrosis prediction represents a significant step forward in the management of SAP, allowing for earlier interventions and improved outcomes [58, 59].

7.3.3 Sepsis and Intensive Care Unit (ICU) admission

Sepsis and ICU admission are critical outcomes in SAP, often indicating the need for immediate and intensive medical interventions. Predictive models using advanced machine learning algorithms have shown remarkable efficacy in identifying high-risk patients early [60].

Light Gradient Boosting Machines (LightGBM):

- Integrated into hospital information systems (HIS), LightGBM models provide real-time predictions for critical outcomes, such as sepsis and ICU admission.
- These models achieved outstanding AUC values of 0.961 for sepsis prediction and 0.973 for ICU admission, significantly outperforming traditional scoring systems like BISAP and APACHE II [60].
- LightGBM models analyse a wide range of data, including vital signs, laboratory results, and dynamic clinical parameters, to deliver rapid and automated predictions of sepsis [60].

Other machine learning models:

Additional models, such as Extreme Gradient Boosting (XGBoost) and Random Forest algorithms, have been applied to ICU admission predictions with similarly high performance. These models utilise a mix of clinical and biochemical data, focusing on early-stage indicators of disease progression [60].

By providing real-time insights, these predictive models empower clinicians to prioritise patients at higher risk, optimise ICU resources, and implement life-saving interventions promptly. Their integration into hospital information systems underscores the transformative potential of AI in managing critical SAP outcomes, improving decision-making processes, and ultimately enhancing patient survival rates.

7.3.4 Mortality prediction

Mortality remains a critical endpoint in AP, particularly among patients with persistent organ failure. Various AI-based models have demonstrated superior predictive capabilities compared to conventional scoring systems:

Gaussian Naive Bayes (GNB):

- GNB models have achieved AUCs ranging from 0.840 to 0.862, outperforming traditional scoring systems such as sequential organ failure assessment (SOFA) and Ranson [61].
- These models effectively integrate clinical and laboratory data, providing precise mortality predictions in both internal and external validations [61].

Artificial Neural Networks (ANNs):

- ANNs trained on large ICU datasets, such as MIMIC-III and MIMIC-IV, have achieved an AUC of 0.769 [62].
- Despite utilising fewer predictive variables, ANNs emphasise impactful markers, allowing for robust predictions tailored to specific patient profiles [62].

Multimodal AI models:

- Advanced models like EASY-APP, NECRO-APP, and PrismSAP combine clinical, laboratory, and imaging data to enhance predictive accuracy [6, 51, 58].
- These models consistently deliver AUC values exceeding 0.91 for complications like severity prediction, necrosis, AKI, ARDS, sepsis, and mortality [53, 55].

7.4 AI in personalised management of acute pancreatitis

The integration of AI into AP management heralds a future of personalised medicine. AI-driven tools can:

- Predict optimal surgical timing: Models like PrismSAP combine clinical data, imaging, and radiomic features to guide the decision-making process for interventions such as drainage or necrosectomy [6].
- Optimise treatment strategies: AI personalises therapy by identifying patient-specific risk factors, thus improving resource allocation, ICU admission protocols, and targeted therapies.

AI and ML have redefined the landscape of acute pancreatitis management by enhancing diagnostic precision, refining risk stratification, and enabling tailored treatment approaches. The incorporation of radiomics and real-time predictive models into clinical workflows promises to revolutionise AP care, reducing morbidity and mortality while improving healthcare efficiency. However, further research, validation, and integration are needed to fully realise the transformative potential of these technologies in routine practice.

8. Conclusions

Acute pancreatitis (AP) continues to present significant clinical challenges due to its diverse manifestations and potential for severe complications. However, advancements in diagnostic accuracy, personalised risk stratification, and therapeutic innovations are transforming the landscape of AP management. Cutting-edge technologies, including artificial intelligence (AI), machine learning (ML), radiomics, and biomarkers, now enable healthcare providers to predict complications, optimise interventions, and tailor treatments to individual patients with unprecedented precision.

The shift towards minimally invasive interventions, early enteral nutrition, and outpatient management of mild AP has not only improved clinical outcomes but also reduced healthcare burdens by enhancing cost-effectiveness and patient satisfaction. Simultaneously, the integration of AI-driven models, such as NECRO-APP, PrismSAP, and LightGBM, into clinical workflows has elevated the standard of care, offering real-time predictions for complications like necrosis, sepsis, and mortality. These tools empower clinicians to make informed decisions, ensuring timely and effective management of AP across all severities.

Looking ahead, the fusion of genomics, proteomics, and AI holds the promise of truly personalised medicine in AP care. By leveraging these technologies, clinicians can identify high-risk patients early, minimise unnecessary interventions, and maximise therapeutic efficacy. Despite these advances, ongoing challenges, such as ensuring equitable access, model validation across diverse populations, and seamless integration into clinical practice, must be addressed.

In conclusion, the future of AP management lies in a multidisciplinary, technology-driven approach that prioritises patient-centred care. By embracing innovation, the medical community is well-positioned to overcome the complexities of AP, reduce complications, and improve outcomes, ultimately ushering in a new era of precision medicine.

Acknowledgements

The authors would like to express their gratitude for the research grant awarded by the 'Acadèmia de Ciències Mèdiques i de la Salut de Catalunya i Balears,' the 'Societat Catalana de Cirurgia,' and the 'Asociación Española de Cirujanos.' Finally, the authors wish to thank The Catalan Pancreatitis Collaborative Group.

Conflict of interest

The authors declare no conflict of interest.

Author details

Elena Ramírez-Maldonado[1,2]*, Sandra López Gordo[3,4] and Rosa Jorba[1,2]

1 General and Digestive Surgery Department, Universitary Hospital of Tarragona Joan XXIII, Tarragona, Spain

2 Biomedicine Department, Rovira i Virgili University, Tarragona, Spain

3 General and Digestive Surgery Department, Maresme Health Consortium, Mataro, Spain

4 Unit of Human Anatomy and Embriology, Department of Morphological Sciences, Faculty of Medicine, Autonomous University of Barcelona, Bellaterra, Spain

*Address all correspondence to: elena.ramirezmaldonado@gmail.com

References

[1] Navarro S. Historical review of our knowledge of acute pancreatitis. Gastroenterología y Hepatología. 2018;**41**(2):143.e1-143.e143143. DOI: 10.1016/j.gastrohep.2017.11.004

[2] Greenberg JA, Hsu J, Bewazeer M, Marshall J, Friedrich JO, Nathes A, et al. Compliance with evidence-based guidelines in acute pancreatitis: An audit of practices in university of Toronto hospitals. Journal of Gastrointestinal Surgery. 2016;**20**(2):392-400. DOI: 10.1007/s11605-015-3023-9

[3] Leppäniemi A, Tolonen M, Tarasconi A, Segovia-Lohse H, Kirkpatrick AW, Ball CB, et al. 2019 WSES guidelines for the management of severe acute pancreatitis. World Journal of Emergency Surgery. 2019;**14**:27. DOI: 0.1186/s13017-019-0247-0

[4] Working Group IAP/APA Acute Pancreatitis Guidelines. IAP/APA evidence- based guidelines for the management of acute pancreatitis. Pancreatology. 2013;**13**(4 Suppl 2):e1-e15. DOI: 10.1016/j.pan.2013.07.063

[5] Tenner S, Baillie J, Vege SS, Sneth SG, Sauer B, Yang A, et al. American College of Gastroenterology guideline: Management of acute pancreatitis. The American Journal of Gastroenterology. 2024;**119**: 419-437. DOI: 10.14309/ajg. 0000000000002645

[6] Yin M, Lin J, Wang Y, Liu Y, Zhang R, Duan W, et al. Development and validation of a multimodal model in predicting severe acute pancreatitis based on radiomics and deep learning. International Journal of Medical Informatics. 2024 Apr;**184**:105341. DOI: 10.1016/j.ijmedinf.2024.105341

[7] Mashayekhi R, Parekh VS, Faghih M, Singh VK, Jakobs MA, Zander A. Radiomic features of the pancreas on CT imaging accurately differentiate functional abdominal pain, recurrent acute pancreatitis, and chronic pancreatitis. European Journal of Radiology. 2020;**123**:108778. DOI: 10.1016/j.ejrad.2019.108778

[8] Strum WB, Boland CR. Advances in acue and chronic pancreatitis. World Journal of Gastroenterology. 2023;**29**(7):1194-1201. DOI: 10.3748/wjg. v29.i7.1194

[9] Li X, Ma F, Jia K. Early enteral nutrition within 24 hours or between 24 and 72 hours for acute pancreatitis: Evidence based on 12 RCTs. Medical Science Monitor. 2014;**17**(20):2327-2335. DOI: 10.12659/MSM.892770

[10] Horibe M, Nishizawa T, Suzuki H, Minami K, Iwasaki E, et al. Timing of oral refeeding in acute pancreatitis: A systematic review and meta-analysis. United European Gastroenterology Journal. 2016;**4**(6):725-732. DOI: 10.1177/2050640615612368

[11] Yao Q, Liu P, Peng S, Xu X, Wu Y. Effects of immediate or early oral feeding on acute pancreatitis: A systematic review and meta-analysis. Pancreatology. 2022;**22**:175-184. DOI: 10.1016/j. pan.2021.11.009

[12] Eckerwall GE, Tingstedt BB, Bergenzaun PE, Andersson RG. Immediate oral feeding in patients with mild acute pancreatitis is safe and may accelerate recovery—A randomized clinical study. Clinical Nutrition. 2007;**26**(6):758-763. DOI: 10.1016/j. clnu.2007.04.007

[13] Teich N, Aghdassi A, Fisher J, Walz B, Caca K, Wallochny T, et al. Optimal timing of oral refeeding in mild acute pancreatitis: Results of an opera randomized multi centre trial. Pancreas. 2010;**39**(7):1088-1092. DOI: 10.1097/MPA.0b013e3181d3ce05

[14] Li J, Xue GJ, Liu YL, Javed MA, Zhao XL, Wan MH, et al. Early oral refeeding wisdom in patients with mild acute pancreatitis. Pancreas. 2013;**42**(1):88-91. DOI: 10.1097/MPA.0b013e3182575fb5

[15] Lariño-Noia J, Lindkvist B, Iglesias-García J, Seijo-Ríos S, Iglesias-Canle J, Domínguez-Muñoz JE. Early and/or immediately full caloric diet versus standard refeeding in mild acute pancreatitis: A randomized open-label trial. Pancreatology. 2014;**14**(3):167-173. DOI: 10.1016/j.pan.2014.02.008

[16] Khan S, Ranjha WA, Tariq H, Nawaz H. Efficacy of early oral referring in patients of mild acute pancreatitis. Pacific Journal of Medical Sciences. 2017;**33**(4):899-902. DOI: 10.12669/pjms.334.12338

[17] Karabulut U, Koynuku MB, Sezgin O, Ucbilek E, Aydin MK, Altintas E. Early oral refeeding and selection of initial diet in mild acute pancreatitis. Japanese Journal of Gastroenterology and Hepatology. 2019;**1**(2):1-5

[18] Lozada-Hernández EE, Barrón-González O, Vázquez-Romero S, Cano-Rosas M, Apolinar-Jimenez E. Non-inferiority comparative clinical trial between early oral refeeding and usual oral refeeding in predicted mild acute biliary pancreatitis. BMC Gastroenterology. 2020;**20**:228. DOI: 10.1186/s12876-020-01363-3

[19] Horibe M, Iwasaki E, Nakagawa A, Matsuzaki J, Minami K, Machida Y, et al. Efficacy and safety of immediate oral intake in patients with mild acute pancreatitis: A randomized controlled trial. Nutrition. 2020;**74**:110724. DOI: 10.1016/j.nut.2020.110724

[20] Ramírez-Maldonado E, Gordo S, Pueyo EM, Sanchez-García A, Mayol S, Gonzalez S, et al. Immediate oral refeeding in patients with mild and moderate acute pancreatitis: A multicentre, randomized controlled trial (PADI trial). Annals of Surgery. 2021;**274**(2):255e63. DOI: 10.1097/sla.0000000000004596

[21] Jacobson BC, Vander Vliet MB, Hughes MD, Maurer R, McManus K, Banks PA. A prospective, randomized trial of clear liquids vs. low-fat solid diet as the initial meal in mild acute pancreatitis. Clinical Gastroenterology and Hepatology. 2007;**5**(8):946-951. DOI: 10.1016/j.cgh.2007.04.012

[22] Sathiaraj E, Murthy S, Mansard MJ, Rao GV, Mahukar S, Reddy DN. Clinical trial: Oral feeding with a soft diet compared with celar liquid diet as initial meal in mild acute pancreatitis. Alimentary Pharmacology & Therapeutics. 2008;**15**(2):777-781

[23] Moraes JM, Felga GE, Chebli LA, Franco MB, Gomes CA, Gaburri PD, et al. A full solid diet as the initial meal in mild acute pancreatitis is sabe and result in a shorter length of hospitalization: Results from a prospective, randomized, controlled, double-blind clinical trial. Journal of Clinical Gastroenterology. 2010;**44**(7):517-522. DOI: 1097/MCG.0b013e3181c986b3

[24] Rajkumar N, Karthikeyan VS, Ali SM, Sistla SC, Kate V. Clear liquid diet vs soft diet as the initial meal in patients with mild acute pancreatitis: A randomized interventional trial. Nutrition in Clinical

Practice. 2013;**28**(3):365-370. DOI: 10.1177/0884533612466112

[25] Qi D, Yu B, Huang J, Peng M. Meta-analysis of early enteral nutrition provided within 24 hours of admission on clinical outcomes in acute pancreatitis. JPEN Journal of Parenteral and Enteral Nutrition. 2018;**42**(7):1139-1147

[26] Nelly DM, Kelly EG, Clarke M, Ridway P. Systematic review with meta-analysis. Nasogastric nutrition is efficacious in severe acute pancreatitis: A systematic review and meta-analysis. The British Journal of Nutrition. 2014;**112**(11):1769-1778. DOI: 10.1017/S0007114514002566

[27] Meng WB, Li X, Li YM, Zhu XL. Three initial diets for management of mild acute pancreatitis: A meta-analysis. World Journal of Gastroenterology. 2011;**17**(37):4235-4241. DOI: 10.3748/wjg.v17.i37.4235

[28] De Lucia SS, Candelli M, Polito G, Maresca R, Mezza T, Schepis T, et al. Nutrition in acute pancreatitis: From the old paradigm to the new evidence. Nutrients. 2023;**15**(8):1939. DOI: 10.3390/nu15081939.3

[29] Liu L-W, Xie Y, Li GQ, Zhang T, Sui Y-H, Zhao Z-J, et al. Gut microbiota-derived nicotinamide mononucleotide alleviates acute pancreatitis by activating pancreatic SIRT3 signalling. British Journal of Pharmacology. 2023;**180**(5):647-666. DOI: 10.1111/bph.15980

[30] Patel BK, Patel KH, Bhatia M, Iyer SG, Madhavan K, Moochhala SM. Gut microbiome in acute pancreatitis: A review based on current literature. World Journal of Gastroenterology. 2021;**27**(30):5019-5036. DOI: 10.3748/wjg.v27.i30.5019

[31] Ince AT, Senturk H, Singh VK, Yildiz K, Danalioglu A, Einar A, et al. A randomized consoled trial of home monitoring versus hospitalization for mild non-alcoholic acute interstitial pancreatitis: A pilot study. Pancreatology. 2014;**14**:174-178. DOI: 10.1016/j.pan.2014.02.007

[32] Serrra Pla S, García Monforte N, García Borobia FJ, Rebasa Cladera P, García Pacheco JC, Romaguera Monzonis A, et al. Early discharge in mild acute pancreatitis. Is it possible observational prospective study in a tertiary-level hospital. Pancreatology. 2017;**17**:669-674. DOI: 10.1016/j.pan.2017.07.193

[33] Kothari DJ, Babineau M, Hall M, Freedman SD, Shapiro NI, Seth SG. Preventing hospitalization in mild acute pancreatitis using a clinical pathway in the emergency department. Journal of Clinical Gastroenterology. 2018;**52**(8):734-741. DOI: 10.1097/MCG.0000000000000954

[34] Kumar VV, Treacy PJ, Li M, Dharmawardane A. Early discharge of patients with acute pancreatitis to enchanted outpatient care. ANZ Journal of Surgery. 2018;**88**(12):1333-1336. DOI: 10.1111/ans.14710

[35] Ahmed A, Kothari DJ, Wardlaw S, Freedman SD, Seth SD. Reducing hospitalization in mild acute pancreatitis: Results of long-term follow-up. Journal of Clinical Gastroenterology. 2021;**55**(2):180-186. DOI: 10.1097/MCG.0000000000001354

[36] Anderson K, Shah I, Yakah W, Cartelle AL, Zuberi SA, McHenry N, et al. Prospective evaluation of an emergency department protocol to prevent hospitalization in mild acute pancreatitis: Outcomes and predictors of discharge. Pancreatology.

2023;**23**(3):299-305. DOI: 10.1016/j.pan.2023.02.006

[37] Sorribas M, Carnaval T, Peláez N, Secanella L, Salord S, Sarret S, et al. Home monitoring vs hospitalization for mild acute pancreatitis. A pilot randomized controlled clinical trials. Medicine (Baltimore). 2023;**102**(20):e33853. DOI: 10.1097/MD.0000000000033853

[38] Ramírez-Maldonado E, Rodrigo-Rodrigo M, Lopez Gordo S, Sanchez A, Coronado Llanos D, Sanchez R, et al. Home care/outpatient versus hospital admission in mild acute pancreatitis: Protocol of a multicentre, randomised controlled trial (PADI_2 trial). BMJ Open. 2023;**13**(6):e071265. DOI: 10.1136/bmjopen-2022-071265

[39] Van Santpoort HC, Basselink MG, Bakker OJ, Hofter HS, Boermeester MA, Dejong CH, et al. A step-up approach or open necrosectomy for necrotizing pancreatitis. The New England Journal of Medicine. 2010;**362**(16):1491-1502. DOI: 10.1056/NEJMoa0908821

[40] van Grinsven J, van Santvoort HC, Boermeester MA, Dejong CH, van Eijck CH, Fockens P, et al. Timing of catheter drainage in infected necrotizing pancreatitis. Nature Reviews. Gastroenterology & Hepatology. 2016;**13**(5):306-312. DOI: 10.1038/nrgastro.2016.23

[41] Van Veldhuisen CL, Sissingh NJ, Boxhoorn L, van Dijk SM, van Grinsven J, Verdonk RC, et al. Long-term outcome of immediate versus postponed intervention in patients with infected necrotizing pancreatitis (POINTER): Multicentre randomized trial. Annals of Surgery. 2024;**279**(4):671-678. DOI: 10.1097/SLA.0000000000006001

[42] Zerem E, Kurtcehajic A, Kunosic S, Zerem Malkocevic D, Zerem O. Current trends in acute pancreatitis: Diagnostic and therapeutic challenges. World Journal of Gastroenterology. 2023;**29**(18):2747-2763. DOI: 10.3748/wjg.v29.i18.2747

[43] Song Y, Lee SH. Recent treatment strategies for acute pancreatitis. Journal of Clinical Medicine. 2024;**13**(4):978. DOI: 10.3390/jcm13040978

[44] Yang Y, Zhang Y, Wen S, Cui Y. The optimal timing and intervention to reduce mortality for necrotizing pancreatitis: A systematic review and network meta-analysis. World Journal of Emergency Surgery: WJES. 2023;**18**(1):9. DOI: 10.1186/s13017-023-00479-7

[45] Khanna AK, Meher S, Prakash S, Tiwary SK, Singh U, Srivastava A, et al. Comparison of Ranson, Glasgow, MOSS, SIRS, BISAP, APACHE-II, CTSI scores, IL-6, CRP, and procalcitonin in predicting severity, organ failure, pancreatic necrosis, and mortality in acute pancreatitis. HPB Surgery. 2013;**2013**:367581. DOI: 10.1155/2013/367581

[46] Silva-Vaz P, Abrantes AM, Castelo-Branco M, Gouveia A, Botelho MF, Tralhao JG. Multifactorial scores and biomarkers of prognosis of acute pancreatitis: Applications to research and practice. International Journal of Molecular Sciences. 2020;**21**:338. DOI: 10.3390/ijms21010338

[47] Tarján D, Szalai LM, Verbói M, Kai T, Eross B, et al. Persistently high procalcitonin and C-reactive protein are good predictors of infection in acute necrotizing pancreatitis: A systematic review and meta-analysis. International Journal of Molecular Sciences. 2024;**25**:1273. DOI: 10.3390/ijms25021273

[48] Ge P, Luo Y, Zhang G, Chen H. The role of proteomics in acute pancreatitis: New and old knowledge. Expert Review

of Proteomics. 2024;**21**(1-3):115-123. DOI: 10.1080/14789450.2024.2320810

[49] Berbís MA, Godino FP, Royuela del Val J, Alcala Mata L, Luna A. Clinical impact of artificial intelligence-based solutions on imaging of the pancreas and liver. World Journal of Gastroenterology. 2023;**29**(9):1427-1445. DOI: 10.3748/wjg.v29.i9.1427

[50] Brown L, Taylor M, Lee C. Critical appraisal of machine learning prognostic models for acute pancreatitis: Protocol for a systematic review. Pancreatic Research Journal. 2022;**28**(2):120-135. DOI: 10.5678/prj.2022.280212

[51] Kui B, Pintér J, Molontay R, Nagy M, Farkas N, Gede N, et al. EASY-APP: An artificial intelligence model and application for early and easy prediction of severity in acute pancreatitis. Clinical and Translational Medicine. 2022;**12**(6):e842. DOI: 10.1002/ctm2.842

[52] Villasante S, Fernandes N, Perez M, Cordobés MA, Piella G, Martinez M, et al. Prediction of severe acute pancreatitis at a very early stage of the disease using artificial intelligence techniques, without laboratory data or imaging tests: The PANCREATIA study. Annals of Surgery. 2024:4. DOI: 10.1097/SLA.0000000000006579

[53] Lu Y, Qiu M, Pan S, Basharat Z, Zippi M, Fiorino S, et al. Comparison of an interpretable extreme gradient boosting model and an artificial neural network model for prediction of severe acute pancreatitis. Polish Archives of Internal Medicine. 2024;**134**(5):16700. DOI: 10.20452/pamw.16700

[54] Lin S et al. Predictive model of acute kidney injury in critically ill patients with acute pancreatitis: A machine learning approach using the MIMIC-IV database. Renal Failure. 2024;**46**(1). DOI: 10.1080/0886022X.2024.2303395.Zhou

[55] Chang CH, Chen CJ, Ma YS, Shen YT, Sung MI, Hsu CC, et al. Real-time artificial intelligence predicts adverse outcomes in acute pancreatitis in the emergency department: Comparison with clinical decision rule. Academic Emergency Medicine. 2024;**31**(2):149-155

[56] Zou K, Ren W, Huang S, Jiang J, Xu H, Zeng X, et al. The role of artificial neural networks in prediction of severe acute pancreatitis associated acute respiratory distress syndrome: A retrospective study. Medicine (Baltimore). 2023;**102**(29):e34399. DOI: 10.1097/MD.0000000000034399

[57] Zhang M, Pang M. Early prediction of acute respiratory distress syndrome complicated by acute pancreatitis based on four machine learning models. Clinics. 2023;**78**:100215. DOI: 10.1016/j.clinsp.2023.100215

[58] Kiss S, Pintér J, Molontay R, Nagy M, Farkas N, Sipos Z, et al. Early prediction of acute necrotizing pancreatitis by artificial intelligence: A prospective cohort-analysis of 2387 cases. Scientific Reports. 2022;**12**(1):7827. DOI: 10.1038/s41598-022-11517-w

[59] Lan L, Guo Q, Zhang Z, Zhao W, Yang X, Lu H, et al. Classification of infected necrotizing pancreatitis for surgery within or beyond 4 weeks using machine learning. Frontiers in Bioengineering and Biotechnology. 2020;**8**:541. DOI: 10.3389/fbioe.2020.00541

[60] Chang CH, Chen CJ, Ma YS, Shen YT, Sung MI, Hsu CC, et al. Real-time artificial intelligence predicts adverse outcomes in acute pancreatitis in the emergency department: Comparison with clinical decision rules. Academic Emergency Medicine. 2024;**31**(2):149-155. DOI: 10.1111/acem.14824

[61] Ren W, Zou K, Huang S, Xu H, Zhang W, Shi S, et al. Prediction of in-hospital mortality of intensive care unit patients with acute pancreatitis based on an explainable machine learning algorithm. Journal of Clinical Gastroenterology. 2024;**58**(6):619-626. DOI: 10.1097/MCG.0000000000001910

[62] Ding N, Goo C, Li C, Zhou Y, Chai X. An artificial neural networks model for early predicting In-hospital mortality in acute pancreatitis in MIMIC-III. BioMed Research International. 2021;**2021**:6638919. DOI: 10.1155/2021/6638919

Chapter 10

Surgical Anatomy of the Pancreas

Armando Di Dato and Riccardo Bellino

Abstract

The pancreas is a retroperitoneal organ and is difficult to access. From an embryological point of view, the pancreas derives from the midgut and has an intimate relationship with the portal and mesenteric vessels. Describing the complexity of pancreas vasculature is of utmost importance for safe pancreatic surgery. It is imperative for the surgeon to know all the peripancreatic vessels, their course, which one to ligate, and which one to preserve in different surgical cases, such as pancreatitis with subversion of the anatomy (when it needs an operation) or pancreatic cancer that infiltrates local vessels.

Keywords: pancreas, pancreatic cancer, pancreatitis, superior mesenteric artery, supramesocolic area

1. Introduction

During millions of years of evolution, the pancreas wandered to the retroperitoneum for a reason; surgeons should think twice before messing with it. It is a citation from Schein's Common Sense.

Doctors who aspire to become pancreatic surgeons must know pancreas anatomy thoroughly in order to make pivotal decisions during preoperative, intraoperative, and post-operative times, such as: "I need to remove another piece of pancreas to perform an adequate oncological resection or I need to perform a total pancreatectomy to do so but making the patient insulin dependent for life, or in the pre-operative time there's a focal portal vein invasion from a pancreas head cancer I know how to perform in a safe way this kind of intervention."

Dreadful consequences derive from poor decision-making, and poor decisions derive from bad judgement or, far worse, bad knowledge of the anatomical relationships of the pancreas. We must respect this organ to offer our patients therapy and relief, but we also need to pay our respect to the great people who have preceded us, and who have paved the way to perform routine pancreatic surgery. From this preface, we delve into an anatomical description of this gland.

The pancreas is a parenchymatous organ, a gland that is anatomically and functionally annexed to the gastrointestinal system with highly important and specific tasks to be performed, firstly and most importantly blood glucose control by insulin secretion and fat and protein digestion [1].

This gland remembers macroscopically and microscopically a salivary gland (**Figure 1**).

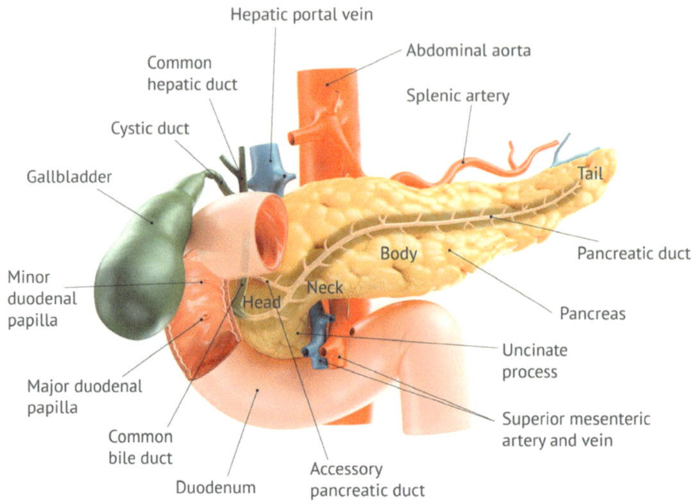

Figure 1.
Anterior vision of the pancreas with duodenum section and vision of pancreatic ducts. 3D model reconstruction. Adobe Stock ® rights reserved with permission.

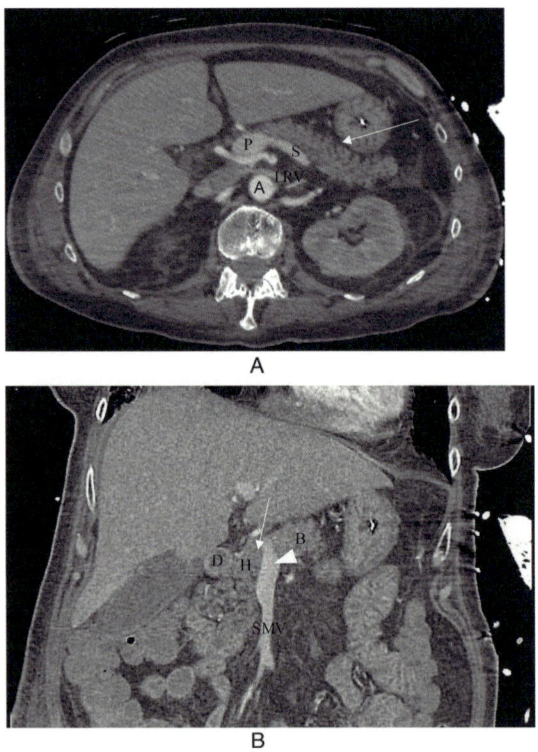

Figure 2.
A. CT scan, transverse section of a 52-year-old woman. This is a portal phase. The body and tail of the pancreas (arrow) are behind the stomach. It is visible the portal vein (P) at the confluence with the splenic vein (S). Further back, the aorta (A) and the relationship with the left renal vein, which normally runs on an anteaortic plane. B. CT scan, coronal section, same patient. Here are visible the head of the pancreas (H), the body (B), and the neck (arrow) right where the superior mesenteric vein continues into the portal vein (arrowhead). The horizontal part of the duodenum is visible (D).

DOI: http://dx.doi.org/10.5772/intechopen.1007049

In the gross description, it remembers a walking cane put horizontally with a pale pink colour [1]. Its surface is lobulated, like a typical exocrine gland, and elastic to the touch, but its consistency can vary depending on the individual characteristics of the person (i.e., in a very old patient, typically the pancreas can be atrophic; in an obese patient can be big and fatty as a cloud, a "*cloudy pancreas*").

It is covered by a single layer of mesothelial cells (posterior parietal peritoneum) except for the tail, where there is an inconstant capsule that makes the gland friable and prone to bleeding [2].

Normally, the gland is 15–23 cm in a male adult in length, 4–5 cm in height and 2–3 cm in width (**Figure 2A** and **B**).

2. Gross description

The pancreas is a single and retroperitoneal organ. It is the second largest gland of our body in terms of size. It lies between the 12th dorsal vertebra and the 2nd lumbar vertebra, so its topographical projection on the abdomen is in the epigastric area. Its major axis is oblique, moving down-up and right to left (**Figure 3**).

As said before, it remembers a walking cane and can be divided into five parts: (A) head; (B) uncinate process; (C) isthmus or neck; (D) body; (E) tail (**Figure 4**) [3].

2.1 Head

It remembers an egg [3]. It lies in the duodenal concavity, which is intimal bound like a fist in the palm of the hand (**Figure 5**). Anteriorly it is covered by a serous lamina that is the parietal peritoneum. On the head, the peritoneum is particularly thick for the insertion of the transverse mesocolon, which divides the head of the pancreas into an upper part that is supramesocolic and a second part that is inframesocolic [4].

This division must be reminded by the surgeon during surgical dissection because of the different anatomical relations that these two parts have with the surroundings.

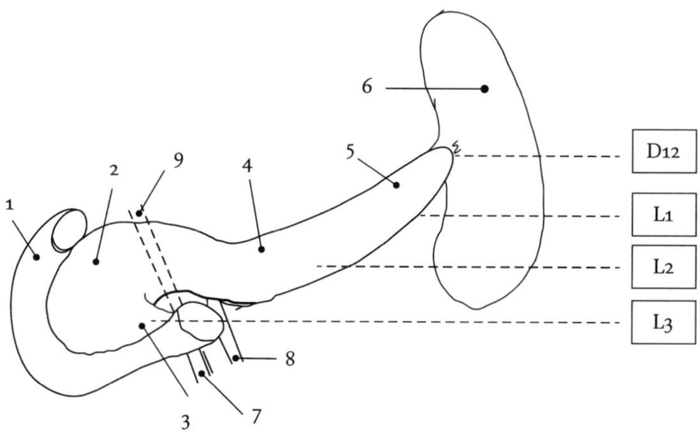

Figure 3.
Drawing scheme with pancreas columnar projection. The most cranial part of the pancreas is the tail at the level of the 12th dorsal vertebra. The most caudal part of the pancreas is the uncinate process at the level of the superior margin of the 3rd lumbar vertebra. (1) duodenum; (2) pancreatic head; (3) uncinate process; (4) pancreatic body; (5) pancreatic tail; (6) spleen; (7) superior mesenteric vein; (8) superior mesenteric artery; (9) portal vein. Personal collection.

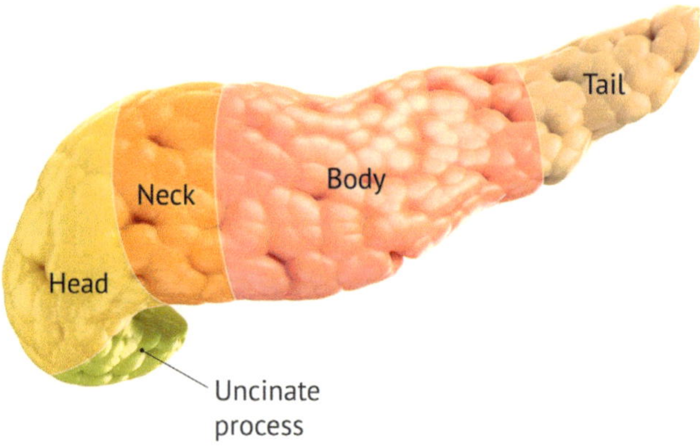

Figure 4.
Pancreas anatomical division. 3D model reconstruction. Adobe Stock ® rights reserved with permission.

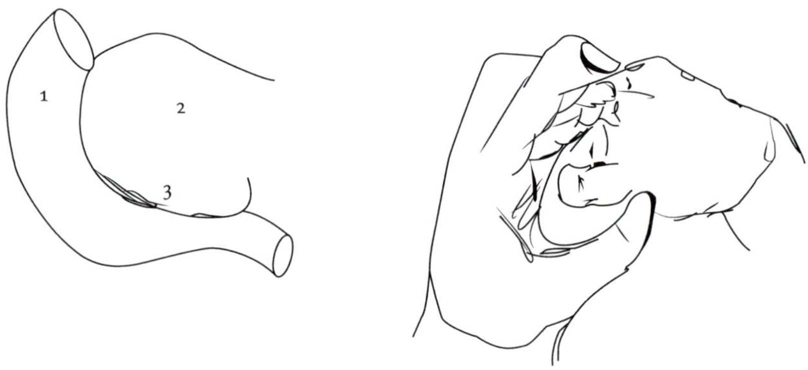

Figure 5.
The drawing depicts the pancreas head and duodenum's intimate relationships, like a fist in the palm of a hand. (1) duodenum; (2) pancreas head; (3) duodenum-pancreatic sulcus. Personal collection.

Posteriorly, the head is in relation to the distal part of the common biliary duct (CBD or *choledochus*), and, mediated by a fibrous fascia (*Treitz fascia*), that derives from the fusion of the meso-duodenum to the retroperitoneum with the inferior cava vein (ICV).

2.2 Uncinate process

It is the extension of the *inframesolic* part of the pancreatic head. It remembers a hook that lies horizontally and encircles posteriorly the superior mesenteric vein (SMV). From this gland, segments emerge as a fibrous layer of tissue, known as *retroportal lamina*, that joins the uncinate process with the posterior wall of the superior mesenteric artery (SMA) and semilunar ganglia [3–5].

This lamina derives from the duodeno-pancreatic-umbilical ligament, the embryological point of fixture of the pancreas [6].

2.3 Neck

It is the thinnest part of the gland and joins the head to the body of the pancreas. Anteriorly it is partially shadowed by the first portion of the duodenum.

Posteriorly, it is modelled by the portal sulcus, an engraving formed by the crossing of the SMV that continues into the Portal vein (PV). The neck of the pancreas is a very important surgical landmark, especially its upper margin; there can be isolated the origin of the gastroduodenal artery (GDA) from the common hepatic artery (CHA) [7].

GDA is the sectioned artery during a pancreas head resection; it vascularises the pancreatic head and the duodenum [2].

2.4 Body

It is the longest part of the pancreas [1–4].

It lies horizontally covered anteriorly by the parietal peritoneum that runs upward to the posterior wall of the stomach. The posterior surface is covered by the *Treitz fascia*; furthermore, it is run by the splenic vein (SV). The upper margin, instead, has an engraving in which lies the splenic artery (SA).

2.5 Tail

It is the leftmost part of the pancreas and the most cranial of all because its projection is on the 12th dorsal vertebra. It is entirely covered by the peritoneum, so it is also the most mobile part of the pancreas [1].

Posteriorly, it is run by the SV and on the upper margin by the SA, as a natural prosecution of the pancreas body. Finally, from the tip of the body derives a thickening of the two epiploon fascias, named the *spleno-pancreatic ligament*, in which can be found splenic vessels and short gastric vessels.

3. Anatomical relationships

Here we synthesise the relationship between the pancreas and its surroundings, making it more memory efficient.

3.1 Head relationships

3.1.1 Anterior relationships

The head is covered by the transverse mesocolon, dividing it into a: (A) supramesocolic part that is in relationship with the pylorus; (B) inframesocolic part, which is, instead by the right colic flexure.

3.1.2 Posterior relationships

The head lies on the *Treitz fascia.* The lateral portion of the head is in relationship with the IVC, particularly with the left renal vein. This kind of relationship is always important to remember for the surgeon because a very deep dissection can result in damage to the left renal vein that causes important bleeding and is difficult to control. The medial portion of the head is in relationship with the lateral part of the PV. The relationship of the head with the CBD is described thoroughly in the dedicated section (see after) (**Figure 6A** and **B**) [8].

3.1.3 Lateral relationships

As said before, the head lies in the concave section of the duodenum like a fist in the palm of the other hand.

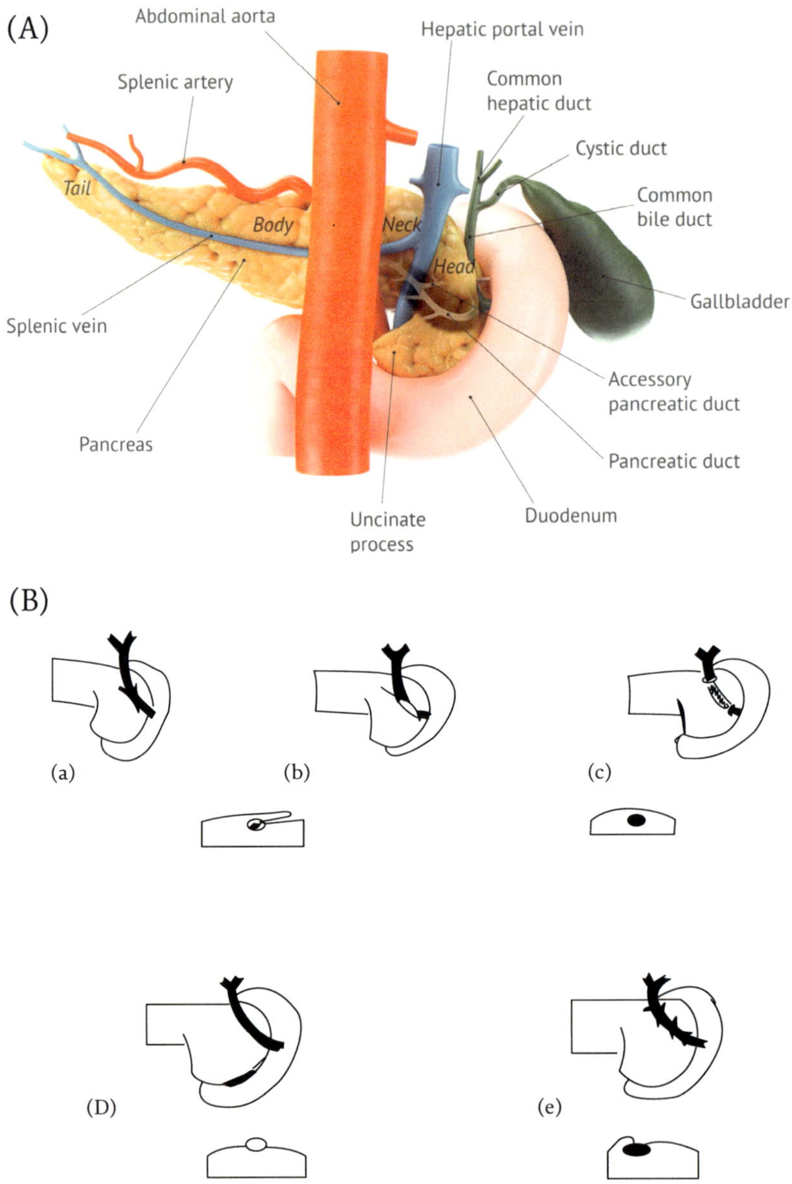

Figure 6.
A. Posterior vision of the pancreas. In this 3D model is visible the CBD tract and its relationship with the pancreatic head. The retro portal lamina is not represented for better vision. 3D model reconstruction. Adobe Stock ® rights reserved with permission. B. Pancreas head and CBD relationships: posterior vision. Typical variants: CBD partially covered by pancreatic head (A) or totally covered (B). CBD intrapancreatic (C), running on the surface (D) or along a tissue engraving (E). Personal collection.

3.1.3.1 Uncinate process

Essentially, it is in relationship with the SMV and SMA, this one with retro portal lamina.

3.1.4 Neck

3.1.4.1 Anterior relationships

It is covered by the posterior wall of the stomach.

3.1.5 Posterior relationships

It is in intimate relation with three important vessels. The SMV runs upward from the uncinate process and goes back to the neck of the pancreas, where it receives the splenic vein into the spleno-mesenteric confluence that continues cranially into the PV, the SMA at the inferior margin, and finally the GDA on the superior margin [7, 9].

3.1.6 Body

3.1.6.1 Anterior relationship

The body is covered by the transverse mesocolic root, which also divides it into two parts: the upper part, covered by peritoneum that continues into the epiploon retro cavity and in relationship with the stomach, and the downward part, covered by inframesocolic peritoneum and in relationship with the 4th part of the duodenum.

3.1.6.2 Posterior relationship

The body lies on the *Treitz fascia* and has relationships with the aorta and its major vessels (celiac trunk and superior mesenteric artery). The SV runs through the gland along its engraving. Finally, the left adrenal gland.

3.1.7 Tail

3.1.7.1 Anterior relationship

The tail is totally covered by the peritoneum. Anteriorly is in relation to the left colic flexure.

3.1.7.2 Posterior relationship

It is in relation to the SV and left renal vein and on the upper margin with the SA.

3.1.7.3 Lateral relationship

The apex of the tail is in relation to the splenic hilum.

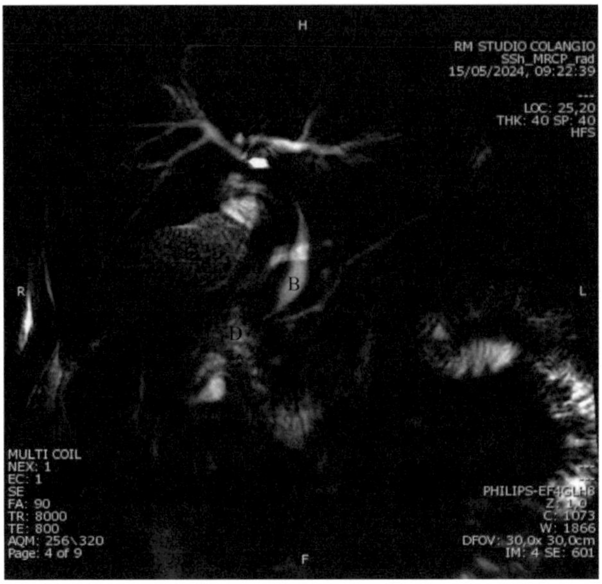

Figure 7.
Magnetic resonance cholangiopancreatography which is visible in the relationship between the Wirsung duct (W) and common bile duct (B) at the Vater papilla in the duodenum (D). It is also visible, that the gallbladder (C), full of stones. Personal collection.

4. Excretion duct

The pancreas has two main ducts for its exocrine function, whose names are the principal pancreatic duct (Wirsung duct) and the accessory pancreatic duct (Santorini duct).

4.1 Wirsung duct

The main pancreatic duct runs through the gland from tail to head and emerges into the duodenum at the *Vater papilla* before fusing with the terminal part of the CBD. Less frequently it emerges alone. (**Figure 7**). It is 20 cm long normally. This exocrine duct originates from the confluence of lesser order ducts at the level of the tail, and then it moves to the head following the pancreas oblique axis [1, 2, 8].

Its progress remembers the profile of an italic S; indeed, at the level of the body, it moves downward when it crosses the head of the pancreas. Along its path, at the level of the neck, it can also drain the accessory pancreatic duct. Of clinical relevance, it is to remember that its diameter varies (1 mm in the tail, 3–4 mm in the head); it goes without saying that if in some parts the Wirsung is dilated, we need to find the cause (i.e., pancreatitis, carcinoma, cystic neoplasm of the pancreas). The diameter grows with ageing.

4.2 Santorini duct

It drains the anterior superior part of the pancreatic head. It is always present but is very thin (almost 1 mm in diameter) and so difficult to note on a celiac trunk (CT) if not dilated. It emerges into the duodenum, 2–3 cm above the *Vater papilla*, at the level of the *minor papilla*. Normally, it drains also into the main pancreatic duct.

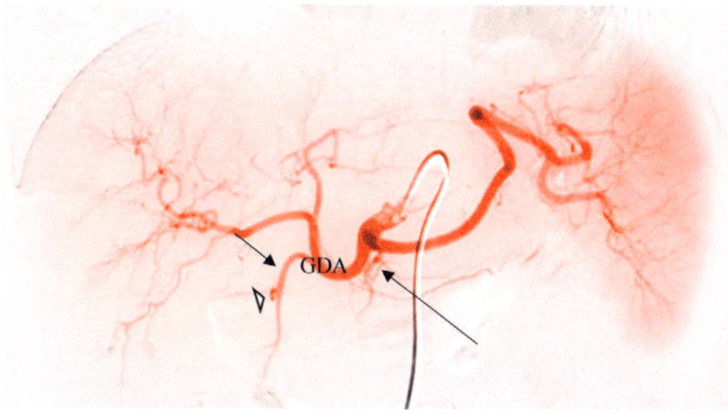

Figure 8.
Celiac arteriography of a patient with HCC of the liver. It is visible in the gastroduodenal artery (GDA) arising from the common hepatic artery. The GDA gives the origin to the ASPDA (little arrow). Right after the origin of the splenic artery rises the dorsal pancreatic artery (long arrow). Adobe Stock ® rights reserved with permission.

5. Pancreas vasculature

The vascular supply of the pancreas is grossly divided into two groups: (A) vascular supply of the pancreatic head; and (B) vascular supply of the body and tail [10].

These two groups are not separate entities but more of an intricate web of anastomoses. These two groups stem from GDA (and so CHA) in the former group and SMA for the latter (**Figure 8**) [11].

On the GDA it is important to remember that derived directly from the common hepatic artery (after GDA origin, the hepatic artery is named *proper hepatic artery* and moves up to the hepatic hilum).

Normally, the GDA is sectioned during pancreatic head resection, but before that, we need to clamp it with a bulldog to evaluate if the hepatic artery flux is GDA-dependent or not [2, 3].

If it is dependent, based on the clinical situation, it is necessary to have an arterial bypass, GDA preservation, or section of the arcuate ligament, which is a fibrous ligament around the aortic ostium of the diaphragm right around the origin of the coeliac trunk. There is a specific clinical condition named Dunbar syndrome, typical of the young woman, that mimics an acute pancreatitis or a peptic ulcer, solely for the occlusion of the celiac trunk (CT) by the arcuate ligament. The treatment is a section of the named ligament to ameliorate CT vasculature.

6. Arteries of the head

The pancreatic head is supplied by two pairs of arteries, the anterior/posterior superior pancreatic-duodenal artery (ASPDA and PSPDA) and the anterior/posterior inferior pancreatic-duodenal artery (AIPDA and PIPDA). The former couple arises from the GDA, 1–2 cm distally from its origin. The latter arises from the SMA or from a common root named the inferior pancreatic-duodenal artery (IPDA), which stems likewise from the SMA [12–14].

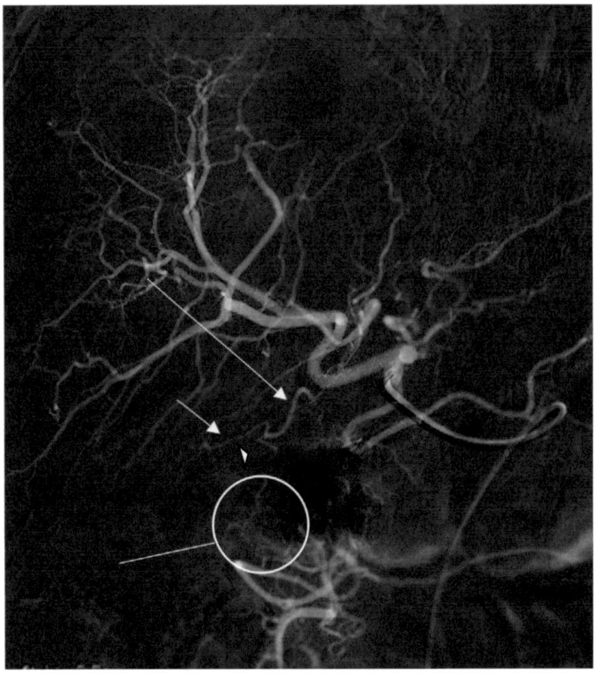

Figure 9.
Detail of a coeliac arteriography. Here is visible the gastroduodenal artery (long arrow), from which originates the posterior superior pancreatic-duodenal artery (short arrow) and the anterior superior pancreatic-duodenal artery (arrowhead). In the circle, we can appreciate the pre-pancreatic arcade between anterior superior and anterior inferior pancreatic-duodenal arteries. Adobe Stock ® rights reserved with permission.

6.1 ASPDA

It is the terminal branch of the GDA. It moves along the *pancreatic-duodenal sulcus* downward, then crosses the third portion of the duodenum to anastomose with the AIPDA (**Figure 9**) [15].

From this artery stems a left branch that anastomoses with the right branch of the dorsal pancreatic artery (DPA), an artery of the pancreatic body, creating the *pre-pancreatic arcade*.

6.2 PSPDA

It arises 1–2 cm distally from the origin of the GDA from CHA. It courses cranially with respect to ASPDA in the back of the pancreatic head and anteriorly to the CBD (**Figure 10**) [15].

There it moves in the *pancreatic-duodenal sulcus* until the third portion of the duodenum, where it runs left and anastomoses with the PIPDA. Its origin can vary; it can arise from CHA or from an accessory right hepatic artery (aRHA) that originates from SMA. It is a thin artery difficult to follow on a CT scan.

6.3 AIPDA and PIPDA

These two arteries originate from a common trunk, named the inferior pancreatic-duodenal artery (IPDA), that arises from the SMA or directly from the SMA. The AIPDA

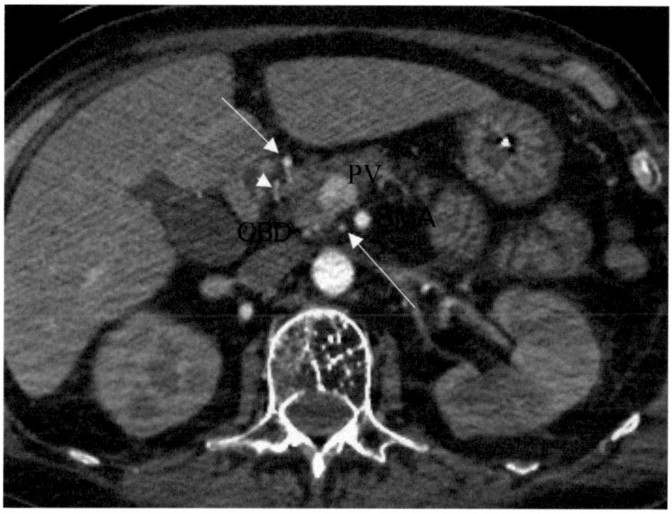

Figure 10.
CT scan, transverse section. Female, 60-year-old patient. Detail of anterior superior pancreatic-duodenal artery (short arrow) and posterior superior pancreatic-duodenal artery right after its origin (arrowhead). The common bile duct (CBD) runs posteriorly to the PSPDA. At the level of the superior mesenteric artery, we can appreciate the origin of the pancreatic dorsal artery (long arrow). Personal collection.

originates as the anterior branch and anastomoses with the ASPDA and forms the anterior arcade of the pancreatic head. The PIPDA is the posterior branch and follows cranially the PSPDA and anastomoses with it, forming the posterior arcade. The anterior and posterior arcades together represent the *pancreatico-duodenal arcade* (Rio-Branco arcade). This vascular anastomotic arcade can supply duodenum and pancreatic head nutritional needs in specific clinical conditions, for example, in a patient with pancreatic cancer that encases and closes CHA, and it is necessary to remove the cancer *en bloc* with CT (modified Appleby procedure or distal pancreatectomy *en bloc* celiac trunk resection) (**Figure 8**) [16].

7. Arteries of the body and tail

7.1 Dorsal pancreatic artery or superior pancreatic artery

This artery regularly originates from the first 2 cm of the splenic artery but can also stem from the CHA, SMA, or CT [17]. The DPA right after its origin divides itself into two branches like an inverted T: (A) the right branch that runs anterior to the pancreatic neck and anastomoses with the left branch of ASPDA; (B) the left branch, also named *transverse pancreatic artery*, that runs along the inferior margin of the pancreatic body [18].

This one also runs inferiorly and anastomoses with the middle colic artery (MCA) (**Figures 8** and **10**).

8. Veins of the pancreas

Similar to the arterial arcades, the pancreatic head vein drainage is formed by an anterior and posterior arcade divided into superior and inferior veins. The body and the tail are drained by multiple left veins that directly drain into the splenic vein and the inferior pancreatic vein that drains into the SMV [19].

8.1 ASPDV

It drains the anterior portion of the pancreatic head and duodenum. It emerges at the *pancreatic-duodenal sulcus* medially to the homologous artery and drains into the *gastrocolic trunk of Henle*, which directly drains into the SMV 3 cm under the confluence with the portal vein (PMC) [19]. The gastrocolic trunk is formed by the confluence of three veins: (A) ASPDV; (B) right gastroepiploic vein (RGEV); (C) middle colic vein (MCV) and runs anteriorly to the pancreatic head. This trunk has great clinical relevance not only in pancreatic surgery but also in colorectal surgery; it is, not by chance, the first cause of intraoperative bleeding during right hemicolectomy. When the retroperitoneal dissection is performed along the duodenal plane, if the dissection is too deep, trunk damage is highly possible, making the bleeding very hard to stop, especially during the laparoscopic procedure (**Figure 11**).

8.2 PSPDV

It drains the posterior part of the pancreatic head and duodenum. It runs behind the CBD and drains into the portal vein, normally 2–3 cm above the PMC [19]. It anastomoses with PIPDV, forming the posterior venous arcade of the pancreatic head (**Figure 12**).

8.3 AIPDV and PIPDV

The AIPDV derives from veins of the uncinate process and directly drains into the 1st jejunal branch of the SMV [19, 20]. The PIPDV derives from little veins running along the upper margin of the 3rd duodenal portion, ending into the 1st jejunal branch or directly into the SMV [20].

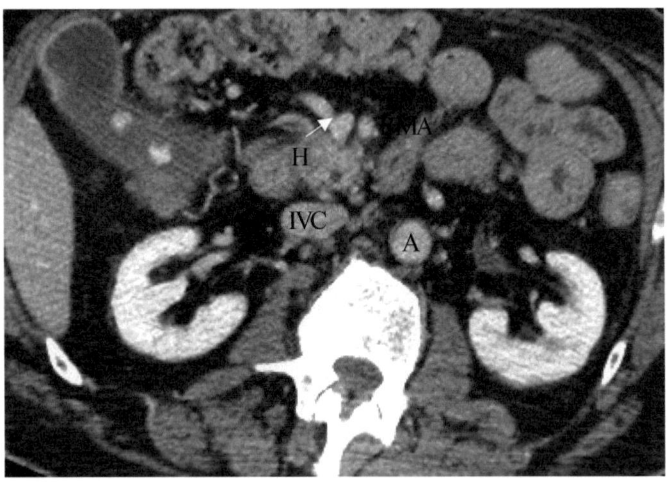

Figure 11.
CT scan, transverse section. Male, 52-year-old patient with pancreatic head tumour. Detail of the gastrocolic trunk of Henle at the confluence of the right gastroepiploic vein and anterior superior pancreatic-duodenal vein (short arrow). The tumour is characteristically hypodense (H). Superior mesenteric artery (SMA), Inferior Vena Cava (ICV), Abdominal Aorta (A). Personal collection.

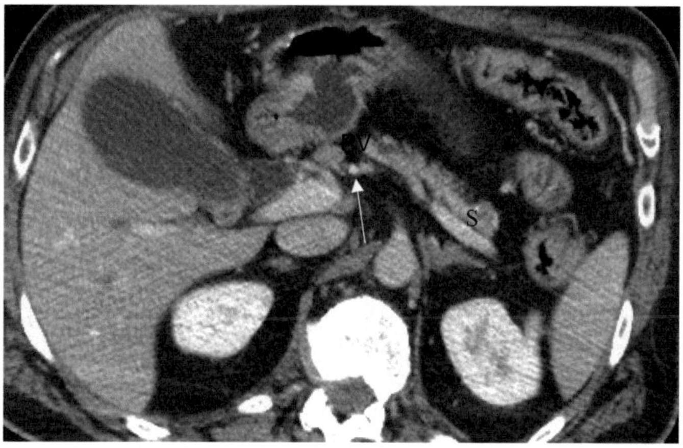

Figure 12.
CT scan, transverse section. Female, 75-year-old patient. Detail of posterior superior pancreatic-duodenal vein (arrow) that is draining into the portal vein (PV). In this section, CBD is not dilated and so not clearly visible and anterior to the vein. It is visible in the splenic vein (S) before its confluence with the portal vein at the neck of the pancreas. Personal collection.

AIPDV and PIPDV anastomosis between themselves in an inconstant arcade. Normally not visible in a CT scan, they are very thin. However, in the case of pancreatic cancer with SMV occlusion, they become visible because they drain directly into PV (via the superior arcade), bypassing the obstacle.

9. Inferior pancreatic vein (IPV) and left pancreatic veins

IPV runs through the inferior border of the pancreas body and drains into the inferior mesenteric vein or left border of the SMV [19]. The left pancreatic veins are small branches that drain exclusively the body and the tail. They are no more than 0.13 mm veins and directly drain into the SV that runs behind the pancreas body and tail.

10. Lymphatic drainage

Pancreatic lymphatic drainage starts in little vases that originate in the pancreatic stroma, and they confluence into bigger lymph vessels that reach the pancreas surface. These vessels connect to the intricate complex of lymph stations that surround the pancreatic space; of great importance are the superior mesenteric lymphatic group and the coeliac group. The nature of pancreatic cancer is to disseminate through lymphatic vessels, so normally the N status (lymphatic metastasis) is of utmost importance in the definition of local oncological status in a pancreatic cancer patient. It is necessary to remove at least 15 nodes during pancreatic resection, and the pancreatic surgeon needs to know all the lymph node stations involved in the neoplastic process. The description and classification of these stations follow the Japanese classification of gastric carcinoma (JGCG 6th edition, 2021) [21].

This description falls outside the purpose of this chapter. Of note is to remember that still today is amply debated on the extent of lymphadenectomy during pancreatic resection, especially during pancreatic head resection. It is stated in the guidelines, that at least 16 nodes need to be removed for a correct pathological staging of pancreatic cancer [21].

Technically, most of the lymph nodes removed during the resection time of the intervention are peripancreatic nodes (station 5, 8a, 8p, 13, 14) and the ones that are removed for the technical movements required for the intervention, such as the pericholecystic nodes (12b), the proper hepatic artery ones (12a), around choledochus (12b), or portal vein (12v). Some pancreas centres in Italy, Germany, and France perform an extended lymphadenectomy as a standard practice, named the artery-first approach [2, 3].

Essentially, after the Kocher manoeuvre of the duodenum, the SMA is isolated and divested from its periadventitial tissue cranially from its emergency at the transverse mesocolic root. This feature makes the intervention more prone to bleeding because, during the divestment, all collaterals of the SMA originate perpendicularly from the vessel. We need to remember the middle colic artery that originates right after the SMA origin from the aorta and the first jejunal branch, normally visible in the left part of the SMA right after its emergence from the retroperitoneum.

11. Innervation

The innervation of the pancreas is supported by the autonomic nervous system, with both sympathetic and parasympathetic fibres thanks to the vagus nerve [1]. Fibres move along periadventitial artery tissue and contain the fibres for gland secretion and fibres for visceral pain. Sympathetic efferent nerves derive from the fifth to tenth dorsal segment of the spinal cord and take synapses with the neurons of the right semilunar ganglion, which is in the right angle between the IVC and left renal vein, and the left semilunar ganglion, located under the splenic artery, at the left of the abdominal aorta. From these ganglia, post-ganglionic fibres depart along and around periadvential tissue on the inferior pancreatic-duodenal arteries and constitute the neurological laminae known as the *right and left superior pancreatic plexus*, which are a fixity element of the pancreatic head. From the gland depart the afferent fibres along the grand splanchnic nerve and lumbar splanchnic nerve that carry pain messages to the central nervous system. This anatomy description explains why, during acute pancreatitis or in the case of locally advanced pancreatic cancer of the body or the neck, the patient complains of epigastric pain irradiated posteriorly. The parasympathetic nerves run along the *vagus nerve*, take synapses with the neurons inside the pancreas parenchyma, and carry secretion and vasoactive commands.

12. Technical aspects

- The pancreas is a retroperitoneal organ, so to be seen and palpated is needed to access the greater omentum by section of the colo-epiploic ligament. Always remember to lower the hepatic flexure/right colic flexure; it gives three advantages: (A) better vision of the surgical field; (B) the *Gerota fascia* is clearly visible and makes the Kocher manoeuvre less prone to bleeding; (C) it can mobilise the ascending colon from the right colic flexure in a lateromedial direction; this dissection is named the Cattel-Braasch manoeuvre and is an essential surgical time if the pancreas head tumour infiltrates the SMV or, worse, the SMA.

- Always advisable to perform an ample Kocher manoeuvre to evaluate the resecability of the pancreatic head. In this way, the tumour can be palpated posteriorly, and the surgeon can understand if there is an extension into the mesenteric root. This situation is, by default, a technical limitation for a safe and oncological resection.

- Cholecystectomy is a good starting point for lymphadenectomy. Simple as that, in open surgery, gallbladder removal gives the surgeon a great hand, because the cystic duct is sectioned at the confluence with the hepatic duct. Practically, we are at the level of the choledochus, and so the lymphadenectomy can be started from here, then moving cranially up to the origin of the hepatic duct; instead, moving medially can be dissected the proper hepatic artery and posteriorly the choledochus, there is the portal vein. In this way, the twelfth station is completely removed in a safe way. Remember to consult the preoperative CT scan and to look out for possible anatomic variants of the hepatic hilum (normally, the triad order is an artery, bile duct, vein, so remember the ABV rule).

- When the gastroduodenal artery is isolated, before its section, always remember to evaluate hepatic flux with a clamp on the gastroduodenal artery. This is a safe way to understand if it is necessary to preserve the gastroduodenal artery or perform an arterial bypass using a vascular graft, such as the saphenous vein or a cadaveric internal iliac artery, or de-rotate the splenic artery in case of total pancreatectomy.

- Wirsung diameter is not only descriptive information for its own sake but is one of the most, if not the most, important elements to foresee pancreatic fistula, the worst surgical complication in pancreatic surgery. During a pancreatic head resection, if the Wirsung is 2–3 mm in diameter, it is better to perform an anastomosis between the jejunum and pancreatic remnant with a tube such as a pigtail into the Wirsung to reduce (unfortunately, not negate) pancreatic fistula. On the other hand, a Wirsung with a diameter greater than 5–6 mm is less prone to leak after anastomosis.

- Biliary anastomosis is normally executed in a single-layer fashion with adsorbable stitches. But it is equally effective as a double-layer technique. It also has the advantage of reducing the risk of post-operative bile leakage. On the other hand, with this technique, a late complication known as biliary stricture is more common. Nevertheless, we must consider that this patient can be treated with percutaneous biliary dilatation or biliary stenting; rarely is a second intervention needed [22].

Author details

Armando Di Dato* and Riccardo Bellino
Ospedale SS. Trinità Borgomanero, Novara, Italy

*Address all correspondence to: a.didato92@gmail.com

References

[1] Lanza GG et al. Trattato di anatomia umana. 4th ed. Via G. Spadolini, Milano, Italy: Edi-Ermes; 2010. ISBN: 9788870514285

[2] Lillemoe KD, Jarnagin W. Master Techniques in Surgery: Hepatobiliary and Pancreatic Surgery. Via Altinate, Padova, Italy: Piccin Nuova Libraria; 2013. ISBN: 9781608311729

[3] Paletto AE et al. Nuovo Trattato di Tecnica Chirurgica. Via G. Spadolini, Milano, Italy: Edra; 2016. ISBN: 9788821442186

[4] Stranding S et al. Gray's Anatomy, the Anatomical Basis of Clinical Practice. Hampshire, Cambridge: Elsevier Inc. (S&T Books and Cell Press); 2020. ISBN: 9780702077050

[5] Cameron JL, Cameron AM. Current Surgical Therapy. 14th ed. Cambridge, MA: Elsevier Inc. (S&T Books and Cell Press); 2022. ISBN: 9780323796835

[6] Skandalakis LJ, Rowe JS, Gray SW, Skandalakis JE. Surgical Embryology and Anatomy of the Pancreas. Surgical Clinics of North America. 1993;**73**(4):661-697. ISSN 0039-6109. DOI: 10.1016/S0039-6109(16)46080-9

[7] Anacker H. Radiological anatomy of the pancreas. In: Anacker H, editor. Efficiency and Limits of Radiologic Examination of the Pancreas. Thieme ed. Acton, MA: Publishing Sciences Group; 1975

[8] Dowdy GS Jr, Waldron GW, Brown WG. Surgical anatomy of the pancreatobiliary ductal system. Archives of Surgery. 1962;**84**:229

[9] Donatini B. A systematic study of the vascularization of the pancreas. Surgical and Radiologic Anatomy. 1990;**12**:173-180

[10] Falconer CWA, Griffiths F. Anatomy of the blood vessels in the region of the pancreas. The British Journal of Surgery. 1950;**37**:334

[11] Ibukuro K. Vascular anatomy of the pancreas and clinical applications. International Journal of Gastrointestinal Cancer. 2001;**30**:87-104. DOI: 10.1385/IJGC:30:1-2:087

[12] Hong KC, Freeny PC. Pancreaticoduodenal arcades and dorsal pancreatic artery. AJR. 1999;**172**:925-931

[13] Woodburne RT, Olsen LL. The arteries of the pancreas. The Anatomical Record. 1951;**111**:255-270

[14] Bertelli E, DiGregorio F, Bertelli L, Mosca S. The arterial blood supply of the pancreas: A review I. The superior pancreaticoduodenal and the anterior superior pancreaticoduodenal arteries. An anatomical and radiological study. Surgical and Radiologic Anatomy. 1995;**17**:97-106

[15] Bertelli E, DiGregorio F, Bertelli L, Civeli L, Mosca S. The arterial blood supply of the pancreas: a review III. The inferior pancreaticoduodenal artery. An anatomical and radiological study. Surgical and Radiologic Anatomy. 1996;**18**:67-74

[16] Bertelli E, DiGregorio F, Bertelli L, Orazioli D, Bastianini A. The arterial blood supply of the pancreas: A review IV. The anterior inferior and posterior pancreaticoduodenal aa., and minor sources of blood supply for the head of the pancreas. An anatomical and radiological study. Surgical and Radiologic Anatomy. 1997;**19**:203-212

[17] Bertelli E, DiGregorio F, Mosca S, Bastianini A. The arterial blood supply of the pancreas: a review V. The dorsal pancreatic artery. An anatomical and radiological study. Surgical and Radiologic Anatomy. 1998;**20**:445-452

[18] Matsumura H. The significance of the morphology of the dorsal pancreatic artery in determining the presence of the accessory right hepatic artery passing behind the portal vein. Acta Anatomica Nipponica. 1998;**73**:517-527

[19] Mourad N, Zhang J, Rath AM, Chevrel JP. The venous drainage of the pancreas. Surgical and Radiologic Anatomy. 1994;**16**:37-45

[20] Crabo LG, Conley DM, Graney DO, Freeny PC. Venous anatomy of the pancreatic head. AJR. 1993;**160**:1039-1045

[21] Japanese Gastric Cancer Association. Japanese Gastric Cancer Treatment Guidelines 2021 (6th edition). Gastric Cancer. 2023;**26**:1-25. DOI: 10.1007/s10120-022-01331-8

[22] Napoli N, Kauffmann EF, Caputo R, Ginesini M, Asta F, Gianfaldoni C, et al. Outcomes of double-layer continuous suture hepaticojejunostomy in pancreatoduodenectomy and total pancreatectomy. HPB: The Official Journal of the International Hepato Pancreato Biliary Association. 2022;**24**(10):1738-1747. DOI: 10.1016/j.hpb.2022.05.005. Epub 2022 May 17

Chapter 11

Surgical Update on the Management of Necrotizing Pancreatitis: Step-Up Approach

Betsabé Reyes Correa, Javier Padilla Quintana and Alicia Goya Pacheco

Abstract

Acute pancreatitis (AP) is an inflamatory condition of the pancreatic gland with or without involvement of peripancreatic tissues and distant organs. The incidence of AP is 20–35 cases per 100,000 inhabitants per year, with an overall mortality of 2–10%. In recent decades, the incidence of AP has increased globally. Most cases follow a mild, self-limiting course, but 10–20% of patients develop a severe form with systemic and local life-threatening complications of pancreatic, and peripancreatic necrosis come about 20–40% of patient with severe AP and aggravate organ functions. The traditional approach to the treatment of necrotizing pancreatitis with secondary infection of necrotic tissue is open necrosectomy to remove the infected necrotic tissue. But this is associated with high rates of complications, death, and pancreatic insufficiency. The benefits of sequential treatment in cases of infected necrosis ("Step an approach") compared to traditional open necrosectomy, showing less morbidity and lower costs. The sequential treatment is an alternative to open necrosectomy, including percutaneous drainage, endoscopic (transgastric) drainage, and minimally invasive retroperitoneal necrosectomy. With this approach, up to 35% of patients can be treated only with drainage, to avoid necrosectomy and to reduce the percentage of complications.

Keywords: necrotizing pancreatitis step-up approach, acute pancreatitis, percutaneous, endoscopic, necrosectomy

1. Introduction

Acute pancreatitis (AP) is one of the most common causes for gastrointestinal-related office visits and admissions to hospital pancreatitis. AP is an inflammatory condition of the pancreas that may or may not involve surrounding tissues and distant organs [1]. The incidence of AP ranges from 20 to 35 cases per 100,000 people annually, with an overall mortality rate of 2–10% [1]. Over the past few decades, the global incidence of AP has risen and is expected to continue increasing. The most common cause is gallstone disease, responsible for approximately 40–50% of cases, followed by alcohol use, particularly in males, which accounts for over 30%. In 10–25% of cases, the cause remains unidentified.

Regardless of the underlying etiology, precipitating factors elicit supraphysiological intracellular signaling pathways that culminate in the premature activation of trypsin within zymogen granules. This aberrant enzyme activation leads to acinar cell injury and necrosis, subsequently triggering a cascade of local and systemic inflammatory responses. Most patients experience a mild, self-limiting form of the condition, but 10–20% develop severe pancreatitis [2–6], leading to life-threatening complications such as pancreatic and peripancreatic necrosis. This severe form occurs in 20–40% of cases and can lead to further organ dysfunction.

Infected pancreatic necrosis remains one of the most challenging and potentially life-threatening complications of acute pancreatitis. The progressive nature of this condition, characterized by the presence of necrotic pancreatic tissue and infection, often leads to multi-organ failure and high mortality rates if not properly managed. Surgical intervention holds a critical role in the treatment, particularly when conservative measures, such as antibiotics and drainage, are insufficient.

In recent years, the approach to managing infected pancreatic necrosis has evolved significantly. Advances in imaging techniques, minimally invasive surgery, and endoscopic interventions have revolutionized the way we address this complex condition. The step-up approach, which advocates for a staged escalation of treatment, has become the gold standard for many patients, with initial drainage followed by debridement when necessary. However, selecting the appropriate surgical strategy remains a subject of ongoing debate, as each patient presents unique challenges related to the location and extent of the necrosis.

Infected necrosis [7] is identified by the presence of Gram-positive bacteria in necrotic pancreatic or peripancreatic tissue, detected either by fine-needle aspiration or during initial drainage or surgery, or by the presence of gas in the fluid collection on contrast-enhanced computed tomography (CT). Suspected infected necrosis is characterized by ongoing sepsis or worsening clinical conditions in the intensive care unit without confirmed infected necrosis. Organ failure affects 40% of patients with pancreatic necrosis, though it can occasionally occur in cases without necrosis. Mortality rates rise to 30% when infection is present in the pancreatic or peripancreatic necrosis. Over the past decade, there have been significant advances in understanding the disease's presentation and progression. An expert consensus panel has also redefined how pancreatic fluid collections are categorized (Appendices A and B).

This chapter aims to provide an updated overview of the surgical management of infected pancreatic necrosis, focusing on the latest advancements in techniques, timing, and patient selection. We will explore current evidence-based practices, discuss the benefits and limitations of various surgical approaches, and examine the role of novel technologies in improving patient outcomes. As the field continues to evolve, a comprehensive understanding of these strategies is essential for optimizing.

2. Step-up approach

The "step up" strategy is nowadays the strategy validated by several consensus conferences for the treatment of necrosis infection occurring in severe acute pancreatitis as described [3]. Multicenter randomized clinical trial PANTER [7] demonstrated that a step-up approach for the treatment of necrotizing pancreatitis reduces mortality, multi-organ failure, healthcare costs, and late surgical complications. The step-up approach involves percutaneous catheter drainage or endoscopic transluminal drainage, followed by minimally invasive necrosectomy only when clinically indicated [8], and is currently the standard of care.

The surgical step-up approach has demonstrated [2] a reduction in the composite outcome of mortality and major complications in patients with infected necrotizing pancreatitis when compared to primary open necrosectomy. Notably, approximately 35% of patients achieve clinical resolution with catheter drainage alone. Despite initial concerns that minimally invasive techniques might lead to higher rates of reintervention due to residual necrotic collections or delayed complications, subsequent long-term follow-up by the same research group has countered this notion, reinforcing the advantages of a step-up approach. It is important to recognize the significant heterogeneity of necrotizing pancreatitis, which necessitates individualized therapeutic strategies and may still warrant open necrosectomy in select cases. Nevertheless, national data continue to support the long-term efficacy and superiority of minimally invasive step-up interventions [9, 10] in the management of infected necrotizing pancreatitis.

2.1 Percutaneous catheter drainage

Infected pancreatic or peripancreatic necrosis can develop within the first 3 weeks following the onset of acute necrotizing pancreatitis. For patients in the early stages of the disease (within 2 to 4 weeks) who have either suspected or confirmed infected necrosis without a walled-off collection and are not responding to conservative treatment, percutaneous drainage may be an effective and safe method for drainage and controlling the infection.

The preferred technique for percutaneous drainage involves accessing the retroperitoneal space on the left side, as this allows for easier minimally invasive surgical intervention if necessary (**Figure 1**). Current data suggests that around 35% of

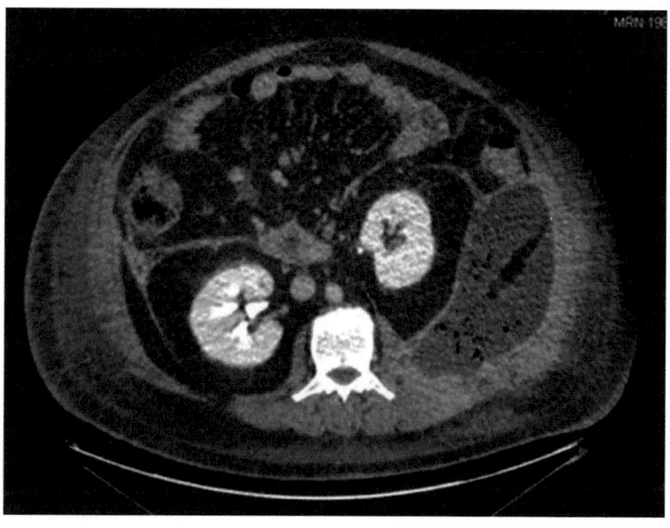

Figure 1.
CT scan revealing a left retroperitoneal collection, which is easily accessible for percutaneous drainage and permits a retroperitoneal laparoscopic approach.

patients receiving percutaneous drainage during the walled-off necrosis (WON) phase do not require further surgical intervention [8]. In some cases, where the drainage catheter size is gradually increased, success rates can reach up to 50%. The necrotic cavity is typically irrigated with saline 3 to 4 times a day, relying on gravity for drainage. Depending on the number, size, and connection of the collections, multiple drainage tubes may be placed. A large multicenter cohort study revealed that 35% of patients managed with primary percutaneous drainage did not need any further treatment [10]. Additionally, two prospective randomized trials [11, 12] comparing various management strategies for symptomatic WON found that percutaneous drainage was successful in 35 and 51% of patients, respectively.

Based on recent evidence, current guidelines recommend using percutaneous drainage when endoscopic options are not available, unsuccessful, or technically infeasible. Another key advantage of percutaneous drainage is that it can serve as an entry point for other minimally invasive debridement procedures, such as video-assisted retroperitoneal debridement (VARD).

The POINTER study [13] is a multicenter, randomized clinical trial comparing long-term outcomes of two treatment approaches in patients with infected necrotizing pancreatitis: immediate drainage and delayed drainage. The objective is to compare long-term outcomes of immediate drainage versus delayed drainage in patients with infected necrotizing pancreatitis. In this study, 104 patients with infected necrotizing pancreatitis were randomly assigned to two groups: Immediate Drainage: Catheter drainage within 24 hours of diagnosis or Delayed Drainage: Initial treatment with antibiotics and catheter drainage only if necessary later. The delayed drainage approach, utilizing antibiotics, resulted in fewer interventions compared to immediate drainage and should be the preferred approach for treating infected necrotizing pancreatitis. Additionally, no significant differences were observed in pancreatic function and long-term quality of life between the two groups. The study suggests that antibiotic treatment may be effective for many patients, reducing the need for invasive interventions.

2.2 Transgastric endoscopic drainage

Endoscopic procedures are especially beneficial for treating central pancreatic collections and pancreatic necrosis (**Figure 2**). Necrosis can occur in the head, body, or tail of the pancreas and can be approached endoscopically either through the stomach (transgastrically) or the duodenum (transduodenally), depending on the size and positioning of the necrotic area relative to these structures. The step-up approach, whether performed surgically or endoscopically, has been evaluated in two major randomized studies. In the TENSION trial [11], it was found that the endoscopic step-up approach did not show superiority over surgery in terms of major complications or mortality; however, the endoscopic group had fewer pancreatic fistulas and a shorter length of hospital stay. Similarly, the MISER trial [14] demonstrated that an endoscopic transluminal approach for infected necrotizing pancreatitis led to fewer complications, reduced costs, and improved quality of life when compared to minimally invasive surgery.

The timing for drainage in patients with walled-off necrosis (WON) remains an area of active research. Traditionally, waiting 4 weeks for necrotic tissue to mature and wall off has been standard practice, influenced by surgical guidelines. Newer evidence, however, supports initiating endoscopic step-up therapy before the four-week mark when appropriate, and this approach has been associated with lower mortality when patients are managed in this manner [15]. As a result, endoscopic management has become the

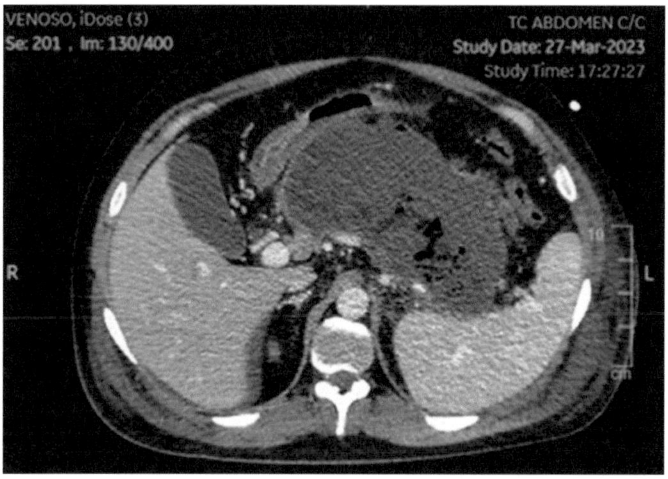

Figure 2.
Abdominal CT scan showing a large retrogastric collection, amenable to transgastric drainage.

recommended approach for infected necrotizing pancreatitis in recent years [16–20]. Large-bore percutaneous drainage, combined with either standard or therapeutic endoscopy, allows for direct removal of necrotic tissue, promoting quicker debridement and less invasive procedures. Nonetheless, this method may not be suitable for all patients, as its effectiveness depends on factors like the anatomical location of necrosis, the availability of specialized equipment, and the expertise of the medical center.

In cases where necrotic collections are large or extend into the pelvic or paracolic regions, a combined approach involving both endoscopic transluminal and percutaneous drainage (dual-modality drainage) may be necessary. Currently, metal stents are most commonly used for endoscopic drainage between the stomach and infected collections. Although originally developed in 2011, these stents have since been replaced by plastic stents, which have a wider lumen that

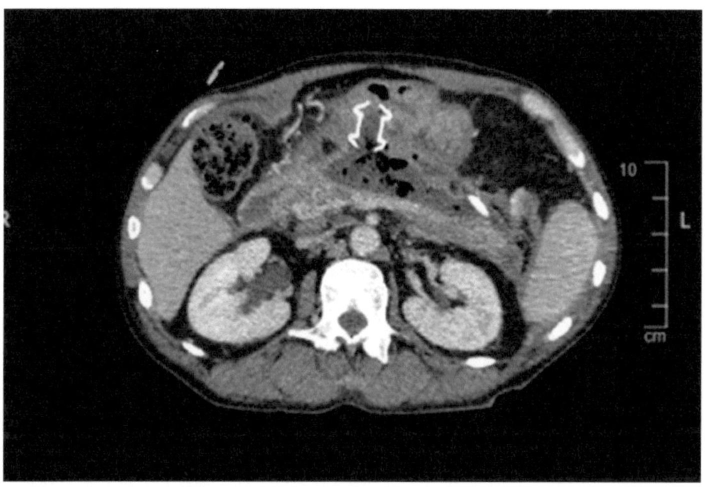

Figure 3.
Abdominal CT image demonstrating transgastric drainage of an acute necrotic collection.

facilitates better drainage and improves access for transluminal necrosectomy. A randomized trial comparing metal and plastic stents (**Figure 3**) for drainage in infected pancreatic necrosis found no significant differences in hospital stay length, readmissions, or procedure numbers [21]. However, metal stents were more costly and associated with complications like stent migration. Therefore, current guidelines [21, 22] recommend the use of either metallic stents or double-pigtail plastic stents for endoscopic drainage, with stent removal typically occurring after 4 weeks to minimize risks.

3. Phased approach in the surgical treatment of necrotizing pancreatitis

For a long time, surgical resections with pancreatic were the first treatment option for acute necrotizing pancreatitis as a desperate measure to change the lethal course of the disease and its high mortality. Over time, scientific evidence showed that despite the aggressiveness of such management, mortality and morbidity rates remained high. This causes a change in the handling towards a more conservative and personalized form creating specific indications for surgical treatment.

3.1 Surgery is needed in the first hours of admission for severe necrotizing pancreatitis

In the early phase of pancreatitis, pancreas surgery is not usually performed, although many visceral complications may require urgent surgery: intestinal necrosis, hemorrhage, and abdominal compartment syndrome.

3.1.1 Abdominal compartment syndrome (ACS)

Abdominal Compartment Syndrome (ACS) is an uncommon but severe complication of acute pancreatitis. Increased intra-abdominal pressure (IAP), or high intra-abdominal pressure (HIAP), refers to the pathological, sustained, or recurrent rise in IAP above 12 mmHg. ACS is characterized by a persistent increase in IAP exceeding 20 mmHg, accompanied by the onset of organ failure. When conservative measures fail, and IAP remains above 25 mmHg with associated organ dysfunction or failure, emergency abdominal surgical decompression is warranted. Common conservative interventions include nasogastric tubes, rectal tubes, epidural catheters for pain management, and percutaneous intra-abdominal catheters. Although percutaneous drainage of pancreatic ascites can temporarily reduce IAP in some instances, surgical decompression [23] remains the definitive approach to relieve HIAP and restore organ function, particularly in the pulmonary, cardiovascular, and renal systems. Laparotomy may be necessary for patients with abdominal hypertension, although conservative management is the preferred approach at present. The DECOMPRESS [24] study aims to assess whether decompressive laparotomy with temporary abdominal closure reduces mortality and major morbidity compared to percutaneous abdominal catheter placement in ACS patients.

There are three primary surgical options for decompression in patients without an incision. The long vertical midline incision is the most employed technique, shown to effectively reduce IAP. It is quick and simple to perform; however, it carries a risk of intestinal fistula formation and often results in failure to close the fascia, necessitating complex reconstructive surgery at a later stage [25]. Transverse laparostomy

[26] offers a promising alternative, with isolated reports demonstrating its efficacy in lowering IAP and improving access to pancreatic tissue for necrosectomy when necessary. Although it requires slightly more time to perform than a midline laparostomy, the same principles for managing the open abdomen apply.

A third option, used primarily in severe acute pancreatitis (SAP), is the subcutaneous linea alba fasciotomy [27], where the fascia is incised through three small skin incisions, leaving the skin and peritoneum intact. However, this approach invariably results in a ventral hernia that will require subsequent repair.

Various temporary abdominal closure (TAC) methods have been proposed for managing an open abdomen [28]. The ideal method should be simple to implement and remove, provide quick access for subsequent surgical procedures, facilitate drainage of abdominal secretions, support primary closure, and result in acceptable morbidity and mortality rates. One of the most straightforward and cost-effective approaches is simply approximating the skin with a continuous running suture or using towel clips. Another common method is the plastic silo, often referred to as the Bogotá bag (**Figure 4**), which involves a non-adherent plastic sheet, typically derived from a sterile 3-liter urology irrigation bag, being sutured between the fascial edges or over the skin.

In 1995, Barker and his team introduced the vacuum pack technique [8], where a perforated plastic sheet is placed over the viscera, with sterile surgical towels filling the wound and a drain attached to continuous negative pressure. This system was further refined with the introduction of a polyurethane sponge and an adjustable pump (**Figure 5**), allowing for precise control of negative pressure. This modification has several benefits, including fewer dressing changes, improved vascularization of the wound, reduced bacterial growth, and prolonged opportunities for definitive closure of the fascia.

A further advancement involved the use of a spider-like sponge, which not only enhances fluid drainage but also improves wound contraction. This technique has been associated with a primary fascial closure rate of 89% [29, 30]. Acosta, in turn, described a combined approach that utilized the VAC system alongside a polypropylene mesh placed along the fascial edges to maintain traction, leading to a fascial closure rate of 76.6% [31]. While many modifications of these techniques have been

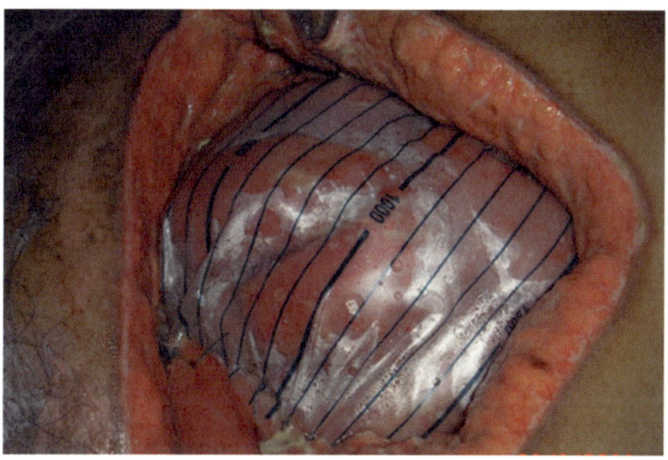

Figure 4.
Temporary closure of abdominal wall by means of bogota bag is shown.

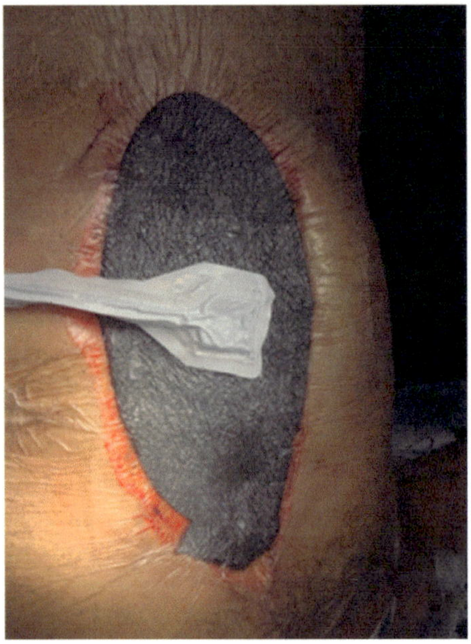

Figure 5.
Temporary open abdomen closure system type VAC is shown.

documented, a standardized approach for managing patients with an open abdomen remains elusive.

3.1.2 Visceral complications: Intestinal necrosis and perforations

The anatomical relationships between the large intestine and the pancreas (**Figure 6**) play a significant role in the development and localization of related lesions. Enzymatic inflammation and ischemic processes are frequently implicated

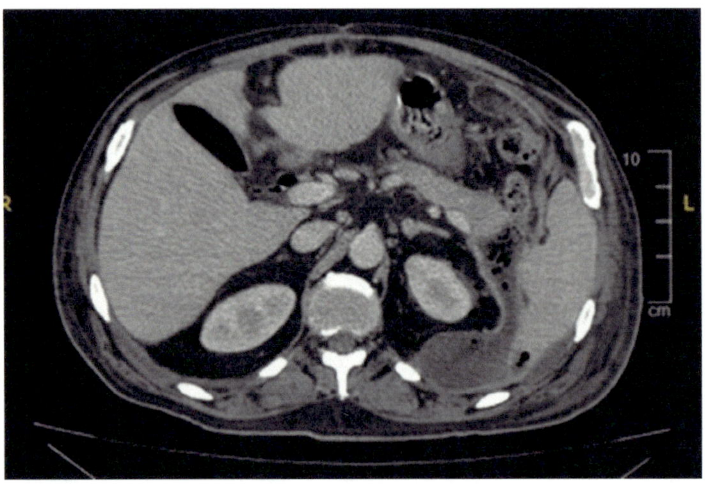

Figure 6.
Abdominal CT scan revealing a collection in the left flank with air, secondary to perforation of the splenic flexure of the colon, due to its proximity to the pancreatic tail.

in most theoretical models. Acute necrotizing pancreatitis can lead to a range of complications, with colonic perforation being a relatively rare occurrence [32]. The site of perforation can involve nearly any segment of the colon, although it is most seen at the splenic flexure [33, 34]. In addition to colonic perforation, other instances of perforations within the intestinal tract, such as those in the duodenum [35], have been documented, albeit infrequently. In some cases, dual perforations involving both the colon and duodenum have been reported, and there are instances of concomitant gastric and colonic perforations in the same patient.

In the presence of intestinal ischemia or perforation of hollow viscera, laparotomy is essential (**Figures** 7 and **8**). Many patients require ostomies, multiple surgical interventions, and the application of open abdominal techniques.

3.1.3 Hemorrhage

The most frequent cause of hemorrhage in acute pancreatitis is the formation of arterial pseudoaneurysms. An arterial pseudoaneurysm, also known as a false aneurysm, is a collection of blood that forms due to partial disruption of the arterial wall, resulting in hemorrhage contained within a sac formed by perivascular tissue or surrounding structures, rather than by the layers of the arterial wall itself. The development of arterial pseudoaneurysms in the context of pancreatitis is a rare yet serious complication (**Figure 9**) [36]. A ruptured pseudoaneurysm leading to bleeding into the gastrointestinal tract, pancreatic duct, retroperitoneum, or peritoneal cavity constitutes one of the most rapidly fatal complications associated with pancreatitis. Visceral arteries exposed to proteolytic pancreatic enzymes often exhibit localized arteritis and damage to the vessel wall, potentially resulting in pseudoaneurysm formation or hemorrhage into an existing pseudocyst. Arterial complications in pancreatitis are observed in approximately 4–10% of patients, with an untreated mortality rate reaching 90%.

Management options include operative treatment and interventional procedures, either used alone or as a temporizing measure before a definitive operation. Coil embolization should be the first approach, provided the patient is hemodynamically

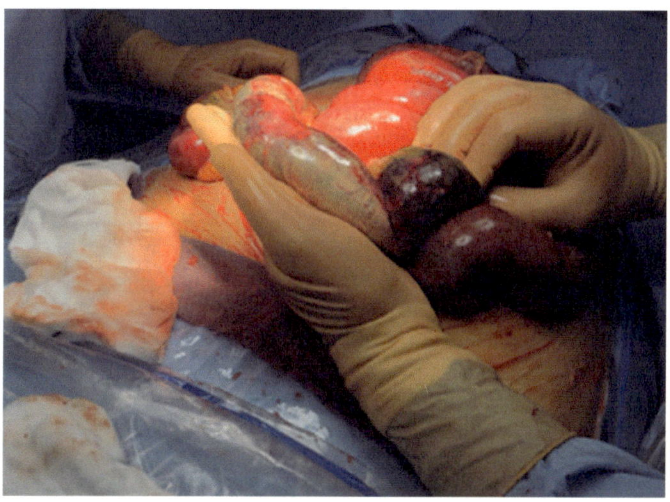

Figure 7.
Ischemic small intestine segment is shown by enzymatic reaction of acute pancreatitis.

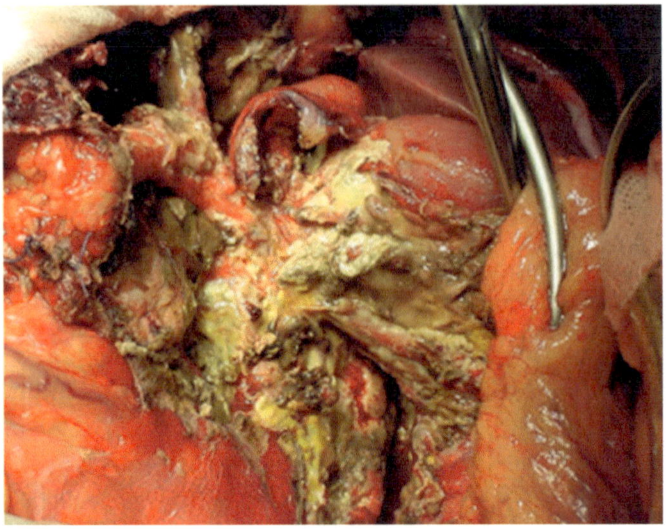

Figure 8.
Is shown enzymatic reaction of pancreatitis that has completely digested the vessels of the meso colon.

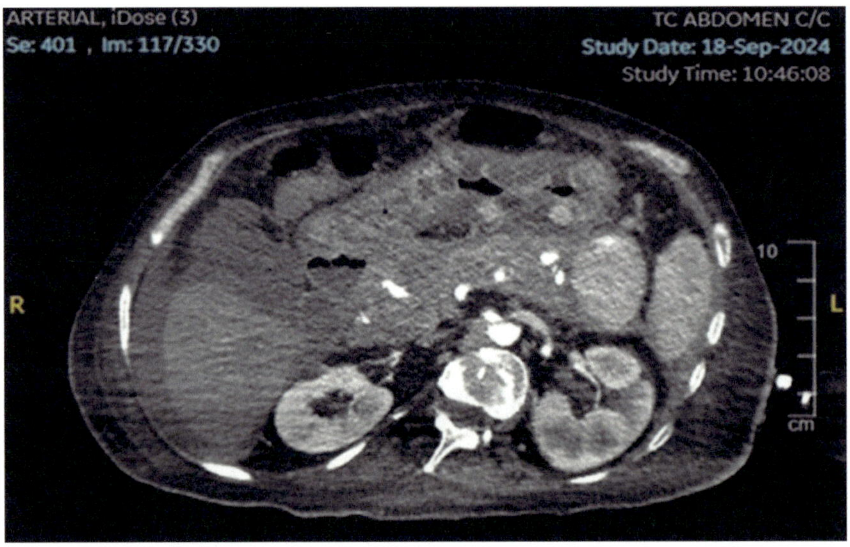

Figure 9.
Abdominal CT scan showing a large pseudosplenic artery aneurysm in the context of necrotizing pancreatitis.

stable (**Figure 10**). If embolization proves successful, no further intervention may be necessary. However, failure of embolization warrants surgical intervention. If the patient's overall condition and the inflammatory state of the pancreas permit, partial pancreatectomy is generally preferred over vessel ligation.

3.2 Surgical necrosectomy

Surgical debridement should be considered for patients with infected pancreatic necrosis or for those with sterile necrosis who develop persistent organ dysfunction.

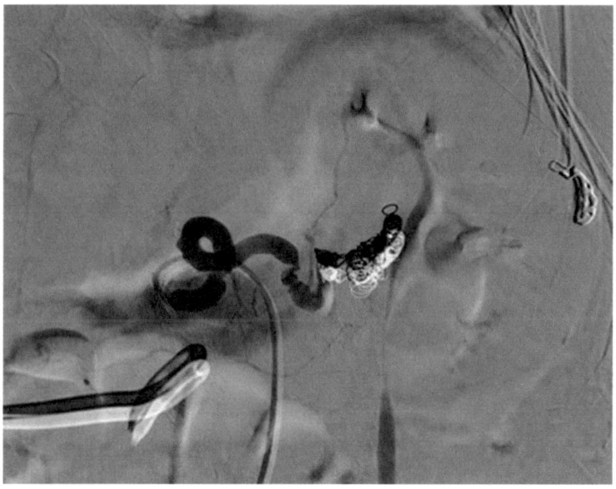

Figure 10.
Aortografía image with pseudoaneurysm of splenic artery embolized by metal coils.

While percutaneous or endoscopic drainage alone may lead to improvement in 23–47% of cases, surgery is often necessary for patients with continuing disease [7, 37, 38]. The primary objectives of debridement are to eliminate the infection source, reduce necrotic tissue, and limit the inflammatory response in critically ill patients. In recent years, there has been a shift towards less invasive techniques. Available surgical options include VARD (step-up approach), laparoscopic or open transgastric debridement, and traditional open debridement. Each approach offers its own set of benefits and challenges, which should be assessed individually for each patient.

The timing of the procedure plays a critical role in patient outcomes [12]. Performing surgery early in the course of acute pancreatitis—before the patient enters the subacute phase (within 2–4 weeks of onset)—has been linked to higher mortality rates compared to waiting for the disease to stabilize. Ultimately, the goal of surgical debridement is to manage infection, alleviate necrotic tissue, and minimize the inflammatory response to the procedure.

3.2.1 Video-assisted retroperitoneal debridement (VARD) in infected necrotizing pancreatitis

How we have seen so far: The step-up approach includes percutaneous drainage combined with other minimally invasive techniques such as endoscopic necrosectomy or video-assisted retroperitoneal debridement (VARD).

Several techniques have been described, including video-assisted retroperitoneal access, which has been associated with significantly lower rates of abdominal complications compared to more traditional methods. This technique utilizes radiological drainage as a guide to the collection, with an emphasis on positioning the drainage on the left side whenever possible. The tract formed by the anterior drain is then used to access the retroperitoneal space for intracavitary video-assisted necrosectomy (**Figure 11**). A 15 mm optical trocar, equipped with a zero-degree, 5 mm or 10 mm scope, is used. The trocar is advanced into the retroperitoneum, following the path of the drain, which remains in place. When pancreatic necrosis is encountered and resistance to advancing the trocar is lost, this indicates entry into the necrotic cavity. Traditional laparoscopic instruments are then used under direct visualization (**Figure 12**). Cavity insufflation may

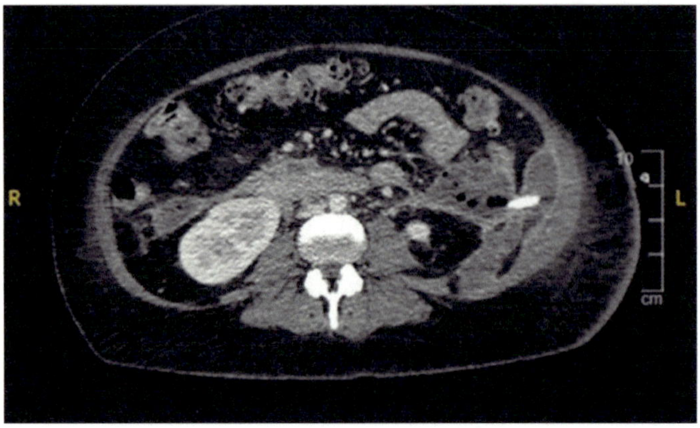

Figure 11.
Abdominal CT scan image showing percutaneous drainage within the necrotic collection, which serves as a guide for performing the VARD procedure.

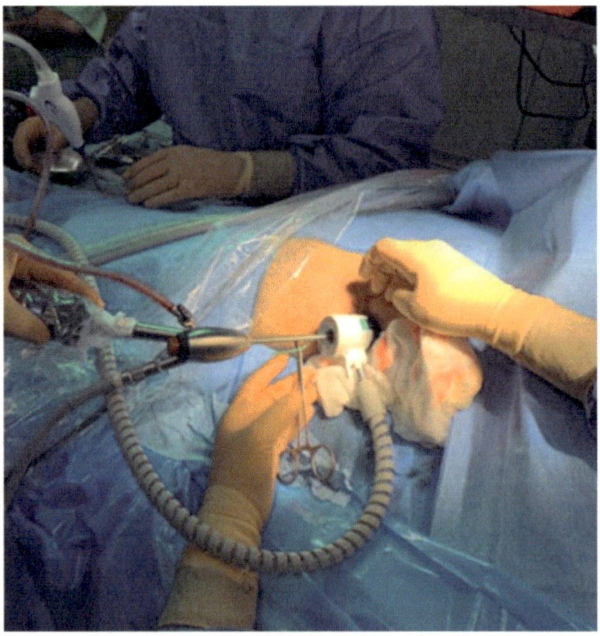

Figure 12.
Guided by left retroperitoneal percutaneous drainage, we can access the area using a minimally invasive approach. A laparoscopic trocar was observed through which we introduced the camera, suction device, and laparoscopic forcep.

be employed during debridement but is typically intermittent, mainly used for inspection. Laparoscopic forceps are inserted through the trocar alongside the scope and used to gently debride the necrotic pancreatic tissue. Direct observation should be maintained during the debridement whenever possible. Once satisfactory debridement is achieved, a Silastic® drain is placed in the cavity (**Figure 13**). This drain is anchored to the skin with a nonabsorbable suture to prevent displacement. Irrigation should be initiated as soon as possible to avoid drain occlusion and ensure proper drainage. Well-positioned drains allow effective washing, and the procedure may be repeated if necessary to further remove infected pancreatic necrosis.

It is important to note that the VARD approach is more effective for treating infected pancreatic necrosis located centrally or extending into the left paracolic gutter. Accessing necrosis located to the right of the mesenteric vessels is more challenging, although our team has successfully performed the procedure on right-sided collections with increased complexity and caution required (**Figure 14**) (is explained in detail in **Figure C1** of Annex C).

The Dutch Pancreatitis Study Group compared the step-up approach with open necrosectomy in a prospective randomized multicenter trial (PANTER) [7] and found equivalent mortality rates between the two approaches. However, the open necrosectomy group had a higher incidence of multiple-organ failure (40 vs. 12%). The VARD technique is particularly suitable for patients with centrally distributed necrosis [40] extending into the left paracolic gutter.

The VARD technique is not without complications. VARD is accompanied with the risk of vascular injury, external pancreatico-cutaneous, or enterocutaneous fistulae. Some authors have included fluorescence imaging with indocyanine green (ICG) during VARD [41]. This modified technique—ICG-guided video-assisted retroperitoneal debridement (VARD)—offers enhanced visualization of tissue planes during necrosectomy, potentially reducing the risk of vascular or enteric injury. By delineating viable and necrotic tissues more clearly, ICG guidance may enable surgeons to perform debridement with greater precision and safety in the management of severe acute necrotizing pancreatitis.

3.2.2 Surgical transgastric debridement

The concept is analogous to endoscopic transgastric drainage and can be performed either via an open or laparoscopic approach. A gastrostomy is made on the anterior wall of the stomach to access its posterior aspect and subsequently the infected cavity. This approach is particularly beneficial for central collections that do not extend to the flanks (**Figure 15**). Studies with small sample sizes [42–44] have demonstrated the efficacy of the technique, showing low morbidity rates.

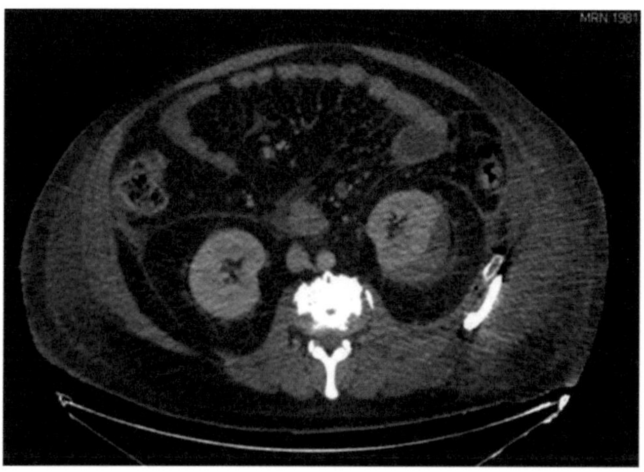

Figure 13.
Image of CT scan that objective retroperitoneal necrotic collection with drainage inside placed by laparoscopic retroperitoneal access.

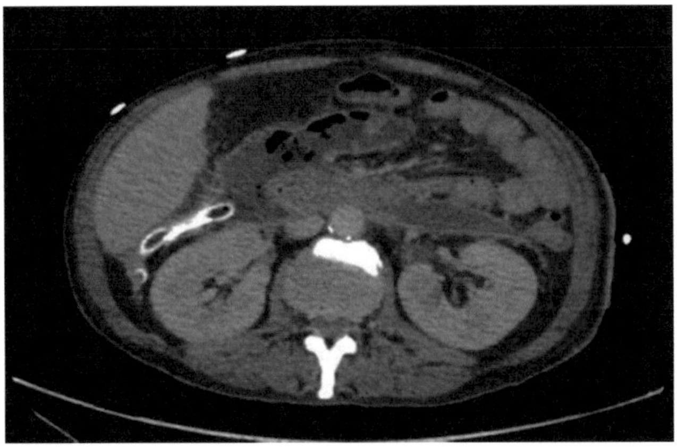

Figure 14.
CT scan demonstrating surgical drainage on the right flank via laparoscopic retroperitoneal access.

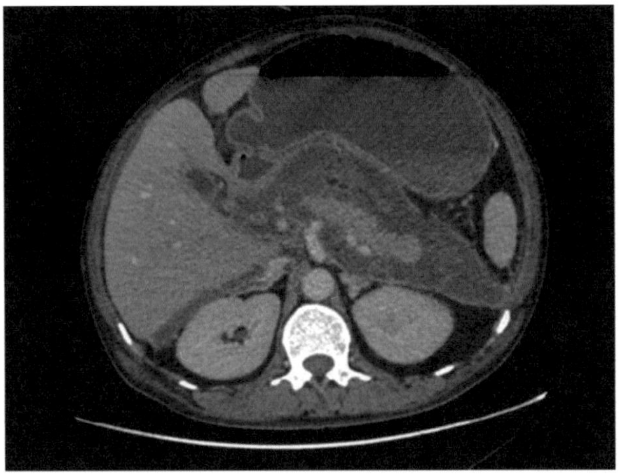

Figure 15.
CT scan image showing collection near the gastric posterior wall that would allow a transgastic approach.

Additionally, simultaneous cholecystectomy can be performed in patients with biliary pancreatitis. In cases of disconnected pancreatic duct syndrome, the relatively large size of the cystgastrostomy offers the potential advantage of providing a durable route for enteric drainage of a pancreatic fistula.

A clinical trial [45] published in 2020 compared endoscopic and laparoscopic transgastric debridement, concluding that both techniques exhibit similar efficacy for internal drainage of appropriate pancreatic fluid collections with less than 30% debris. The choice of procedure should be based on available expertise and tailored to the individual characteristics of each case.

A current randomized controlled trial [46] compared transperitoneal laparoscopic drainage with endoscopic drainage, using either lumen-apposing metal stents (LAMS) or plastic stents, depending on the amount of necrotic tissue. The trial found that laparoscopic drainage was not superior to endoscopic transmural drainage with stent placement, but the hospital stay was shorter with the endoscopic approach.

Our technique involves a standard laparoscopic approach with the patient in the French position. An optical umbilical trocar is inserted, along with two paraumbilical trocars of 11 or 12 mm. The anterior surface of the stomach is incised, and endoscopic drainage is performed if necessary. Intraoperative ultrasound may be used for guidance. The drainage hole is enlarged, and the necrotic tissue is removed. The procedure then proceeds with irrigation, drainage, and necrosectomy. Finally, the anterior stomach wall is closed with a 3/0 barbed suture, and a nasogastric tube is placed near the transgastric communication (**Figure 16**).

3.2.3 Open surgical necrosectomy

If the methods fail to control the infectious process, and the patient continues to deteriorate despite adequate drainage, including minimally invasive techniques, an open surgical approach should be considered. The mortality rate for patients with infected pancreatic necrosis exceeds 30%. As previously mentioned, delaying surgery as long as possible tends to be more beneficial for the patient in terms of reducing both mortality and morbidity. Early surgical intervention [35, 36], particularly in cases of sterile necrosis, has been associated with a significant increase in mortality. Thus, these surgical techniques are typically reserved for situations where all other options have proven ineffective.

A retrospective study conducted at Helsinki University Hospital [47], which analyzed 109 patients who underwent open necrosectomy over a 12-year period, revealed that the mortality rate was 10.6% when necrosectomy was delayed for 4 weeks following the onset of symptoms. Risk factors for 90-day mortality included age over 60, preexisting comorbidities, necrosectomy within 4 weeks, multiorgan failure, elevated white blood cell count, and prolonged organ failure or deterioration, which necessitated necrosectomy. In contrast, when fewer risk factors were present, open necrosectomy did not lead to increased mortality.

Another study [48] explored an innovative approach combining open necrosectomy with continuous positive drainage and prophylactic ileostomy for managing late-stage infected pancreatic necrosis. This strategy resulted in faster recovery of

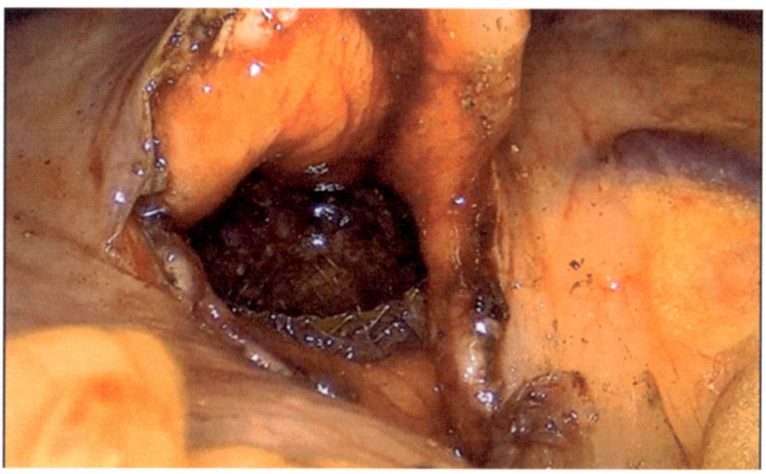

Figure 16.
Intraoperative image by laparoscopic approach, anterior face opening with transgastric endoscopic drainage exposure.

organ function, fewer colonic complications, shorter hospital stays, and reduced costs when compared to other groups.

Open surgical debridement continues to play a critical role in the management of pancreatic necrosis. A common surgical approach involves an upper transverse subcostal laparotomy, providing optimal exposure to the necrotic areas. However, midline laparotomy may be selectively employed, particularly in patients who have undergone laparostomy for abdominal compartment syndrome or when bowel resection is anticipated.

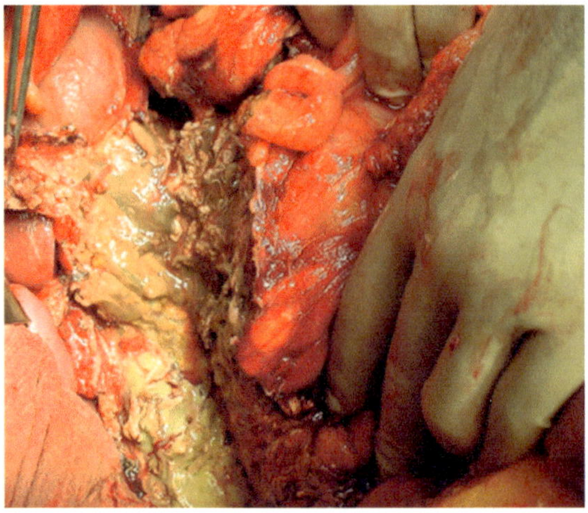

Figure 17.
Surgical image following the opening of the transcavity in epiploic pancreatic necrosis and peripancreatic necrosis.

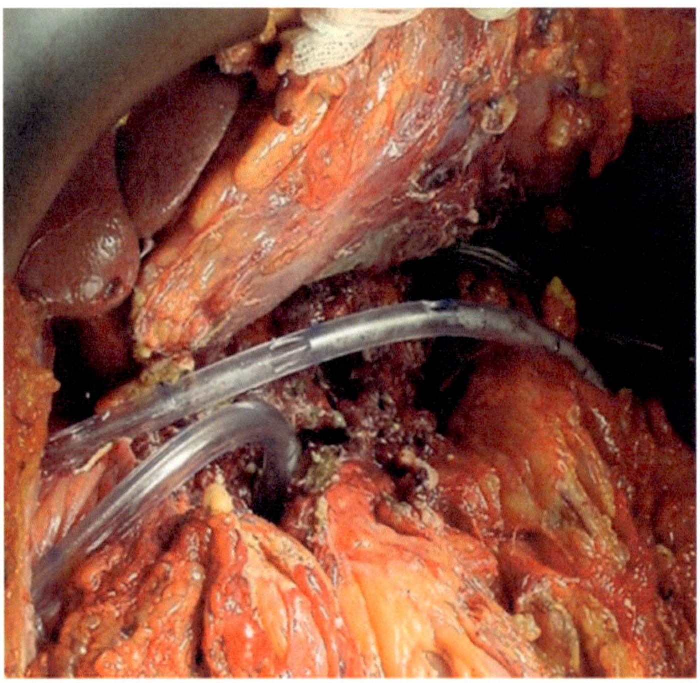

Figure 18.
Following the open necrosectomy, large-bore drains are placed for postoperative drainage.

The necrosis is typically approached through the gastrocolic ligament. Necrosectomy is performed using blunt manual dissection, with careful suction to minimize trauma to surrounding vital tissues (**Figure 17**). Microbiological samples from necrotic tissue are routinely collected during the procedure. In cases of biliary pancreatitis, cholecystectomy can be performed concurrently. Large-bore drains are left in place postoperatively for lavage and to manage potential fistulas, if needed (**Figure 18**).

While several open necrosectomy techniques have been described, none have been definitively shown to be superior, largely due to the absence of randomized trials. For localized necrosis, necrosectomy with closure of the abdominal wall may be performed. Most patients will require multiple necrosectomies and external scrubbing in the intensive care unit. The use of open abdomen techniques significantly increases patient morbidity [31]. In cases where abdominal closure is not possible or in instances of abdominal compartment syndrome, Vacuum Assisted Closure therapy is employed as a temporary measure. Open debridement is indicated for patients with extensive necrosis spread diffusely throughout the abdomen, particularly in those who do not respond to staged interventions.

Appendix A

Decision tree outlining the acute- and late-phase management of patients with severe acute pancreatitis and necrosis, including a multidisciplinary approach to drainage and/or debridement when required (**Figure A1**) [13].

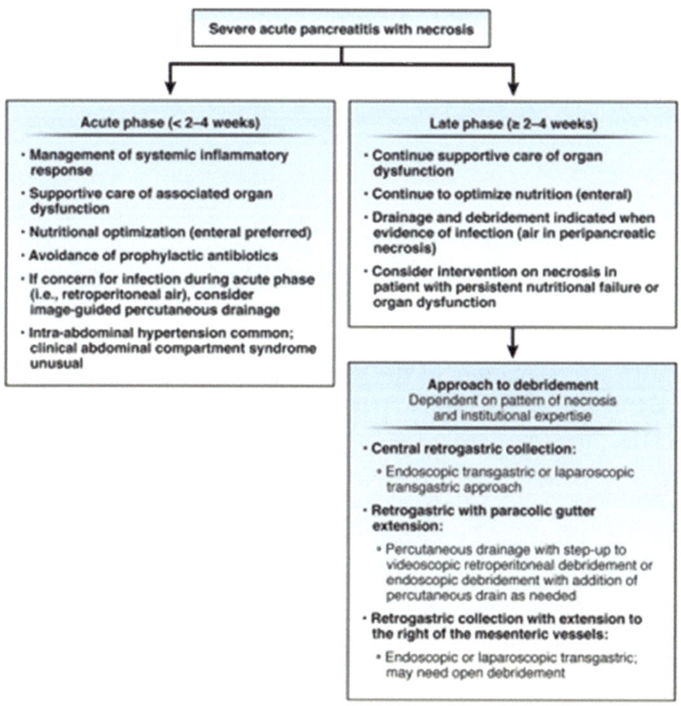

Figure A1.
Clinical decision algorithm detailing the acute and late-phase management of severe acute pancreatitis with necrosis, emphasizing a multidisciplinary approach to interventional drainage and/or surgical debridement as clinically indicated [49].

Appendix B

Classification of acute pancreatitis and associated fluid collections. Based on international consensus according to the Acute Pancreatitis Classification Working Group (revised Atlanta criteria). From Trikudanathan et al. (**Figure B1**) [13, 15].

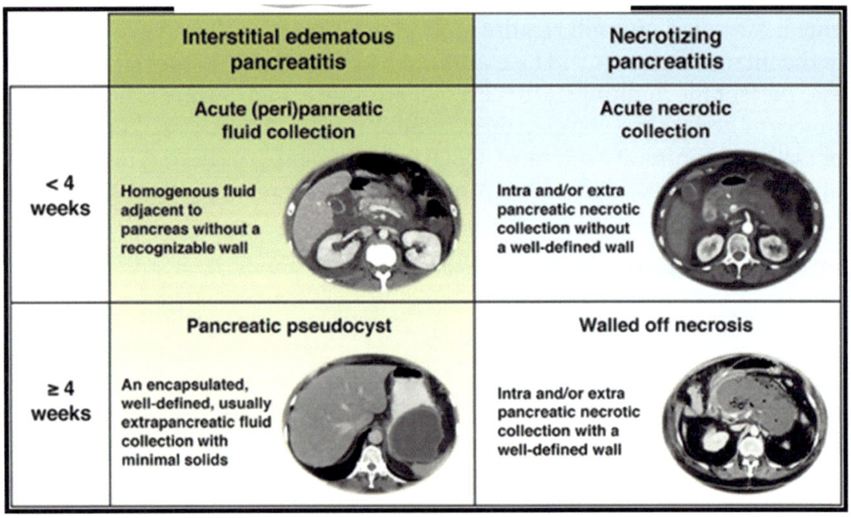

Figure B1.
Classification of acute pancreatitis and related fluid collections, based on the international consensus established by the Acute Pancreatitis Classification Working Group (revised Atlanta criteria) [49].

Appendix C

Video-assisted retroperitoneal debridement (VARD) and laparoscopic-assisted pancreatic necrosectomy (LAPN)operative techniques(a). Pancreatic necrosum with a percutaneous drain in place, the initial component of step-up approach for necrotizing pancreatitis (b). Depiction of the VARD operative approach, utilizing a 5cm incision; (c). Depiction of the LAPN operative approach, utilizing a 12 mm trocar (**Figure C1**) [41].

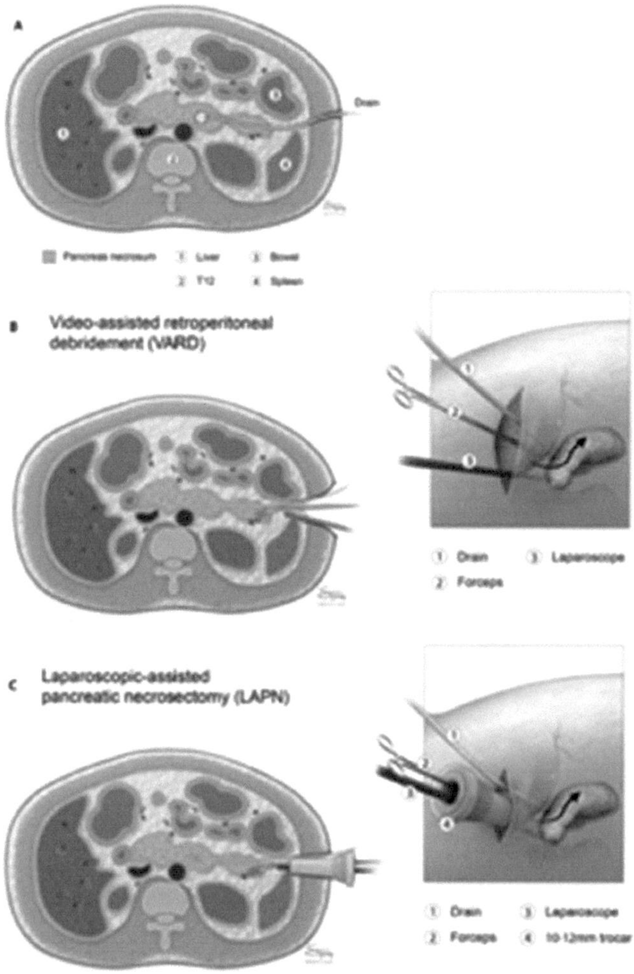

Figure C1.
Operative techniques for video-assisted retroperitoneal debridement (VARD) and laparoscopic-assisted pancreatic necrosectomy (LAPN): (a) Pancreatic necrosis with a percutaneous drain in place, representing the initial step of the step-up approach for necrotizing pancreatitis; (b) illustration of the VARD technique, performed through a 5 cm incision; (c) illustration of the LAPN technique, utilizing a 12 mm trocar [39].

Author details

Betsabé Reyes Correa*, Javier Padilla Quintana and Alicia Goya Pacheco
Virgen de La Candelaria University Hospital, Spain

*Address all correspondence to: bereyes86@hotmail.com

References

[1] Leppäniemi A, Tolonen M, Gamberini ATE, et al. 2019 WSES guidelines for the management of severe acute pancreatitis. World Journal of Emergency Surgery. 2019;**14**:27

[2] Banks PA, Freeman ML. Practice guide- lines in acute pancreatitis. The American Journal of Gastroenterology. 2006;**101**:2379-2400

[3] Whitcomb DC. Acute pancreatitis. The New England Journal of Medicine. 2006;**354**:2142-2150

[4] Uhl W, Warshaw A, Imrie C, et al. IAP guidelines for the surgical management of acute pancreatitis. Pancreatology. 2002;**2**:565-573

[5] Nathens AB, Curtis JR, Beale RJ, et al. Management of the critically ill patient with severe acute pancreatitis. Critical Care Medicine. 2004;**32**:2524-2536

[6] Forsmark CE, Baillie J, AGA Institute Clinical Practice and Economics Committee, AGA Institute Governing Board. AGA Institute technical review on acute pancreatitis. Gastroenterology. 2007;**132**:2022-2044

[7] van Santvoort HC, Besselink MG, Bakker OJ, et al. For the Dutch pancreatitis study group. A step-up approach or open Necrosectomy for necrotizing pancreatitis. The New England Journal of Medicine. 2010;**362**:1491-1502

[8] van Grinsven J, van Brunschot S, Bakker OJ, et al. Diagnostic strategy and timing of intervention in infected necrotizing pancreatitis: An international expert survey and case vignette study. HPB: The Official Journal of the International Hepato Pancreato Biliary Association. 2016;**18**:49-56

[9] Hollemans RA, Bakker OJ, Boermeester MA, Bollen TL, Bosscha K, Bruno MJ, et al. Superiority of step-up approach vs open Necrosectomy in long-term follow-up of patients with necrotizing pancreatitis. Gastroenterology. 2019;**156**(4):1016-1026. DOI: 10.1053/j.gastro.2018.10.045. Epub 2018 Nov 2

[10] van Santvoort HC, Bakker OJ, Bollen TL, et al. A conservative and minimally invasive approach to necrotizing pancreatitis improves outcome. Gastroenterology. 2011;**141**:1254-1263

[11] van Brunschot S, van Grinsven J, van Santvoort HC, et al. Endoscopic or surgical step-up approach for infected necrotising pancreatitis: A multicentre randomised trial. Lancet. 2018;**391**:51-58

[12] Baron TH, DiMaio CJ, Wang AY, Morgan KA. American Gastroenterological Association clinical practice update: Management of pancreatic necrosis. Gastroenterology. 2020;**158**:67-75

[13] Van Veldhuisen CL, Sissingh NJ, Boxhoorn L, van Dijk SM, van Grinsven J, Verdonk RC, et al. Long-term outcome of immediate versus postponed intervention in patients with infected necrotizing pancreatitis (POINTER): Multicenter randomized trial. Annals of Surgery. 2024;**279**(4):671-678. DOI: 10.1097/SLA.0000000000006001. Epub 2023 Jul 17

[14] Bang JY, Arnoletti JY, Holt JP, et al. An endoscopic transluminal approach, compared to minimally invasive surgery,

reduces complications and costs for patients with necrotizing pancreatitis. Gastroenterology. 2019;**156**:1027-1040

[15] Trikudanathan G, Tawfik P, Amateau SK, et al. Early (<4 weeks) versus standard (≥4 weeks) endoscopically centered step-up interventions for necrotizing pancreatitis. The American Journal of Gastroenterology. 2018;**113**:1550-1558

[16] Nemoto Y, Attam R, Arain MA, et al. Interventions for walled off necrosis using an algorithm based endoscopic step-up approach: Outcomes in a large cohort of patients. Pancreatology. 2017;**17**:663-668

[17] Ross AS, Irani S, Gan SI, et al. Dual-modality drainage of infected and symptomatic walled-off pancreatic necrosis: Long-term clinical outcomes. Gastrointestinal Endoscopy. 2014;**79**:929-935

[18] Ross A, Gluck M, Irani S, et al. Combined endoscopic and percutaneous drainage of organized pancreatic necrosis. Gastrointestinal Endoscopy. 2010;**71**:79-84

[19] Gluck M, Ross A, Irani S, et al. Dual modality drainage for symptomatic walled-off pancreatic necrosis reduces length of hospitalization, radiological procedures, and number of endoscopies compared to standard percutaneous drainage. Journal of Gastrointestinal Surgery. 2012;**16**:248-257

[20] Sahar N, Kozarek R, Kanji ZS, et al. Do lumen-apposing metal stents (LAMS) improve treatment outcomes of walled-off pancreatic necrosis over plastic stents using dual-modality drainage? Endoscopy International Open. 2017;**5**:E1052-E1059

[21] Bang JY, Navaneethan U, Hasan MK, Sutton B, Hawes R, Varadarajulu S. Nonsuperiority of lumen-apposing metal stents over plastic stents for drainage of walled-off necrosis in a randomised trial. Gut. 2019;**68**:1200-1209

[22] Arvanitakis M, Dumonceau J-M, Albert J, et al. Endoscopic management of acute necrotizing pancreatitis: European Society of Gastrointestinal Endoscopy (ESGE) evidence-based multidisciplinary guidelines. Endoscopy. 2018;**50**:524-546

[23] Robin-Lersundi A, Abella Álvarez A, Cruz Cidoncha A, López-Monclús J, Gordo Vidal F, García-Ureña MA. Pancreatitis aguda grave y síndrome compartimental abdominal: tratamiento mediante laparotomía descompresiva y cierre abdominal temporal con malla de politetrafluoroetileno expandido. Medicina Intensiva. 2013;**37**(4):301-302. DOI: 10.1016/j.medin.2012.08.011

[24] Radenkovic DV, Bajec D, Ivancevic N, Bumbasirevic V, Milic N, Jeremic V, et al. Decompressive laparotomy with temporary abdominal closure versus percutaneous puncture with placement of abdominal catheter in patients with abdominal compartment syndrome during acute pancreatitis: Background and design of multicenter, randomised, controlled study. BMC Surgery. 2010;**10**:22. DOI: 10.1186/1471-2482-10-22

[25] De Waele JJ, Hoste EAJ, Malbrain MLNG. Decompressive laparotomy for abdominal compartment syndrome– A critical analysis. Critical Care. 2006;**10**:R51

[26] Leppäniemi A, Mentula P, Hienonen P, Kemppainen E. Transverse laparostomy is feasible and effective in the treatment of abdominal compartment syndrome in severe acute pancreatitis. World Journal of Emergency Surgery : WJES. 2008;**3**:6

[27] Leppäniemi AK, Hienonen PA, Siren JE, Kuitunen AH, Lindström OK, Kemppainen EA. Treatment of abdominal compartment syndrome with subcutaneous anterior abdominal fasciotomy in severe acute pancreatitis. World Journal of Surgery. 2006;**30**:1922-1924

[28] Coccolini F, Biffl W, Catena F, Ceresoli M, Chiara O, Cimbanassi S, et al. The open abdomen, indications, management and definitive closure. World Journal of Emergency Surgery: WJES. 2015;**10**:32. DOI: 10.1186/s13017-015-0026-5

[29] Lindstedt S, Malmsjö M, Hlebowicz J, Ingemansson R. Comparative study of the microvascular blood flow in the intestinal wall, wound contraction and fluid evacuation during negative pressure wound therapy in laparostomy using the V.A.C. Abdominal dressing and the ABTheraopen abdomen negative pressure therapy system. International Wound Journal. 2013;**12**:83-88. DOI: 10.1111/iwj.12056

[30] Frazee RC, Abernathy SW, Jupiter DC, Hendricks JC, Davis M, Regner JL, et al. Are commercial negative pressure systems worth the cost in open abdomen management? Journal of the American College of Surgeons. 2013;**216**(4):730-733

[31] Petersson U, Acosta S, Björck M. Vacuum-assisted wound closure and mesh-mediated fascial traction–a novel technique for late closure of the open abdomen. World Journal of Surgery. 2007;**31**(11):2133-2137

[32] Calleja SMC, Urien Blázquez LM. Perforación colónica, una rara complicación de pancreatitis aguda necrotizante. Anales de Medicina Interna (Madrid) [Internet]. 2006;**23**(5):235-237

[33] Chao HG, Chung JP, Yum JS, Park HJ, Lee KS, Chon CY, et al. Spontaneous bowel perforation during the course of acute pancreatitis, a case report. Yonsei Medical Journal. 1996;**37**:158-164

[34] Yang WG, Wang SS, Lee FY, Chao Y, Chen CC, Chang FY, et al. Severe colonic complications in acute pancreatitis. Zhonghua Yi Xue Za Zhi. 1998;**61**:59-64

[35] Sakorafas GH, Tsiotos GG, Sarr MG. Experience with duodenal necrosis. A rare complication of acute necrotizing pancreatitis. International Journal of Pancreatology. 1999;**25**:147-149

[36] Bergert H, Hinterseher I, Kersting S, Leonhardt J, Bloomenthal A, Saeger HD. Management and outcome of hemorrhage due to arterial pseudoaneurysms in pancreatitis. Surgery. 2005;**137**(3):323-328. DOI: 10.1016/j.surg.2004.10.009

[37] Freeny PC, Hauptmann E, Althaus SJ, et al. Percuta- neous CT-guided catheter drainage of infected acute necrotizing pancreatitis: Techniques and results. AJR. American Journal of Roentgenology. 1998;**170**:969-975

[38] Horvath K, Freeny P, Escallon J, et al. Safety and efficacy of video-assisted retroperitoneal debridement for infected pancreatic collections: A multicenter, prospective, single-arm phase 2 study. Archives of Surgery. 2010;**145**:817-825

[39] Eng NL, Fitzgerald CA, Fisher JG, et al. Laparoscopic-assisted pancreatic necrosectomy: Technique and initial outcomes. The American SurgeonTM. 2022;**89**(11):4459-4468

[40] Eng NL, Fitzgerald CA, Fisher JG, Small WC, Willingham FF, Galloway JR, et al. Laparoscopic-assisted

pancreatic necrosectomy: Technique and initial outcomes. The American Surgeon. 2023;**89**(11):4459-4468. DOI: 10.1177/00031348221101495. Epub 2022 May 16

[41] Huang L, Chen W, Chen J, Chen D, Zhang K, Cai J, et al. Indocyanine green-guided intraoperative imaging to facilitate video-assisted retroperitoneal debridement for treating acute necrotizing pancreatitis. Journal of Visualized Experiments. 8 Sep 2022;**187**. DOI: 10.3791/63236

[42] Munene G, Dixon E, Sutherland F. Open transgastric debridement and internal drainage of symptomatic noninfected walled-off pancreatic necrosis. HPB: The Official Journal of the International Hepato Pancreato Biliary Association. 2011;**13**:234-239

[43] Gibson SC, Robertson BF, Dickson EJ, et al. 'Step-port' laparoscopic cystgastrostomy for the management of organized solid predominant post-acute fluid collections after severe acute pancreatitis. HPB: The Official Journal of the International Hepato Pancreato Biliary Association. 2014;**16**:170-176

[44] Worhunsky DJ, Qadan M, Dua MM, et al. Laparoscopic transgastric necrosectomy for the management of pancreatic necrosis. Journal of the American College of Surgeons. 2014;**219**:735-743

[45] Garg PK, Meena D, Babu D, Padhan RK, Dhingra R, Krishna A, et al. Endoscopic versus laparoscopic drainage of pseudocyst and walled-off necrosis following acute pancreatitis: A randomized trial. Surgical Endoscopy. 2020;**34**(3):1157-1166. DOI: 10.1007/s00464-019-06866-z. Epub 2019 May 28

[46] Angadi S, Mahapatra SJ, Sethia R, Elhence A, Krishna A, Gunjan D, et al. Endoscopic transmural drainage tailored to quantity of necrotic debris versus laparoscopic transmural internal drainage for walled-off necrosis in acute pancreatitis: A randomized controlled trial. Pancreatology. 2021;**21**(7):1291-1298. DOI: 10.1016/j.pan.2021.06.006. Epub 2021 Jun 21

[47] Husu HL, Kuronen JA, Leppäniemi AK, Mentula PJ. Open necrosectomy in acute pancreatitis-obsolete or still useful? World Journal of Emergency Surgery : WJES. 2020;**15**(1):21. DOI: 10.1186/s13017-020-00300-9

[48] Niu DG, Li WQ, Huang Q, Yang F, Tian WL, Li C, et al. Open necrosectomy combined with continuous positive drainage and prophylactic diverting loop ileostomy for late infected pancreatic necrosis: A retrospective cohort study. BMC Gastroenterology. 2020;**20**(1):212. DOI: 10.1186/s12876-020-01343-7

[49] Baron TH, DiMaio CJ, Wang AY, Morgan KA. AGA clinical practice update: Expert review. Gastroenterology. 2020;**158**:67-75

Chapter 12

Acute Pancreatitis

Yi-Hua Wu

Abstract

Acute pancreatitis is an acute inflammatory condition of the pancreas with varying severity. It is primarily caused by gallstones and alcohol consumption, with other etiologies including hypertriglyceridemia, medications, and autoimmune disease. Diagnosis typically requires at least two of the following: characteristic abdominal pain, serum amylase or lipase levels elevated more than three times the upper normal limit, and imaging findings consistent with pancreatitis. Management is largely supportive, emphasizing fluid resuscitation, pain control, and early nutritional support. Most cases are self-limiting; however, a subset of patients may develop severe complications such as pancreatic necrosis, systemic inflammatory response, and multiorgan failure. Early recognition and appropriate supportive care are essential for improving outcomes. Chronic pancreatitis (CP) is a progressive fibroinflammatory disease characterized by irreversible morphological changes leading to exocrine and endocrine insufficiency. Histological diagnosis is limited in clinical practice; thus, diagnosis primarily relies on clinical features, imaging, and pancreatic function tests. CP may lead to serious complications including pseudocysts, biliary and duodenal obstruction, pancreatic fistula, vascular events, diabetes mellitus, and increased risk of pancreatic cancer. Pain is the predominant symptom and remains therapeutically challenging. Management is multidisciplinary and stepwise, encompassing medical, endoscopic, and surgical approaches based on ductal anatomy and disease severity. In select patients with small duct disease, total pancreatectomy with islet autotransplantation may be considered.

Keywords: pancreatitis, acute, chronic, diagnosis, management, prognosis

1. Introduction

Patients with severe acute pancreatitis may display hypoxemia, hypotension, tachypnea, tachycardia, fever, and an abrupt onset of severe pain in the upper abdomen; some patients also experience nausea and vomiting simultaneously. During physical examinations, patients frequently report feeling abdominal pain when the doctor probes them [1, 2].

2. Definition

Acute pancreatitis is characterized by a patient fulfilling two of the following three criteria: (1) acute onset of epigastric and/or left upper quadrant pain,

 IntechOpen

frequently radiating to the back; (2) serum amylase or lipase levels exceeding three times the upper limit of the laboratory's reference range; and (3) radiologic imaging indicative of pancreatitis, typically evaluated *via* CT or MRI. Pancreatitis is deemed acute until imaging studies, such as CT, MRI, EUS, or ERCP, reveal evidence of chronic pancreatitis. Consequently, pancreatitis is classified as chronic, with each subsequent episode of acute pancreatitis regarded as an exacerbation of the chronic condition. Patients may undergo an episode of acute on chronic pancreatitis, fulfilling all three criteria [3–5].

3. Pathogenesis

The majority of our understanding of acute pancreatitis's etiology comes from research conducted on animal models. Acute pancreatitis due to gallstones or alcohol may account for up to 60% of human cases; however, no animal model can reproduce these symptoms at this time (**Table 1**). The chemicals cerulein and taurocholate, which cause pancreatitis in animals, have less of an impact on humans. Acute pancreatitis models in animals have many anatomical and biochemical features similar to those of human patients, despite these limitations [6, 7]. Acute pancreatitis (AP) causes a similar cascade of events that manifests locally and systemically regardless of the cause. Because a pharmaceutical treatment may be most useful in halting the course of the illness at its early stages if administered quickly upon its availability, this is of the utmost importance.

The most common side effect of medicines is mild pancreatitis that goes away on its own. If the patient is of legal drinking age, they should first rule out malignancy, hypertriglyceridemia, hypercalcemia, gallstones, and alcohol. Some medications,

Obstruction
Gallstones
Tumors
Parasites
Duodenal diverticula
Annular pancreas
Choledochocele
Alcohol/other toxins/drugs
Ethyl alcohol
Methyl alcohol
Scorpion venom
Organophosphorus insecticides
Drugs
Metabolic abnormalities
Hypertriglyceridemia
Diabetes mellitus
Hypercalcemia
Infection

Vascular disorders
Vasculitis
Emboli to pancreatic blood vessels
Hypotension/ischemia
Trauma
Postoperative state
Post-ERCP
Hereditary/familial/genetic
Controversial
Pancreas divisum
SOD
Miscellaneous
Idiopathic

Table 1.
Conditions that predispose to acute pancreatitis.

such as 6-mercaptopurine (3–5% frequency) and didanosine (5–10% frequency), have a substantial connection with acute pancreatitis (AP), according to randomized trials. Sadly, a lot of prescriptions are mistakenly attributed to AP and then discontinued

Mechanical	Gallstones, biliary sludge, ascariasis, periampullary diverticulum, pancreatic or periampullary cancer, ampullary stenosis, duodenal stricture or obstruction
Toxic	Ethanol, methanol, scorpion venom, organophosphate poisoning
Metabolic	Hyperlipidemia (types I, IV, V), hypercalcemia
Drugs	Didanosine, pentamidine, metronidazole, stibogluconate, tetracycline furosemide, thiazides, sulphasalazine, 5-ASA, L-asparaginase, azathioprine, valproic acid, sulindac, salicylates, calcium, estrogen
Infection	Viruses-mumps, coxsackie, hepatitis B, CMV, varicella-zoster, HSV, HIV
	Bacteria-mycoplasma, Legionella, Leptospira, Salmonella
	Fungi-aspergillus
	Parasites-toxoplasma, cryptosporidium, Ascaris
Trauma	Blunt or penetrating abdominal injury, iatrogenic injury during surgery, or ERCP (sphincterotomy)
Congenital	Cholodochocele type V, pancreas divisum*
Vascular	Ischemia, atheroembolism, vasculitis (polyarteritis nodosa, SLE)
Miscellaneous	Post ERCP, pregnancy, renal transplantation, alpha-1-antitrypsin deficiency
Genetic	CFTR, PRSS1, SPINK1, and other genetic mutations

**Whether pancreas divisum causes pancreatitis or is an incidental finding is controversial. 5-ASA: 5-aminosalicylic acid; CMV: cytomegalovirus; HSV: herpes simplex virus; HIV: human immunodeficiency virus; ERCP: endoscopic retrograde cholangiopancreatography; PRSS: protease serine; SPINK: serine protease inhibitor Kazal type; SLE: systemic lupus erythematosus; CFTR: cystic fibrosis transmembrane conductance regulator.*

Table 2.
Etiology of acute pancreatitis.

since the irate doctor could not come up with any other potential reasons. Some medications (like statins) may not react well to such a sudden discontinuation of treatment (**Table 2**).

When diagnosing drug-induced acute pancreatitis, doctors should exercise caution since there is no known etiology and only a tiny number of instances. Chronic pancreatitis has not been shown to be caused by any medicine (**Table 3**).

Acetaminophen
5-Aminosalicylic acid compounds (sulfasalazine, azodisalicylate, and mesalamine)
L-Asparaginase
Azathioprine
Benazepril
Bezafibrate
Cannabis
Captopril
Carbimazole
Cimetidine
Clozapine
Codeine
Cytosine arabinoside
Dapsone
Didanosine
Dexamethasone
Enalapril
Erythromycin
Estrogen
Fluvastatin
Furosemide
Hydrochlorothiazide
Hydrocortisone
Ifosfamide
Interferon-α
Isoniazid
Lamivudine
Lisinopril
Losartan
Meglumine
Methimazole
Methyldopa
Metronidazole
6-Mercaptopurine

Nelfinavir
Norethindrone/mestrol
Pentamidine
Pravastatin
Procainamide
Pyritinol
Simvastatin
Sulfamethazine
Sulfamethoxazole
Stibogluconate
Sulindac
Tetracycline
Trimethoprim/sulfamethoxazole
Valproic acid

Table 3.
Drugs associated with acute pancreatitis.

4. Diagnosis and assessment

Once a patient is diagnosed with acute pancreatitis, their condition is further categorized according to its severity. In extreme cases of acute pancreatitis, organ failure lasts more than 48 hours. Acute collections of fluid or necrosis, walled-off necrosis, infectious or sterile pancreatic and peripancreatic necrosis, and pseudocyst formation are all problems that may occur on a local level. In addition to an APACHE-II score of 8 or above, severe pancreatitis is also indicated by satisfying three out of eleven of Ranson's criteria for nongallstone pancreatitis [8–10].

Hemorrhagic pancreatitis and phlegmon are two terminologies that have varying meanings depending on who you ask in the medical field; neither of them was part of the original Atlanta classification. Two types of pancreatitis, hemorrhagic and necrotizing, are distinct from one another [11].

Venous hemorrhage, which may cause bleeding early in the process, can happen during the acute inflammatory phase. Therefore, cases of significant bleeding are associated with an increased risk of pseudoaneurysm development, which might result in hemoperitoneum or hemorrhagic collections. Individuals with interstitial pancreatitis, which constitutes about 75–80% of all cases, do not show any non-perfused, low attenuation patches on contrast-enhanced CT scans of the pancreas [12–15]. Both mild pancreatitis and interstitial pancreatitis refer to a gradual deterioration of the condition, hence the two phrases are interchangeable.

The Atlanta categorization includes pancreatic and surrounding tissue necrosis. Both pancreatic and peripancreatic tissues are involved in almost half of the instances with necrotizing pancreatitis, whereas peripancreatic necrosis alone is characterized in nearly half of those cases [16].

Pure pancreatic necrosis affects about 5% of patients. About 15.

Pancreatic necrosis may be detected by a CT scan when at least 30% of the pancreatic parenchyma does not show enhancement or has poor attenuation.

The pancreas is encircled by low attenuation zones, which cause a sudden accumulation of fluid around it. If these collections cross fascial planes like Gerota fascia, the right diagnosis should be acute peripancreatic necrotic collections, not fluid [17–25].

4.1 Laboratory results

Enzymes produced by the pancreas are released into the circulation by acinar cell leakage when acute pancreatitis first starts. Acute pancreatitis patients may have abnormally high amounts of pancreatic enzymes, breakdown products, inflammatory mediators, and lipase and amylase in their blood. Serum lipase is a somewhat more sensitive indication of acute pancreatitis than amylase because elevations in the former happen faster and last longer. Patients who will be seeing a doctor in the future will benefit greatly from serum lipase. When it comes to alcohol-induced pancreatitis, serum lipase is more sensitive than amylase. In about 85% of cases of acute pancreatitis, a condition called acute interstitial edematous pancreatitis, a contrast-enhanced abdominal computed tomography (CT) scan will show a larger pancreas. Around 15% of instances of necrotizing pancreatitis include necrotic pancreatic parenchyma, peripancreatic tissue, or both [26, 27].

4.2 Diagnosis

Two of the following must be present for a diagnosis of acute pancreatitis to be made: (1) sudden onset of severe epigastric pain that radiates to the back; (2) a rise in serum lipase or amylase levels three times or more above the upper limit of normal; or (3) imaging findings on contrast-enhanced computed tomography, magnetic resonance imaging, or transabdominal ultrasonography that are indicative of acute pancreatitis.

An imaging test is not necessary to confirm a diagnosis of acute pancreatitis in patients who exhibit the classic abdominal pain symptoms in addition to serum lipase or amylase levels three times or higher than the upper limit of normal.

Balthazar grades	**Definition**	**Points**
A	Normal pancreas consistent with mild pancreatitis	0
B	Focal or diffuse enlargement of the gland, including contour irregularities and inhomogeneous attenuation, but without peripancreatic inflammation	1
C	Grade B plus peripancreatic inflammation	2
D	Grade C plus associated single fluid collection	3
E	Grade C plus 2 or more peripancreatic fluid collections or gas in the pancreas or retroperitoneum	4
CTSI = Balthazar grade points plus necrosis score*		
	Necrosis score	**Points**
	Absence of necrosis	0
	Necrosis of up to 33% of the pancreas	2
	Necrosis of 33–50%	4
	Necrosis of >50%	6

**Highest attainable CTSI score: 4 (Balthazar grade E) + 6 (necrosis of >50%) = 10 points.*

Table 4.
CT grading system of Balthazar and the CT severity index (CTSI).

We conduct a contrast-enhanced abdominal CT scan (**Table 4**) to diagnose acute pancreatitis and rule out other possible causes of acute abdominal pain in patients who display symptoms that are not typical of the condition or who have serum amylase and/or lipase levels that are less than three times the upper limit of normal. "Differential Diagnosis" and "Abdominal Computed Tomography" are the relevant parts to consult [28–30].

Most cases of acute pancreatitis are minor, according to the disease's natural history and progression, and patients usually recover in 3 to 5 days without problems or organ failure. While most people recover well from acute pancreatitis, 20% have moderate to severe cases, which may lead to organ failure or other problems [31–33].

How acute pancreatitis is classified: Acute pancreatitis is characterized by a rapid onset of pancreatic inflammation. Two primary forms of acute pancreatitis are edematous interstitial and necrotizing, respectively. Organ failure and systemic or local consequences are not seen in mild acute pancreatitis. If there are local problems, organ failure that lasts less than 48 hours, or both, then the acute pancreatitis is considered moderately severe. Organ failure that does not go away within 48 hours, affecting one or more organs, is a hallmark of severe acute pancreatitis [34–39].

4.3 Preliminary assessment

A clinical examination is necessary for the first assessment of acute pancreatitis in order to determine its severity. This examination should concentrate on early fluid losses, organ failure, and the SIRS score. Patients presenting with acute pancreatitis should not get a routine abdominal CT scan at initial presentation unless the diagnosis is in doubt (**Tables 4** and 5).

Patients with acute pancreatitis who are very ill or who fulfill any combination of the following criteria must be admitted to an intensive care unit or monitoring unit.

Ranson (alcoholic or other)	Ranson (biliary)
At admission	At admission
Age > 55 years	Age > 70 years
GB > 16,000/mm^3	GB > 18,000/mm^3
LDH > 350 U/L	LDH > 250 U/L
AST > 250 U/L	AST > 250 U/L
Glycemia > 200 mg/dL	Glycemia > 220 mg/dL
In 48 hours	**In 48 hours**
Drop in hematocrit > 10%	Drop in hematocrit > 10%
BUN increase > 5 mg/dL	BUN increase > 2 mg/dL
Calcium < 8 mg/dL	Calcium < 8 mg/dL
PO^2 < 60 mmHg	PO^2 < 60 mmHg
Bases deficit > 4 mEq/L	Bases deficit > 5 mEq/L
Fluid loss > 6 L	Fluid loss > 4 L
Each item worth 1 point (0 to 11 points)	

Table 5.
Ranson criteria.

- Pulse <40 or >150 beats per minute
- Systolic arterial pressure < 80 mmHg, mean arterial pressure < 60 mmHg, or diastolic arterial pressure > 120 mmHg
- Respiratory rate exceeding 35 breaths per minute
- Serum sodium <110 mmol/L or >170 mmol/L, serum potassium <2.0 mmol/L or >7.0 mmol/L, serum glucose >800 mg/dL, serum calcium >15 mg/dL
- PaO_2 < 50 mmHg
- pH <7.1 or > 7.7
- Anuria
- Coma

5. Treatment

5.1 Fluid replacement

Pain management, accurate intravenous fluid administration (particularly in the first 24 hours), and correction of metabolic and electrolyte imbalances are all components of supportive therapy for acute pancreatitis [40–42]. Patients with moderate acute pancreatitis may only need a lower volume of normal saline than what was previously recommended (250 to 500 mL/hour, or 5 to 10 mL per kilogram of body weight per hour), according to randomized controlled trials. Both intense fluid resuscitation (a 20 mL/kg bolus of lactated Ringer's solution followed by 3 mL/kg/hour) and moderate resuscitation (1.5 mL/kg/hour with a 10 mL/kg bolus administered only to hypovolemic patients) were used in a randomized experiment including 249 individuals with acute pancreatitis. Fluid overload was assessed with a first physical examination 3 hours after ingestion in all groups, and goal-directed resuscitation was modified at 12, 24, 48, and 72 hours according to volume status [43, 44]. Fluid overload was more common in the vigorous resuscitation group (20% vs. 6%), which led to the trial's early termination despite no difference in the incidence of moderately severe or severe pancreatitis or length of hospitalization between the two groups [45–48].

5.2 Pain management

People suffering from acute pancreatitis often report severe stomach pain as their primary symptom. Injecting opioids like hydromorphone and fentanyl intravenously, often with the use of a patient-controlled analgesia pump, is the gold standard for pain therapy [49, 50].

Patients with mild pancreatitis often make a speedy recovery, eliminating the need for additional nourishment. Within 24 hours, you may begin a soft diet if you feel well enough to do so [51]. If you are not experiencing ileus, severe nausea, or vomiting, it is usually OK to start on a low-fat, soft diet with little residue.

In patients with moderate to severe pancreatitis, we advise against starting parenteral nutrition and instead encourage enteral feeding by a nasojejunal tube that has been inserted endoscopically or radiologically. Additional parenteral nourishment should be administered if the goal rate is not reached within 48 to 72 hours and severe acute pancreatitis persists [52–57].

5.3 Criteria for subsequent imaging

To evaluate for pancreatic or extrapancreatic necrosis and related local consequences, a contrast-enhanced CT scan should be performed on patients with moderately severe or severe acute pancreatitis, indications of sepsis, or a worsening of clinical status 72 hours after first presentation. Referral to specialized facilities is necessary for patients with prolonged organ failure and significant local consequences [58].

People who have acute pancreatitis run the risk of developing either localized or systemic problems. **Table 3** shows that acute pancreatitis may have a variety of local consequences, such as a pancreatic pseudocyst, acute necrotic collection (ANC), and walled-off necrosis (WON). Although pancreatic pseudocysts and walled-off necrosis often do not show up until after 4 weeks have passed from the start of acute pancreatitis, acute necrotic collections and acute peripancreatic fluid collections may occur within that time frame [59, 60].

5.4 Individuals with infected necrosis

Even though they start off sterile, walled-off necrosis (WON) and acute necrotic collections (CNCs) may develop infections. Among those suffering from acute necrotizing pancreatitis, pancreatic infection ranks high in terms of mortality and morbidity. A patient with pancreatic or extrapancreatic necrosis should be considered for infected necrosis (picture 4) if they show signs of clinical deterioration (instability or septic physiology, high leukocyte count, fever) or do not show signs of recovery after 7–10 days of hospitalization. Instead of CT-guided fine needle aspiration, we recommend empiric antibiotics for patients with suspected infected necrosis [61].

If a patient's infected necrosis is not improving after treatment or if their condition is very precarious, pancreatic debridement may be necessary. We want to wait 4 weeks from the first presentation before intervening in order to encourage the encapsulation of the infected necrosis. Endoscopic, percutaneous, and laparoscopic necrosectomy are our go-to minimally invasive procedures; we only resort to open surgical debridement when all other options fail [62].

If cholangitis is visible, patients with gallstone pancreatitis must have sphincterotomy and endoscopic retrograde cholangiopancreatography within 24 hours. After all operable patients with gallstone pancreatitis or biliary sludge have recovered from acute pancreatitis, a cholecystectomy should be done, unless another reason is found [63].

6. Interventional treatments

6.1 Cholecystectomy

This includes both elective ERCP in the days leading up to cholecystectomy and urgent ERCP in the first 24 to 72 hours after gallstones are detected. Failing to have a cholecystectomy during the first episode of biliary pancreatitis increases the risk of further episodes of acute pancreatitis by 18% within 6 weeks. Because of concerns about abdominal inflammation during the operation, surgeons used to be uneasy about operating on the gallbladder when the patient was experiencing an acute pancreatitis episode. Current guidelines support same-admission cholecystectomy in cases with mild and interstitial pancreatitis, and cholecystectomy approaches have evolved to better manage these patients. For patients with moderate to severe (necrotizing) pancreatitis, these guidelines also suggested delaying and thereafter doing interval cholecystectomy. The suggested timeframes varied from 6 weeks after the incident to when the inflammation has subsided and fluid collections have returned to normal. Cholecystectomy within 72 hours of randomization reduced the incidence of pancreaticobiliary complications and readmissions in patients with acute biliary pancreatitis compared to cholecystectomy performed after 25 to 30 days, according to a recent randomized controlled trial (RCT). However, there was no difference in mortality rates, as mentioned earlier. The number of patients who had an open cholecystectomy did not change [64–66].

When a cholecystectomy is not an option or when a patient has necrotizing pancreatitis and is waiting for interval cholecystectomy, a biliary sphincterotomy can prevent additional acute pancreatitis episodes; however, it will not prevent biliary problems like biliary pain or acute cholecystitis. According to a recent study, patients who were misdiagnosed with mild interstitial pancreatitis and had cholecystectomy on the same admission had worse outcomes when their necrotizing pancreatitis progressed (such as infected pancreatic necrosis) compared to patients of the same age and sex who did not undergo the same procedure on the same admission [67–69].

An elevated white blood cell count prior to cholecystectomy in patients with interstitial acute biliary pancreatitis who are being evaluated for the procedure during the same admission requires a repeat CT scan to detect any necrotizing pancreatitis that might not have been visible on the first scan.

6.2 Interventions for pancreatic fluid accumulations

By the conclusion of the second week, pancreatic fluid collections often solidify into a wall. This procedure often takes around 4 weeks. The existence of a wall around a collection of acute (peri-)pancreatic fluid indicates the likelihood of a walled-off necrosis (WON) rather than pseudocysts, since these collections often resolve around that period. Action is not obligatory only due to the presence of specific local challenges. Approximately 66% of individuals with necrotizing pancreatitis recover independently. Additional clarification indicates that minimally invasive drainage or debridement is essential in instances of infected (peri)pancreatic necrosis, biliary or gastrointestinal obstruction, chronic illness accompanied by hypothyroidism and weight loss, disconnected pancreatic duct syndrome, and complications including perforation of a hollow viscus or fistulous tract. A randomized controlled trial indicated that although endoscopic therapy was not more effective than surgical cyst gastrostomy for symptomatic pseudocysts in acute pancreatitis, it resulted in shorter hospital stays, improved patient mental and physical health, and decreased costs. Historically, persons exhibiting symptoms of infection or deteriorating clinical conditions were treated by open necrosectomy in cases of pancreatic fluid accumulation. Therefore, it is advisable to postpone intervention until fluid collections have developed a wall, generally around 4 weeks post-surgery, as a randomized controlled trial has demonstrated that early surgery (within 2 weeks) elevates mortality and morbidity rates [70].

The three predominant types of necrosectomy procedures are open packing, closed drainage without irrigation, and closed continuous irrigation utilizing indwelling catheters. Due to the reduced risk of complications and death, several studies have preferred less invasive therapies such as percutaneous, laparoscopic, endoscopic, video-assisted retroperitoneal, and hybrid methods over open surgical necrosectomy. A randomized controlled study indicated that the minimally invasive step-up technique, which involves initial percutaneous drainage followed by video-assisted retroperitoneal drainage, is superior to surgical necrosectomy. The meta-analysis revealed that although the less invasive method offers benefits over open necrosectomy, further rigorous research is necessary due to the variability observed in one randomized controlled trial and three additional reports.308 Subsequently, the same team conducted a second randomized controlled trial that validated the superiority of endoscopic intervention over surgical necrosectomy. The subsequent randomized controlled trial by the same group demonstrated that endoscopic intervention diminished complications such as fistula formation and shortened hospital stay relative to videoscopic retroperitoneal intervention. Nonetheless, mortality and other major complications were similar [71].

Severe pancreatic necrosis that separates the pancreatic duct (PD) into proximal and distal segments results in a condition termed disconnected pancreatic duct (PD) syndrome. A diagnosis is typically established when ERCP identifies obstruction of the pancreatic duct at the correct location, ongoing fluid accumulation in the necrotic area, and a viable, enhancing distal pancreas. Supplementary data have corroborated the hypothesis that this condition requires prolonged pigtail catheter drainage into the fluid collections, following prior studies that suggested this should be performed transgastrically or transduodenally. According to a recent extensive study involving 167 participants, patients with a detached pancreatic duct (PD) were more likely to require hybrid treatments (endoscopic ultrasound-guided multigate/dual modality approach, endoscopic/percutaneous sinus tract necrosectomy) compared to those without a PD. A self-expanding metal stent may be utilized for a brief duration of 3 weeks; thereafter, pigtail catheters would be incorporated into the treatment, potentially involving a singular gastric entry into the fluid accumulation or multiple routes to enhance the drainage of pancreatic secretions [72].

Globally, percutaneous drainage is the benchmark for minimally invasive drainage and debridement of pancreatic fluid accumulation. The endoscopic technique has become more common in the last many years.

There is a dearth of literature on laparoscopic cholecystectomy and the technique has not been extensively used by laparoscopic surgeons, despite the fact that it enables the treatment to be completed in a single session and the simultaneous management of other conditions. It is still unclear whether the approach is better: doing debridement and necrosectomy upfront to cut down on treatment sessions, or starting with drainage and then debridement and necrosectomy.

Following an acute pancreatitis episode, exocrine and endocrine insufficiency are common. Fifteen percent of those who had acute pancreatitis had new-onset diabetes mellitus within a year following the event, and that risk more than doubled after 5 years, according to a meta-analysis. Forty percent of those with newly diagnosed prediabetes or diabetes mellitus who have acute pancreatitis also have pancreatic exocrine insufficiency. Ten percent of patients with acute pancreatitis (AP) and 36% of patients with recurrent AP developed chronic pancreatitis, according to a recent meta-analysis [73].

Author details

Yi-Hua Wu[1,2]

1 Center for Digestive Medicine, Department of Internal Medicine, China Medical University Hospital, Taichung, Taiwan

2 School of Medicine, College of Medicine, China Medical University, Taichung, Taiwan

*Address all correspondence to: qtilovesleep@gmail.com

References

[1] Peery AE, Dellon ES, Lund J, et al. Burden of gastrointestinal diseases in the United States: 2012 update. Gastroenterology. 2012;**143**:1179-1187

[2] Fagenholz PJ, Fernandez-del Castillo C, Harris NS, et al. Direct medical costs of acute pancreatitis hospitalizations in the United States. Pancreas. 2007;**35**:302-307

[3] Fagenholz PJ, Castillo CF, Harris NS, et al. Increasing United States hospital admissions for acute pancreatitis, 1988-2003. Annals of Epidemiology. 2007;**17**:491-497

[4] Yadav D, Lowenfels AB. Trends in the epidemiology of the first attack of acute pancreatitis: A systemic review. Pancreas. 2006;**33**:323-330

[5] Bradley EL. A clinically based classification system of acute pancreatitis. Archives of Surgery. 1993;**128**:586-590

[6] Banks PA, Bollen TL, Dervenis C, et al. Classification of acute pancreatitis—2012: Revision of Atlanta classification and definitions by international consensus. Gut. 2013;**62**:102-111

[7] Busquets J, Fabregat J, Pelaez N, et al. Factors influencing mortality in patients undergoing surgery for acute pancreatitis: Importance of peripancreatic tissue and fluid infection. Pancreas. 2013;**42**:285-292

[8] Marshall JC, Cook DJ, Christou NV, et al. Multiple organ dysfunction score: A reliable descriptor of complex clinical outcome. Critical Care Medicine. 1995;**23**:1638-1652

[9] Wall I, Badalov N, Baradarian R, et al. Decreased morbidity and mortality in patients with acute pancreatitis related to aggressive intravenous hydration. Pancreas. 2011;**40**:547-550

[10] Gardner TB, Vege SS, Pearson RK, et al. Fluid resuscitation in acute pancreatitis. Clinical Gastroenterology and Hepatology. 2008;**6**:1070-1076

[11] Guyatt GH, Oxman AD, Vist GE, et al. GRADE: An emerging consensus on rating quality of evidence and strength of recommendations. BMJ. 2008;**336**:924-926

[12] Clavien PA, Robert J, Meyer P, et al. Acute pancreatitis and normoamylasemia. Not an uncommon combination. Annals of Surgery. 1989;**210**:614-620

[13] Winslet M, Hall C, London NJM. Relation of diagnostic serum amylase levels to aetiology and severity of acute pancreatitis. Gut. 1992;**33**:982-986

[14] Malka D, Rosa-Hezode I. Positive and etiological diagnosis of acute pancreatitis. Gastroentérologie Clinique et Biologique. 2001;**25**:1S153-11S68

[15] UK guidelines for the management of acute pancreatitis. Gut. 2005;**54**:1-9

[16] Shah AM, Eddi R, Kothari ST, et al. Acute pancreatitis with normal serum lipase: A case series. Journal of the Pancreas: JOP. 2010;**11**:369-372

[17] Steinberg WM, DeVries JH, Wadden T, et al. Longitudinal monitoring of lipase and amylase in adults with type 2 diabetes and obesity: Evidence from two phase 3 randomized clinical trials with the once-daily GLP-1 analog liraglutide. Gastroenterology. 2012;**121**:A246

[18] Kiriyama, Gabata T, Takada T, et al. New diagnostic criteria of acute pancreatitis. Journal of Hepato-Biliary-Pancreatic Sciences. 2010;**17**:24-36

[19] Lippil G, Valentino M, Cervellin G. Laboratory diagnosis of acute pancreatitis: In search of the Holy Grail. Critical Reviews in Clinical Laboratory Sciences. 2012;**49**:18-31

[20] Balthazar EJ. Acute pancreatitis: Assessment of severity with clinical and CT evaluation. Radiology. 2002;**223**:603-613

[21] Arvanitakis M, Delhaye M, Maertelaere VD, et al. Computed tomography and MRI in the assessment of acute pancreatitis. Gastroenterology. 2004;**126**:715-723

[22] Zaheer A, Singh VK, Qureshi RO, et al. The revised Atlanta classification for acute pancreatitis: Updates in imaging terminology and guidelines. Abdominal Imaging. 2013;**38**:125-136

[23] Bollen TL, Singh VK, Maurer R, et al. Comparative evaluation of the modified CT severity index and CT severity index in assessing severity of acute pancreatitis. AJR. American Journal of Roentgenology. 2011;**197**:386-392

[24] Stimac D, Miletic D, Radic M, et al. The role of non enhanced magnetic resonance imaging in the early assessment of acute pancreatitis. The American Journal of Gastroenterology. 2007;**102**:997-1004

[25] Lankisch PG, Assmus C, Lehnick D, et al. Acute pancreatitis: Does gender matter? Digestive Diseases and Sciences. 2001;**46**:2470-2474

[26] Gullo I, Migliori M, Olah A, et al. Acute pancreatitis in five European countries: Etiology and mortality. Pancreas. 2002;**24**:223-227

[27] Lowenfels AB, Maisonneuve P, Sullivan T. The changing character of acute pancreatitis: Epidemiology, etiology, and prognosis. Current Gastroenterology Reports. 2009;**11**:97-103

[28] Johnson C, Lévy P. Detection of gallstones in acute pancreatitis: When and how? Pancreatology. 2010;**10**:27-32

[29] Moreau JA, Zinsmeister AR, Melton LJ, et al. Gallstone pancreatitis and the effect of cholecystectomy. Mayo Clinic Proceedings. 1988;**63**:466

[30] Yadav D, O'Connell M, Papachristou GI. Natural history following the first attack of acute pancreatitis. The American Journal of Gastroenterology. 2012;**107**:1096-1103

[31] Ammann RW. The natural history of alcoholic chronic pancreatitis. Internal Medicine. 2001;**40**:368-375

[32] Steinberg W, Tenner S. Medical progress: Acute pancreatitis. The New England Journal of Medicine. 1994;**330**:1198-1210

[33] Whitcomb DC. Genetic polymorphisms in alcoholic pancreatitis. Digestive Diseases and Sciences. 2005;**23**:247-254

[34] Rebours V, Vullierme MP, Hentic O, et al. Smoking and the course of recurrent acute and chronic alcoholic pancreatitis: A dose-dependent relationship. Pancreas. 2012;**41**:1219-1224

[35] Badalov N, Baradarian R, Iswara K, et al. Drug induced acute pancreatitis: An evidence based approach. Clinical Gastroenterology and Hepatology. 2007;**101**:454-476

[36] Fortson MR, Freeman SN, Webster PD. Clinical assessment of

hyperlipidmeic pancreatitis. The American Journal of Gastroenterology. 1995;**90**:2134-2139

[37] Parenti DM, Steinberg W, Kang P. Infectious causes of acute pancreatitis. Pancreas. 1996;**13**:356-371

[38] Farmer RG, Winkelman EI, Brown HB, et al. Hyperlipoproteinemia and pancreatitis. The American Journal of Medicine. 1973;**54**:161-165

[39] Toskes PP. Hyperlipidmic pancreatitis. Gastroenterology Clinics of North America. 1990;**19**:783-791

[40] Yadav D, Pitchumoni CS. Issues in hyperlipidemic pancreatitis. Journal of Clinical Gastroenterology. 2003;**36**:54-62

[41] Simpson WF, Adams DB, Metcalf JS, et al. Nonfunctioning pancreatic neuroendocrine tumors presenting as pancreatitis: Report of four cases. Pancreas. 1988;**3**:223-231

[42] Kohler H, Lankisch PG. Acute pancreatitis and hyperamylasaemia in pancreatic carcinoma. Pancreas. 1987;**2**:117-119

[43] Tandon M, Topazian M. Endoscopic ultrasound in idiopathic acute pancreatitis. The American Journal of Gastroenterology. 2001;**96**:705-709

[44] Al-Haddad M, Wallace MB. Diagnostic approach to patients with acute idiopathic pancreatitis, what should be done? World Journal of Gastroenterology. 2008;**14**:1007-1010

[45] Robertson JF, Imrie CW. Acute pancreatitis associated with carcinoma of the ampulla of Vater. The British Journal of Surgery. 1987;**74**:395-397

[46] Bank S, Indaram A. Causes of acute and recurrent pancreatitis. Clinical considerations and clues to diagnosis. Gastroenterology Clinics of North America. 1999;**28**:571-589, viii

[47] Banks PA. Epidemiology, natural history, and predictors of disease outcome in acute and chronic pancreatitis. Gastrointestinal Endoscopy. 2002;**56**:S226-S230

[48] DiMagno MJ, Dimagno EP. Pancreas divisum does not cause pancreatitis, but associates with CFTR mutations. The American Journal of Gastroenterology. 2012;**107**:318-320

[49] Steinberg WM, Chari ST, Forsmark CE, et al. Controversies in clinical pancreatology: Management of acute idiopathic recurrent pancreatitis. Pancreas. 2003;**27**:103-117

[50] Badalov N, Tenner S, Baillie J. Prevention and treatment of post-ERCP pancreatitis. Journal of the Pancreas: JOP. 2009;**10**:88-97

[51] Tenner S. Initial management of acute pancreatitis: Critical decisions during the first 72 hours. The American Journal of Gastroenterology. 2004;**99**:2489-2494

[52] Cote GA, Imperiale TF, Schmidt SE, et al. Similar efficacies of biliary, with or without pancreatic, sphincterotomy in treatment of idiopathic recurrent acute pancreatitis. Gastroenterology. 2012;**6**:1502-1509

[53] Banks PA, Freeman ML. Practice guidelines in acute pancreatitis. The American Journal of Gastroenterology. 2006;**101**:2379-2400

[54] Freeman MF, Werner J, van Santvoort HC, et al. Interventions for necrotizing pancreatitis. Summary of a multi-disciplinary consensus conference. Pancreas. 2012;**8**:1176-1194

[55] Perez A, Whang EE, Brooks DC, et al. Is severity of necrotizing pancreatitis increased in extending necrosis and infected necrosis? Pancreas. 2002;**25**:229-233

[56] Bakker OJ, van Santvoort H, Besselink MG, et al. Extrapancreatic necrosis without pancreatic parenchymal necrosis: A separate entity in necrotising pancreatitis? Gut. 2012;**18**:143-149

[57] Ranson JH, Pasternack BS. Statistical methods for quantifying the severity of clinical acute pancreatitis. The Journal of Surgical Research. 1977;**22**:79-91

[58] Knaus WA, Draper EA, Wagner DP, et al. APACHE II: A severity of disease classification system. Critical Care Medicine. 1985;**13**:818-829

[59] Wu BU, Johannes RS, Sun X, et al. The early prediction of mortality in acute pancreatitis: A large population-based study. Gut. 2008;**57**:1698Y1703

[60] Papachristou GI, Muddana V, Yadav D, et al. Comparison of BISAP, Ranson's, APACHE-II, and CTSI scores in predicting organ failure, complications, and mortality in acute pancreatitis. The American Journal of Gastroenterology. 2010;**105**:435-441

[61] Wu BU, Johannes RS, Sun X, et al. Early changes in blood urea nitrogen predict mortality in acute pancreatitis. Gastroenterology. 2009;**137**:129-135

[62] Mounzer R et al. Comparison of existing clinical scoring systems to predict persistent organ failure in patients with acute pancreatitis. Gastroenterology. 2012;**142**:1476-1482

[63] Brown A, Orav J, Banks PA. Hemoconcentration is an early marker for organ failure and necrotizing pancreatitis. Pancreas. 2000;**20**:367-372

[64] Lankisch PG, Mahlke R, Blum T, et al. Hemoconcentration: An early marker of severe and/or necrotizing pancreatitis? A critical appraisal. The American Journal of Gastroenterology. 2001;**96**:2081-2085

[65] Frossard JL, Hadengue A, Pastor CM. New serum markers for the detection of severe acute pancreatitis in humans. American Journal of Respiratory and Critical Care Medicine. 2001;**164**:162-170

[66] Papachristou GI, Whitcomb DC. Inflammatory markers of disease severity in acute pancreatitis. Clinics in Laboratory Medicine. 2005;**25**:17-37

[67] Balthazar EJ, Robinson DL, Megibow AJ, et al. Acute pancreatitis: Value of CT in establishing prognosis. Radiology. 1990;**174**:331-336

[68] van Santvoort HC, Besselink MG, Bakker OJ, et al. A step-up approach or open necrosectomy for necrotizing pancreatitis. The New England Journal of Medicine. 2013;**362**:1491-1502

[69] Tran DD, Cuesta MA. Evaluation of severity in patients with acute pancreatitis. The American Journal of Gastroenterology. 1992;**87**:604-608

[70] Mofidi R, Duff MD, Wigmore SJ, et al. Association between early systemic inflammatory response, severity of multiorgan dysfunction and death in acute pancreatitis. The British Journal of Surgery. 2006;**93**:738-744

[71] Buter A, Imrie CW, Carter CR, et al. Dynamic nature of early organ dysfunction determines outcome in acute pancreatitis. The British Journal of Surgery. 2002;**89**:298-302

[72] Papachristou GI, Muddana V, Yadav D, et al. Increased serum

creatinine is associated with pancreatic necrosis in acute pancreatitis. The American Journal of Gastroenterology. 2010;**105**:1451-1452

[73] Heller SJ, Noordhoek E, Tenner SM, et al. Pleural effusion as a predictor of severity in acute pancreatitis. Pancreas. 1997;**15**:222-225

Chapter 13

Causes and Management of Acute Pancreatitis Pain in the Intensive Care Unit

Sándor Márton

Abstract

AP is a mild to severe, potentially life-threatening condition caused by inflammation of the pancreas. Most common causes are excessive alcohol consumption and gallstone disease. For patients in intensive care, pain relief is a priority, as one of the main symptoms of AP is severe, often unbearable abdominal pain. Adequate pain management not only improves patients' comfort but also reduces the systemic stress response and the risk of late complications. The mechanism of pain is complex, with several factors contributing: enzymatic autodigestion, inflammation, oedema, ischaemia and neuronal sensitivity. Intense pain increases the incidence of SIRS, which may also lead to the development of MODS. The main methods of analgesia include: nonopioid analgesics (paracetamol, NSAIDs); opioids: (fentanyl, remi and sufentanyl but their long-term use should be avoided due to their known complications and side effects. Lidocaine infusion, a potent anti-inflammatory and analgesic, is not currently in daily use due to its dangerousness. Epidural analgesia is the most effective and commonly used procedure for severe pain. Appropriate pain management can reduce complications of AP, including sepsis and long hospital stays, and improve patients' chances of survival and quality of life.

Keywords: Opioidok, NSAID, acute pancreatitis, epidural analgesia, acute pain relief

1. Introduction

AP is a serious, potentially life-threatening condition caused by inflammation of the pancreas. Pain management for patients admitted to intensive care units [1] is central to the management of this disease. The most common symptom is severe, often unbearable abdominal pain. Adequate pain relief not only improves patient comfort, but also reduces the systemic stress response and can prevent serious complications that may develop later. The disease is one of the most common acute abdominal conditions, ranging from mild to severe, with life [2] threatening complications. The prevalence of AP varies worldwide, with an average of 13–80 cases per 100,000 population per year between 1990 and 2019 [3]. Because of the risk of serious complications or even fatal outcomes, early recognition of patients at high risk of severe progression is essential, and they require close monitoring and immediate appropriate intervention and treatment. The disease most commonly affects the age group 30–50 years, with an unequal gender distribution due to the aetiology. The cost of care for mild, moderate and especially severe AP patients also differs dramatically, placing a heavy burden on funding systems. In the United States, more than $2 billion is spent annually on hospitalisation for AP [4]. A 2021 study estimates that the median cost of hospitalisation for AP is $13,187, increasing in proportion to the severity of the disease [5]. Treatment costs are influenced by a number of factors, including length of hospital stay, need for intensive care unit care, development of complications, and their management. The average cost of endoscopic treatment for pancreatic necrosis is $57,486, with the largest cost factor being the length of hospital stay, thus limiting the ability to care for patients due to funding difficulties [6].

2. The most common causes of AP

At admission, establishing the cause of AP is essential (previous AP, known gallstones, alcohol abuse, drug and medication abuse, known hyperlipidemia) is of primary importance because it determines the type of therapeutic procedures.

2.1 Alcoholic pancreatitis

AP is an inflammatory disease of the pancreas that occurs suddenly and can range in severity from mild to severe and life-threatening [7]. One of the most common causes is alcohol consumption, which is responsible for a significant proportion of cases in Western societies. The most common complications are necrosis, abscess, pseudocysts and the development of chronic pancreatitis. Pathomechanism: Alcohol damages the pancreas both directly and indirectly: Direct cell damage: Alcohol and its metabolites (e.g. acetaldehyde) have a toxic effect on pancreatic acinar cells. Oxidative stress: during the breakdown of alcohol reactive oxygen species (ROS) are generated, which trigger inflammatory processes. Activation of zymogens: Alcohol can alter the secretion of pancreatic enzymes, causing premature activation of trypsinogen, leading to self-digestion and cell damage. Ductal dysfunction: alcohol increases protein precipitation in the pancreatic ducts, leading to obstruction, increased pressure and inflammation [8]. Clinical signs: the symptoms of alcohol-induced acute pancreatitis are similar to those caused by other aetiological factors, severe epigastric pain radiating to the back nausea, vomiting, fever and tachycardia, hypotension, in severe cases shock jaundice if biliary involvement is also present. Treatment: fluid replacement (Isotonic solutions). Analgesia: paracetamol, opioid analgesics as needed, antiemetics in case of vomiting, enteral feeding recommended after short fasting in mild cases, nasojejunal tube or parenteral feeding in severe cases. Alcohol withdrawal and lifestyle changes. Treatment of complications: if necrotizing pancreatitis develops, antibiotics (carbapenems) and surgical intervention [9].

Chronic pancreatitis: persistent inflammation that develops gradually over time. Symptoms: recurrent abdominal pain, weight loss, indigestion, fatty stools, development of diabetes. Often leads to irreversible damage and exocrine and endocrine failure. Mechanism of development: Alcohol has a direct cell-damaging effect on the acinar cells of the pancreas [8]. It contributes to the obstruction of pancreatic ducts and the development of fibrosis. Symptoms: severe, belt-like abdominal pain, worsening after meals. Nausea, vomiting, bloating, indigestion (fatty, foul stools), weight loss and malnutrition, and in chronic cases, the development of diabetes mellitus. Diagnosis: laboratory tests: elevated amylase and lipase levels in acute cases. Imaging studies: abdominal ultrasound—to exclude gallstones, pancreatic structure: endoscopic ultrasound—to detect subtle abnormalities. Treatment: strict alcohol prohibition! Hospitalisation if necessary: infusion therapy to maintain fluid and electrolyte balance. Pain relief NSAIDs, opioids, in severe cases surgical or interventional intervention required [9].

2.2 Gallstone disease

AP caused by gallstones is a sudden inflammation of the pancreas, triggered by bile duct obstruction caused by gallstones [10]. This condition can result in a severe clinical picture and requires appropriate diagnosis and prompt treatment. Pathophysiology and causes: gallstones develop in the gallbladder or bile ducts and can cause obstruction if they enter the bile duct. This blockage prevents proper drainage of bile and pancreatic fluids, can lead to premature activation of pancreatic enzymes and self-digestion of the gland. Ultrasound is the primary imaging modality for the detection of gallstones and biliary obstruction. If necessary, CT or MRCP (magnetic resonance cholangiopancreatography) can be used to examine the pancreas and bile ducts in more detail. Treatment: Fluid therapy: Intravenous fluid replacement is essential to maintain haemodynamic stability. Analgesia: Opioids may be necessary to relieve severe pain, if possible in combination with "multimodal analgesia". Early enteral feeding is recommended if tolerated by the patient, may reduce the risk of complications. Endoscopic intervention: endoscopic retrograde cholangiopancreatography is recommended to remove biliary obstruction, especially if cholangitis or persistent biliary obstruction is present. Surgical treatment: cholecystectomy is recommended after the first biliary pancreatitis to prevent recurrence. Prognosis: in the majority of cases, biliary pancreatitis is mild and patients recover completely with appropriate treatment. However, in severe cases, complications such as necrosis, infection or organ failure may develop, which increase mortality. The prevalence of gallstone disease varies worldwide [11], depending on a number of factors such as age, sex and geographical location. In general, it affects about 10–20% of the adult population in developed countries. it is more common in women and increases with age. The prevalence of gallstone disease increases with age: up to 20% of men and 35% of women have gallstones by the age of 75 [12]. The incidence of gallstone in relatives of affected individuals is 2–4 times higher than the average population. Among men and women aged 75 years, the incidence of gallstones can vary considerably. In general, gallstones are more common in women, especially those of childbearing age, where the incidence is two to three times higher than in men. This rate decreases after menopause, but the risk of gallstones increases with age in both sexes. People over 60 are more likely to develop gallstones than younger people. Some studies estimate that the prevalence of gallstones in Western countries is about 7.9% in men and 16.6% in women. Another study estimates that in the United States, about 6.3 million men and 14.2 million women aged 20–74 years have gallbladder disease. The risk of developing gallstones depends on many factors, including age, gender, genetic predisposition, diet and other health conditions. Being obese is also a risk factor. There is a linear relationship between body mass index (BMI) and the development of gallstones. However, sudden weight loss is also a risk, especially if it results from surgical intervention - bariatric surgery - presumably due to disruption of the normal enterohepatic biliary circulation [12].

2.3 Older age

Several studies have concluded that older age has a worse prognosis, although the age cut-off has varied between 55 and 75 years in different publications [12]. In an illustrative study, patients over 75 years were more than 15 times more likely to die within 2 weeks and more than 22 times more likely to die within 91 days than patients aged 35 years or younger [13].

2.4 Morbid obesity

Several studies have found that obesity, BMI greater than 30, is a risk factor for severe AP [14]. There is a strong association between circular obesity (central, abdominal-type obesity) and acute pancreatitis (acute pancreatitis). Obesity, especially visceral fat accumulation, increases the severity and complications of AP. Inflammatory state: visceral fat shows increased inflammatory activity, which contributes to more severe pancreatitis. Obese patients have higher levels of proinflammatory cytokines (e.g. TNF-α, IL-6), which increase systemic inflammation. Higher BMI is associated with a higher incidence of pancreatic necrosis. Activation of lipase enzyme from adipocytes may exacerbate necrotic processes. Obese patients require longer hospitalisation, and mortality from severe AP is also higher in those with significant visceral obesity.

3. Definition of AP

The disease is defined on the basis of meeting the "two out of three" criterion

1. Clinical signs (upper abdominal pain

2. Laboratory abnormalities (serum amylase or lipase elevation of at least three times the upper limit of normal)

3. Characteristic abnormalities seen on imaging computed tomography, magnetic resonance imaging, or ultrasound [15]

3.1 Mortalisation of AP

Mild AP < 1%, Severe AP mortality 15–30%, Multiorgan dysfunction syndrome (MODS) mortality up to 50–80% [16].

3.2 Main causes of death

Early phase (week 1)—SIRS and MODS, Late phase (>2 weeks)—sepsis complicating pancreatic necrosis [17]. Modern intensive therapeutic procedures (organ support treatments, targeted antibiotic therapy, minimally invasive surgery) can significantly reduce mortality, but in the most severe cases it remains high. Severe cases of acute pancreatitis (AP) often require intensive care unit (ICU) admission and are associated with a significant mortality rate. The mortality rate in patients with severe acute pancreatitis is approximately 20%, especially when pancreatic necrosis is also present [18]. Several clinical scoring systems, such as the Ranson criteria and APACHE II (Acute Physiology and Chronic Health Evaluation) scores, are used to predict prognosis. These systems combine demographic and laboratory data to estimate disease severity and mortality risk. During treatment, intensive fluid replacement and early enteral feeding with vasopressor therapy if necessary, are key to improving outcome. Recent research has shown that the one-year survival rate for patients with severe acute pancreatitis requiring ICU treatment is approximately 67%.

4. Systemic consequences of pain in AP

Pain during acute pancreatitis not only causes local discomfort, but can also have systemic consequences that affect the patient's general condition and the course of the disease. Severe pain triggers a stress response in the body, leading to activation of the sympathetic nervous system, increasing heart rate, blood pressure and respiratory rate. This places a greater strain on the cardiovascular system, SIRS can contribute to the development of organ dysfunctions, including cardiovascular and respiratory complications. Furthermore, the pain-induced stress response increases the release of inflammatory cytokines, which can exacerbate pre-existing inflammatory conditions and contribute to the development of SIRS. SIRS increases the risk of multi-organ failure and mortality in patients with AP [19].

5. Indications for ICU treatment in AP

ICU admission is region and unfortunately capacity dependent. According to the Society of Critical Care Medicine recommendation, patients diagnosed with AP who are found to have one or more of the following parameters on admission should be admitted urgently to the ICU: 1. heart rate < 40/min or > 150/min; 2. Systolic arterial pressure < 80, mm Hg or mean arterial pressure < 60 mm Hg or diastolic arterial pressure > 120 mm Hg; 3. respiratory rate > 35/min; 4. serum sodium <110 mmol/l or > 170 mmol/l; 5. serum potassium <2.0 mmol/l or > 7.0 mmol/l; 6. paO2 < 50 mm Hg; 7. pH <7.1 or > 7.7; 8. serum glucose >44.4 mmol/l; 9. serum calcium >3.75 mmol/l; 10. anuria; or 11. coma. Addition, severe AP (persistent organ failure) as defined by the modified Atlanta classification is also recommended to be managed in an ICU setting [18].

6. Causes and mechanisms of pain in AP

The mechanism of pain during AP is complex and is the result of a combination of factors. The pain mainly results from inflammation of the pancreatic parenchyma, enzymatic autodigestion and associated tissue damage [20].

6.1 Inflammation and oedema

In acute pancreatitis, inflammation triggers a cytokine cascade (IL-1, IL-6, TNF-α) that increases tissue oedema and inflammatory cell infiltration. Edema tensions the pancreatic capsule and surrounding tissues, leading to activation of nociceptors.

6.2 Enzymatic autolysis and tissue damage

Activation of proteases produced by the pancreas (trypsin, elastase, phospholipase) causes tissue destruction and cell death. Cellular damage increases the release of substance P and bradykinin, which act as inflammatory mediators to amplify the sensation of pain.

6.3 Visceral and somatic pain transmission

The splanchnic nerves and the celiac plexus are involved in the innervation of the pancreas. Inflammation and oedema increase the excitability of afferent visceral nerve fibres. Pain may radiate to the back and chest as pancreatic innervation overlaps with Th6-Th10 segments. In severe cases, inflammation of the peritoneum (peritoneal irritation) may also result in somatic pain.

6.4 Ischaemia and microcirculatory disorder

Local ischaemia due to oedema and microvascular thrombosis can also be a source of pain. Oxidative stress and hypoxia can lead to damage to nerve fibres, which further increases the pain sensation.

6.5 Neuropathic component

Neuropathic pain in pancreatitis is associated with a number of neuronal changes during acute inflammation. It is classically described as sharp, intense and hot pain, and a number of questionnaires have been designed to identify and guide the management of patients with marked neuropathic pain [18]. Neuropathic pain is caused by damage to the peripheral or central nervous system. This can result in damage to nerve endings, leading to the development of chronic pain conditions. In pancreatitis, neuropathic pain is thought to play an important role in the development of pain.

6.6 Neurogenic inflammation

Substances released during the inflammatory process, such as bradykinin and prostaglandins, stimulate nociceptors (pain receptors) in the pancreas and surrounding tissues. This stimulation transmits pain signals to the central nervous system, leading to the sensation of pain.

7. Mechanism of inflammatory response in acute pancreatitis

The inflammatory response to acute pancreatitis occurs in several steps. Initial injury and enzymatic activation: injury to the acinar cells of the pancreas leads to abnormal activation of digestive enzymes, which induces cell damage and inflammation. They attract white blood cells, such as neutrophils and macrophages, to the site of inflammation. These cells further enhance the inflammatory response and promote the removal of damaged tissue. Systemic inflammatory response: In severe cases, SIRS can lead to multiple organ systems being affected and cause serious complications. The pathophysiology of AP involves activation and release of pancreatic enzymes in the interstitium, pancreatic autodigestion, and multi-organ dysfunction following their release into the systemic circulation. The SIRS syndrome (SIRS) is one of the most important complications of acute pancreatitis, which presents as a severe form of the disease [19].

8. Consequences and pain relief of AP

In severe cases: ileus and intestinal necrosis may occur, pain-induced stress and inflammation: increases the production of proinflammatory cytokines (IL-6, TNF-α), promotes the development of SIRS, contributes to the development of MODS. In severe cases: persistent pain may contribute to the development of sepsis and infected pancreatic necrosis, increasing mortality.

9. Pharmacological analgesia

9.1 Non-opioid analgesics

The literature in English on the use of paracetamol (acetaminophen) in the treatment of pancreatitis is limited until 2000. Paracetamol is generally considered to be a safe analgesic, but caution is needed because of its hepatotoxic effects, especially in people with liver disease or alcoholics. Opioids are often used to treat the pain of acute pancreatitis, but paracetamol may also play a role in milder cases or as adjunctive therapy. However, the literature before 2000 does not contain extensive research on the specific use of paracetamol in acute pancreatitis. The use of paracetamol in acute pancreatitis remains a matter of debate and treatment guidelines have evolved since then. For the most up-to-date and comprehensive information, a review of the recent literature is recommended [20].

The role of diclofenac, an NSAID, in the treatment of acute pancreatitis has been investigated in several areas. Preventing post-ERCP pancreatitis: a 2003 randomised controlled trial showed that 100 mg diclofenac administered rectally significantly reduced the incidence of pain after endoscopic retrograde cholangiopancreatography. Pain relief in AP: A 2019 study found that both diclofenac and tramadol were effective, with no significant difference. A 2021 systematic review and meta-analysis concluded that NSAIDs, such as diclofenac, may be effective in relieving pain in acute pancreatitis and their use is supported in the absence of acute gastric renal injury [21].

9.2 Lidocaine in acute pancreatitis

In the treatment of (AP), lidocaine is of increasing interest, particularly for its analgesic and anti-inflammatory effects. Although treatment has traditionally been based on support (fluid therapy, analgesia, nutrition), in recent years a number of studies have investigated the intravenous use of lidocaine as a potential adjunctive therapy. Lidocaine may be beneficial in the treatment of acute pancreatitis through several mechanisms of action: analgesia, reducing pain transmission by inhibiting voltage-dependent sodium channels, and thus also having an opioid-sparing effect. Anti-inflammatory effect: reduces levels of pro-inflammatory cytokines (e.g. TNF-α, IL-6), which may reduce the development of systemic inflammatory response syndrome. Effect on intestinal motility: may improve intestinal function, reduce the incidence of ileus. Improving microcirculation: may support pancreatic microcirculation, thereby reducing organ damage. May shorten the length of hospital stay. May reduce the risk of complications (e.g. organ failure) by reducing the inflammatory response. Larger randomised controlled trials are still lacking, so the use of lidocaine in AP is not currently considered a standard therapy. Initial bolus: 1–1.5 mg/kg intravenously, administered slowly (1 min). Continuous infusion: 1–2 mg/kg/hour, to maintain analgesia [22].

9.3 Opioid analgesics

Reserved for non-opioid treatment of refractory severe or severe pain. The use of opioids for pain relief in severe pancreatitis is common [23]. However, the use of opioids in this context may be associated with several potential side effects that may affect the course of the disease and the patient's condition. These are: gastrointestinal effects: opioids often cause constipation, which can exacerbate the symptoms of pancreatitis. They can also reduce bowel movements and delay gastric emptying, which can increase the risk of intestinal obstruction (ileus): High doses of opioids can cause respiratory depression, which can be particularly dangerous in patients with severe conditions. Immune system effects: opioids may affect the immune response, potentially increasing the risk of infections, including those associated with pancreatitis Addiction and tolerance: there is a risk of addiction and tolerance with long-term opioid use, which may make pain management more difficult. Although a number of recent studies have questioned the side effects of AP. Opioid treatment only increased the risk of more severe acute pancreatitis when given for 6 days or more after the day of admission. Future randomised trials should reassess whether opioids can be safe in acute pancreatitis. Preferred agents: Fentanyl: Preferred in critically ill patients because of its haemodynamic stability and short half-life. Hydromorphone and morphine: Effective but associated with hypotension and ileus. It is recommended to avoid meperidine: due to neurotoxicity and seizure risk. Remifentanyl AP treatment is key for analgesia. Remifentanil is a short-acting opioid that is often used to relieve intense pain, especially in situations where a rapid onset of action and easy dosing are required. Due to its pharmacokinetic properties, remifentanil is rapidly metabolised, allowing for precise dose control and minimisation of side effects: remifentanil's rapid onset and short duration of action may make it advantageous in the treatment of severe pain associated with AP. It allows rapid relief of pain and fine-tuning of dosage according to patient needs. Side effects: as with other opioids, respiratory depression, nausea or constipation. However, due to their short duration of action, these side effects usually disappear quickly. Sufentanil is a potent opioid analgesic that is often used for the analgesia and sedation of intensive care unit patients. There is limited direct evidence on the use of sufentanil in the treatment of acute pancreatitis. One study found that the combination of midazolam and sufentanil improved sedation and analgesia and reduced levels of inflammatory cytokines such as tumour necrosis factor-alpha (TNF-α), which may potentially benefit patients with acute pancreatitis. Pass after stopping the drug [24].

9.4 Complementary agents

1. Gabapentinoids (gabapentin, pregabalin): their use for the modulation of neuropathic pain is currently not widespread [25].

2. Ketamine infusion: Provides opioid-sparing analgesia, especially for severe or opioid-refractory pain. Epidural analgesia: Considered for refractory pain, especially in patients with severe AP requiring long-term opioid therapy.

3. Alpha-2 agonists (dexmedetomidine, clonidine): provide sedative and analgesic effects without significant respiratory depression

10. Regional analgesia

10.1 Epidural analgesia

Effective pain relief, benefits in acute pancreatitis currently "Gold Standard" for intolerable pain. EA provides potent, controllable analgesia, reducing the need for systemic opioids [26]. It provides better haemodynamic stability than systemic opioids as it does not cause a significant drop in blood pressure. Improves splanchnic perfusion EA induces vasodilation, which may improve blood flow to abdominal organs (including the pancreas). Respiratory benefits. Improvement in intestinal motility. Ileus is common in acute pancreatitis, but EA may promote a return of intestinal motility, reducing the duration of intestinal paralysis.

10.2 Potential risks and disadvantages

Hypotension: Epidural blockade may cause hypotension through a decrease in sympathetic tone, which may impair perfusion in patients with volume deficits. Adequate volume replacement and monitoring is important. Coagulopathy and bleeding risk. AP is often associated with coagulation disturbances (DIC, thrombocytopenia), so careful coagulation monitoring is required before the introduction of EA. Contraindicated in active bleeding or INR >1.5. Risk of infection. In severe acute pancreatitis, sepsis or systemic inflammatory response syndrome (SIRS) may develop, increasing the risk of epidural infection or epidural abscess [27]. Medications used: Topically administered anaesthetics (e.g. bupivacaine or ropivacaine), mainly amide types low-dose opioids (fentanyl or sufentanil) and dexmedetomidine may be administered as adjuvant, Dexmedetomidine is a selective $\alpha 2$-adrenergic agonist widely used for sedation and analgesia in anaesthesiology. During epidural analgesia, the use of dexmedetomidine may enhance the efficacy of analgesia and reduce postoperative opioid requirements [28]. A 2024 systematic review and meta-analysis found that the addition of dexmedetomidine to local anaesthetics in epidural obstetric analgesia significantly reduced pain scores in the first 90 min without prolonging the duration of labour. However, it did increase the incidence of bradycardia among mothers.

11. Nondrug pain relief

Nasogastric or nasogastric tube feeding, early enteral feeding can reduce inflammation and help relieve pain. Percutaneous catheter drainage: Infected or sterile pancreatic necrosis can aggravate pain and drainage can provide symptomatic relief.

Psychological support and reassurance: anxiety exacerbates pain and anxiolytic agents such as benzodiazepines or dexmedetomidine may be beneficial in selected patients.

12. Delirium and psychological effects

Intense and untreated pain and its aetiology. Can lead to delirium and acute agitation (especially in elderly alcohol-dependent and ICU patients).

Increase anxiety and depression, may lead to Post Traumatic Stress Syndrome in ICU patients. In severe cases: delirium increases mortality and risk of long-term cognitive decline.

13. Conclusion

AP ranges from mild to severe and life-threatening, so its adequate recognition and treatment is the first line of treatment. The most common symptom of AP is pain of varying intensity. Untreated or inadequately treated pain increases the risk of complications and mortality, increases the development of SIRS and MODS, and thus increases in-hospital mortality and hospitalisation costs, so appropriate pain management is vital in AP.

Conflict of interest

The author have declared that no competing interests exist.

Abbreviations

ALP	alkaline phosphatase
BMI	body mass index
AP	acute pancreatitis
SIRS	systemic inflammatory response syndrome
MR	non steroidal analgesics
ROS	reactive oxygen radicals
TNF-α	tumour necrosis alphaintroduction

Author details

Sándor Márton
Medical School, University of Pécs, Hungary

*Address all correspondence to: drsmarton11@gmail.com

References

[1] Leppäniemi A, Tolonen M, Tarasconi A, Segovia-Lohse H, Gamberini E, Kirkpatrick AW, et al. 2019 WSES guidelines for the management of severe acute pancreatitis. World Journal of Emergency Surgery : WJES. 2019;**14**:27. DOI: 10.1186/s13017-019-0247-0

[2] Greenberg JA, Hsu J, Bawazeer M, Marshall J, Friedrich JO, Nathens A, et al. Clinical practice guideline: Management of acute pancreatitis. Canadian Journal of Surgery. 2016;**59**(2):128-140. DOI: 10.1503/cjs.015015

[3] Li CL, Jiang M, Pan CQ, Li J, Xu LG. The global, regional, and national burden of acute pancreatitis in 204 countries and territories. BMC Gastroenterology. 2021;**21**:332

[4] Fagenholz PJ, Fernández-del Castillo C, Harris NS, Pelletier AJ. Direct medical costs of acute pancreatitis hospitalizations in the United States. Pancreas. 2007;**35**(4):302-307. DOI: 10.1097/MPA.0b013e3180cac24b

[5] Pokras S, Ray M, Zheng S, Ding Y, Chen CC. The short- and long-term burden of acute pancreatitis in the United States: A retrospective cohort study. Pancreas. 2021;**50**(3):330-340. DOI: 10.1097/MPA.0000000000001757

[6] Mayerle J, Hlouschek V, Lerch MM. Current management of acute pancreatitis. Nature Clinical Practice Gastroenterology & Hepatology. Oct 2005;**2**(10)

[7] Tsuchiya T et al. The impact of alcohol consumption on pancreatic disease: An update. World Journal of Gastroenterology. 2021;**27**(2):134-151. DOI: 10.3748/wjg.v27.i2.134

[8] Herreros-Villanueva M, Hijona E, Bañales JM, Cosme A, Bujanda L. Alcohol consumption on pancreatic diseases. World Journal of Gastroenterology. 2013;**19**(5):638-647. DOI: 10.3748/wjg.v19.i5.638

[9] Barry K. Chronic pancreatitis: Diagnosis and treatment. American Family Physician. 2018;**97**(6):385-393

[10] Tenner S, Baillie J, DeWitt J, et al. American College of Gastroenterology guideline: Management of acute pancreatitis. The American Journal of Gastroenterology. 2013;**108**(9):1400-1415

[11] Wang X, Yu W, Jiang G, Zhang C, Sun P, Mao M. Global epidemiology of gallstones in the 21st century: A systematic review and meta-analysis. Systematic Reviews and Meta-Analyses. 2024;**22**(8):1586-1595

[12] Wang DQ-H, Afdhal NH. Gallstone disease. In: Feldman M, Friedman LS, Brandt LJ, editors. Sleisinger and Fordtran's Gastrointestinal and Liver Disease, Pathophysiology/Diagnosis/Management. 10th ed. Philadelphia, PA, USA: Elsevier-Saunders; 2016. pp. 1100-1133

[13] Sun H, Tang H, Jiang S, Zeng L, Chen EQ, Zhou TY, et al. Gender and metabolic differences of gallstone diseases. World Journal of Gastroenterology. 2009;**15**(15):1886-1891. DOI: 10.3748/wjg.15.1886

[14] Baeza-Zapata AA, García-Compeán D, Jaquez-Quintana JO. Acute pancreatitis in elderly patients. Gastroenterology. 2025;**168**:2

[15] Shin KY, Lee WS, Chung DW, Heo J, Jung MK, Tak WY, et al. Influence of

obesity on the severity and clinical outcome of acute pancreatitis. Gut Liver. 2011;**5**(3):335-339. DOI: 10.5009/gnl.2011.5.3.335

[16] Giorga A, Hughes M, Parker S, Smith A, Young A. Quality of life after severe acute pancreatitis: Systematic review. BJS Open. 2023;7(4):zrad067. DOI: 10.1093/bjsopen/zrad067

[17] Finkenstedt A, Jaber S, Joannidis M. Ten tips to manage severe acute pancreatitis in an intensive care unit. Intensive Care Medicine. 2023;**49**:1127-1130. DOI: 10.1007/s00134-023-07121-9

[18] Banks PA, Bollen TL, Dervenis C, et al. Classification of acute pancreatitis—2012: Revision of the Atlanta classification and definitions by international consensus. Gut. 2013;**62**(1):102-111. DOI: 10.1136/gutjnl-2012-302779

[19] Magyar Hasnyálmirigy Munkacsoport. Bizonyítékon alapuló ajánlások. Orvosi Hetilap. 2015;**156**(7):244-261

[20] Beiriger A, Khan A, Yan B, Ross H, WangM,CarducciM,et al.Comprehensive review of acute pancreatitis pain syndrome. Gastrointestinal Disorders. 2023;**5**(2):144-166. DOI: 10.3390/gidisord5020014

[21] Petrov MS, Yadav D. Global epidemiology and holistic prevention of pancreatitis. Nature Reviews. Gastroenterology & Hepatology. 2019;**16**(3):175-184

[22] VanDenKerkhof EG, Stitt L, Clark AJ, et al. Sensitivity of the DN4 in screening for neuropathic pain syndromes. The Clinical Journal of Pain. 2018;**34**:30-36

[23] Subramani SS, Berg AC, Kral LA, et al. Analgesia for the treatment of acute pancreatitis: A protocol for a systematic review and network meta-analysis. BMJ Open. 13 May 2024;**14**(5):e081971

[24] Cai W, Liu F, Wen Y, Han C, Prasad M, Xia Q, et al. Advances in the diagnosis and management of acute pancreatitis. Frontiers in Medicine. 2021;**8**:78215. DOI: 10.3389/fmed.2021.78215

[25] Augustinus S, Bieze M, Van Veldhuisen CL, et al. Intravenous lidocaine for refractory pain in patients with pancreatic ductal adenocarcinoma and chronic pancreatitis: A multicenter prospective nonrandomized pilot study. Clinical and Translational Gastroenterology. 2024;**15**(9):e1. DOI: 10.14309/ctg.0000000000000760

[26] Pandanaboyana S, Knoph CS, Olesen SS, et al. Opioid analgesia and severity of acute pancreatitis: An international multicentre cohort study. United European Gastroenterology Journal. 2024;**12**(3):326-338. DOI: 10.1002/ueg2.12542

[27] Sasabuchi Y, Yasunaga H, Matsui H, Lefor AK, Fushimi K, Sanui M. Epidural analgesia is infrequently used in patients with acute pancreatitis: A retrospective cohort study. Acta Gastro-Enterologica Belgica. 2017;**80**(3):367-371

[28] Liu M, Chen X, Guo D. Effect of epidural dexmedetomidine combined with ropivacaine for cesarean section. BMC Anesthesiology. 2024;**24**:134

Chapter 14

Heterotopic Pancreas

Farajee Soheyla

Abstract

Heterotopic pancreas or aberrant pancreas is a congenital anomaly that may affect variant parts of the gastrointestinal tract and lesser other organs, and there is no anatomical or vascular communication between HP and the main pancreas. It is mostly asymptomatic but can present as gastrointestinal manifestations such as abdominal pain or distention, nausea, vomiting and weight loss. It may be mistaken with other common conditions such as gastro-intestinal stromal tumor (GIST), leiomyoma, neoplasms or cysts. So that accurate diagnosis is important that can be facilitated by CT scan and endoscopic ultrasound (EUS) with fine needle aspiration (FNA). Asymptomatic HP usually may be monitored; otherwise, endoscopic or surgical treatment is indicated for symptomatic patients. In order to risk of complication development and adenocarcinoma arising from HP, monitoring and following up in observation management has an important role.

Keywords: heterotopic, pancreas, aberrant, pancreatitis, gastrointestinal

1. Introduction

1.1 Incidence

Heterotopic, aberrant or accessory pancreas is the most common anomaly after pancreatic divisum [1]. It is a part of pancreatic tissue without any vascular and anatomical connection to the main pancreas [2]. It is also a rare congenital malformation that may be found in different parts of the gastrointestinal tract, or even another organs [3]. It was reported in 1727 by Jean-Schultz for the first time and its pathogenesis is still vague [4]. It has an incidence of about 0/6/% to 14% in autopsies [4] and 0/2% in upper abdominal surgeries [5–7]. Sometimes it is possible to be recognized as a GIST in imaging studies [8].

1.2 Histopathology

In 1909, Von Heinrich classification divided HP into three groups histopathologically based on acini, ducts and islet cell elements [9]. Type 1: consists of ducts, acini and islet cells same normal pancreatic tissue. Type 2: pancreatic tissue with exocrine component (acini, ducts but no islet cells). Type 3: pancreatic tissue with frequent ducts, few to no acini and no islet cells. Later, a fourth group was added which consists of pure endocrine heterotopia, islet cells alone [10].

1.3 Etiology

There are some theses around the formation of HP, including metaplasia, misplacement and totipotent cell theory that embody cell alteration [11–13]. In embryonal age, during rotation of the foregut and fusion of dorsal and ventral pancreatic buds, some parts of tissue detached from the main tissue and form an ectopic pancreas and gain separated vasculature and innervation for function and survive [14].

Adjoining of pancreatic buds to foregut structures leads to the most occurrence of HP in upper GI (70–90%) [2, 15]. As it is found in duodenum (30%), stomach (25%), jejunum (15%), Meckel's diverticulum (6%), ileum (3%), mesentery, hepatobiliary system, spleen. And out of the GI system like the adrenal, mediastinum, lungs, fallopian tubes, umbilicus and omentum [6, 16, 17]. However, there are reports of HP in other regions such as adrenal glands that to date only three cases have been recognized, presented by non-adrenal disease and no change in adrenal hormone levels that was recorded as an incidentaloma in CT scan [18].

1.4 Macroscopy

In macroscopic examination, it is usually a yellow to white mass with irregular borders (**Figures 1–3**) [22].

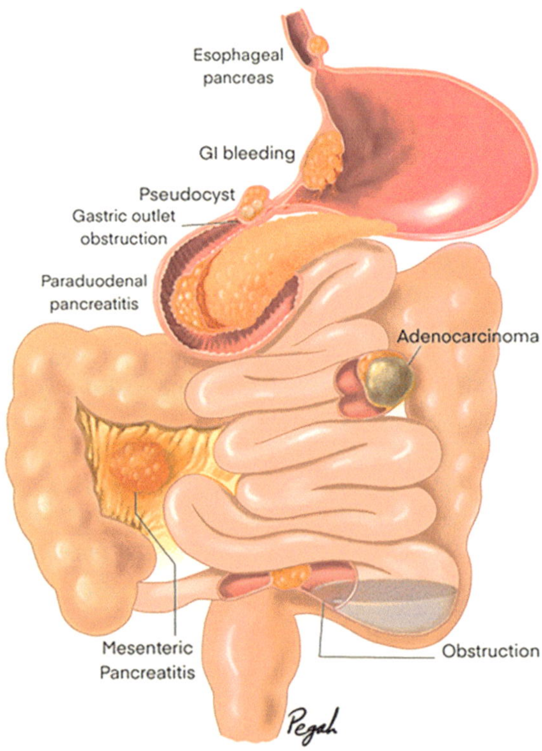

Figure 1.
A schematic view illustrates the most common locations of the heterotopic pancreas [19] including the gastrointestinal tract, Meckel diverticulum, mesentery, hepatobiliary system and spleen, also there are less common extra-gastrointestinal locations such as the mediastinum, lungs, fallopian tubes, umbilicus and omentum [17]. Major gastrointestinal locations of the heterotopic pancreas include the stomach, duodenum and proximal jejunum, probably due to their common embryonal origin [17, 20].

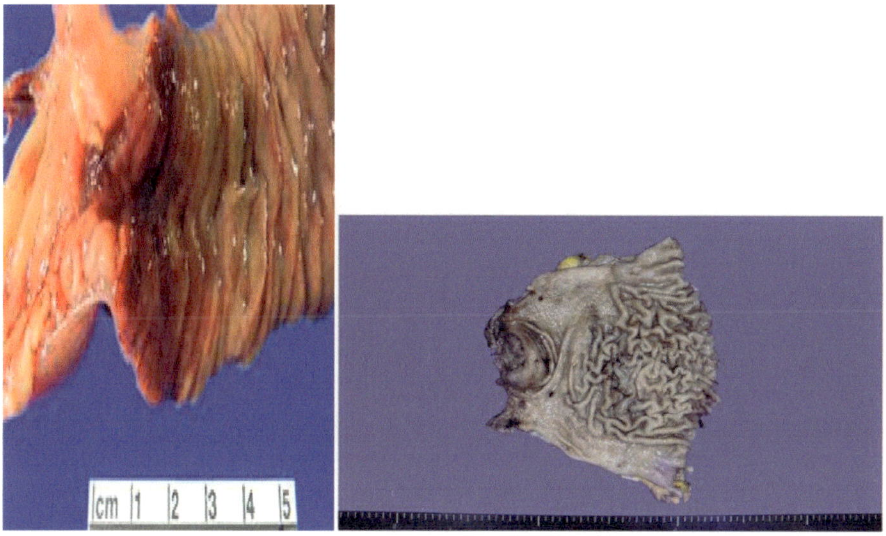

Figure 2.
Gross specimen of HP in duodenal fourth part (left) [21] and bulb with normal mucosa in appearance (right) [6].

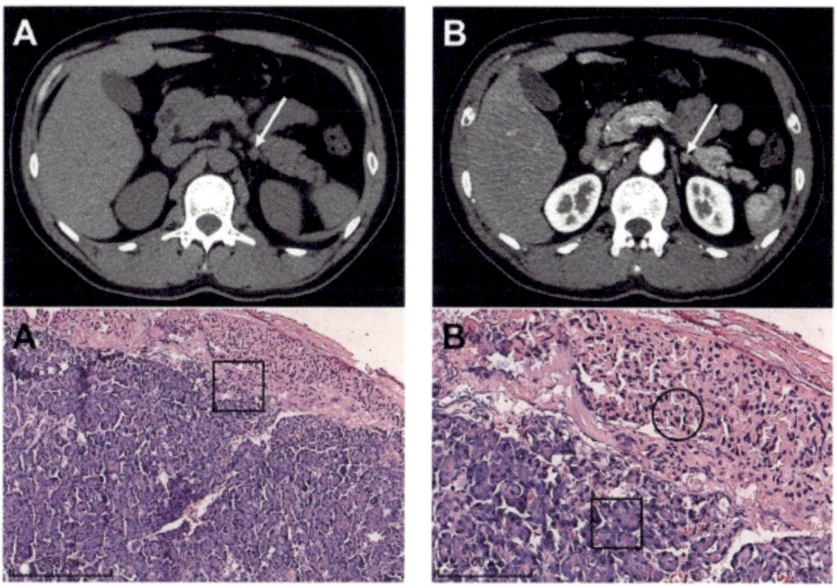

Figure 3.
Left adrenal HP, axial view in abdominal CT scan (above) and histologic examination with a transition zone between the HP and the adrenal gland (A). Acini of ectopic pancreas (black rectangle in B). The adrenal glandular structure (black circle in B) [18].

2. Gastric HP

Mostly it is a single lesion located in the antrum in 85–95% of cases by involving sub mucosal (73%), muscularis (17%) and sub serosal (10%) layers, measuring 3 cm or less in size but may reach to 6 cm [7, 23]. In some studies, it is reported mass in

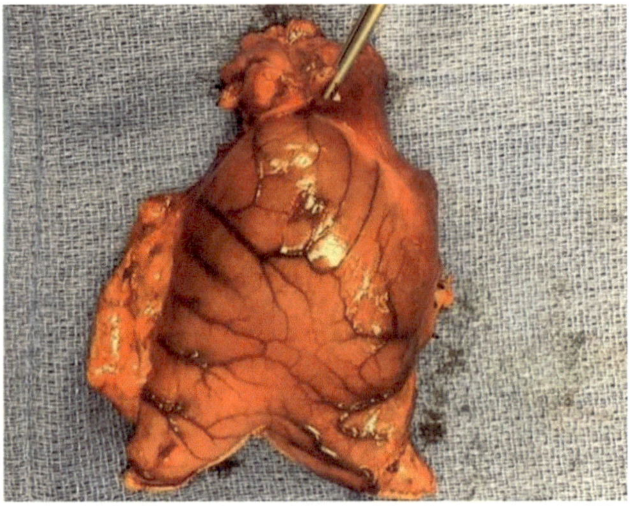
DOI: 10.3748/wjg.v28.i14.1455 Copyright © The Author(s) 2022.

Figure 4.
This is an intramural mass in the gastric antrum diagnosed as a HP [25].

other parts of the stomach as fundous [24]. Following the location of masses, gastric HPs cause obstruction (G.O.O) and nausea, vomiting and anorexia, but epigastric pain is another common presentation associated with mucosal membrane involvement (**Figure 4**) [26].

3. Clinical presentation

Symptoms majorly communicate to the local chemical irritation and inflammation caused by exocrine products [27]. It is thought that symptoms are related to the mucosal involvement extension as in a series by Lai et al., 49% symptomatic patients developed mucosal ulcers while asymptomatic patients lacked objective evidence of ulceration or gastritis [28, 29]. So that complications like perforation can be correlated with the degree of GI tract depth involvement. Extension of the HP lesions through the serosa may be shown in up to 4% of biopsy specimens [23].

But in non-ulcerative cases, the etiology of dyspepsia or abdominal pain is not detected, it is proposed that exocrine excretion of HP affects PH composition and leads to changes in the gastric environment and causes bloating, vomiting and other symptoms [30].

Clinical symptoms may include abdominal pain or distention, nausea, vomiting, dyspepsia, anorexia, weight loss and hematemesis and jaundice (**Table 1**) [31–33].

4. Lab tests

Usually, in the pancreatitis of HP, amylase and even lipase enzyme elevation are mildly because of a small volume of tissue in HP [19, 34].

Years	Total patients	Symptomatic patients	Mean age	Gastric lesions	Duodenal lesions	Location other than foregut	Abdominal pain	Dyspepsia	GI bleeding	pancreatitis	G.O.O(gastric outlet obstruction)	perforation	vomiting	jaundis
1947–2019	1761	978	43	556	378	44	620	445	80	260	80	3	188	37

Table 1.
Review study of 1761 patients from 1947 to 2019. Frequency of symptoms and other features [25].

5. Diagnostic tests

There are some modalities to distinguish HP, including ultrasound, CT scan, upper GI series, MRI, eshophago-gastro-duodenoscopy (EGD) and endoscopic ultrasound (EUS). But the findings of such tools are not completely reliable, so tissue sampling is more valid to determine the lesion [23], but a definitive diagnosis is based on histopathologic examination of the resected tumor [35, 36].

The most common computed tomographic appearance of a heterotopic pancreas is that of a small oval intramural mass with microlobulated margins and an endoluminal growth pattern. The attenuation and enhancement characteristics of these lesions parallel their histologic composition. Acinus-dominant lesions demonstrate avid homogeneous enhancement after intravenous contrast material administration, whereas duct-dominant lesions are hypovascular and heterogeneous. At magnetic resonance imaging, the heterotopic pancreas is isointense to the orthotopic pancreas, with characteristic T1 hyperintensity and early avid enhancement after intravenous gadolinium-based contrast material administration [17].

Appearance in endoscopy is typically smooth borders and central umbilicus [22, 37].

The GI wall is composed of five layers; the epithelium, lamina propria, submucosa, muscularis propria and serosa (advantitia). At usual EUS frequencies (5–12 MHG), these layers are shown in a five stratia pattern from the lumen out: first and second (mucosa and muscularis mucusa), third (submucosa), fourth (muscularis properia) and fifth (serosa and adventitia) [38, 39].

EUS shows focal thickening heterogeneity with inconspicuous margins, mostly in the second and third and less fourth layers of the upper GI with mild hypoechoic or mixed echogenicity in the submucosa [40]. Based on EUS characteristics, HP classifies to two groups: shallow type that derives from mucosal/submucosal layer and the deep type that expand to mascular properia and serosal layer and is difficult to differentiate from other transmural tumors like GIST [41].

A combination of CT scan and EUS has a complementary impression to the diagnosis of HP tumors than CT scan alone [42]. Fine needle aspiration *via* EUS may be indicated as the procedure of choice to achieve tissue from subepithelial lesions in the GI tract specifically in deep lesions [43, 44].

Biopsy should be taken deeply and frequently to achieve a diagnosis, because the lesion mostly located in submucosal layer [22].

Diagnosis of heterotopic pancreas is made by minding all aspects of clinical presentation, radiologic imaging, biochemical evaluations and endoscopic findings [45, 46].

6. Complication

Complications including gastrointestinal bleeding, bowel obstruction, intussusception, acute and chronic pancreatitis, gastric outlet obstruction, pseudo cyst formation, neoplasm, perforation and retention cyst and rarely pericarditis [19, 20, 26, 31]. Pancreatitis is one of the common presentations in symptomatic patients, in normal pancreas, it can be due to variant factors mostly, outflow obstruction and ductal degeneration [47].

As mentioned above, outer layers gastric wall involvement by HP can lead to transmural inflammation, necrosis and even perforation [1, 48] that happens in limited cases.

Paraduodenal pancreatitis is a remnant of HP in the medial duodenal wall that causes abdominal pain or even obstruction or intussusception [17, 49] and mostly affects middle-aged alcoholic-smoking men with chronic and repetitive pancreatitis. Conservative management is the first step (hydration, analgesics, etc.) but surgery is preferred in recurrent epidosed or malignancy concern and achieve complete regression of symptoms in 79% of cases and a 20% rate of complications. Pancreaticoduodenectomy and duodenal resection with pancreatic preservation (PPDR) seem to be the most effective treatment [50].

In esophageal and gastric HP, manifestations are gastro-esophageal reflux, epigastric burning, dysphagia, dyspepsia and possible hemoptysis [24].

Pancreatic enzyme-reached juice leakage can form a cyst that may be mistaken with duplication cyst or mucinous neoplasms and causes G.O.O in the stomach or obstruction in other parts of the GI tract [51–53].

There are few cases of retention cysts in HP, with a higher incidence in middle-aged men, in the stomach and then duodenum (jejunum, mediastinum, esophagus, spleen and kidney lesser) with a median diameter 4 cm [54–56] but sometimes it grows because of pancreatitis or hemorrhage [57]. Concluding neoplasms is challenging in this condition, so it is important to rule out malignancy in retention cyst (**Figures 5** and **6**) [58].

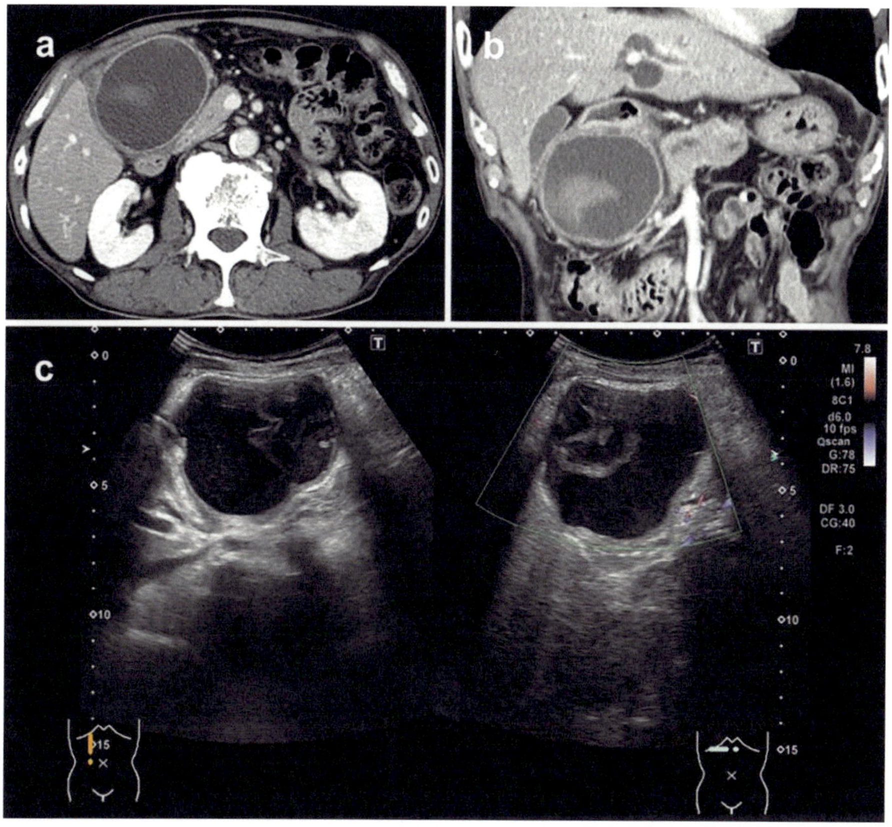

Figure 5.
Retention cyst of HP in the duodenum (figure). Contrast-enhanced CT scan (a, b) and U/S (c) revealed a cyst that has reached to 6 cm due to intra-lesional hemorrhage [57].

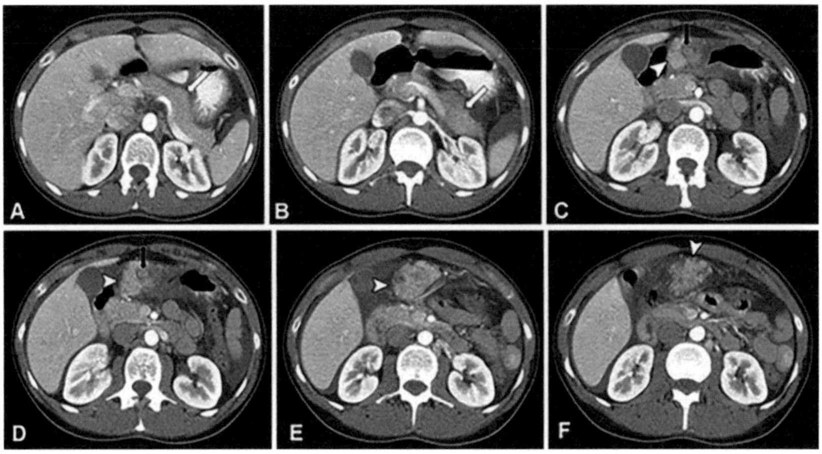

Figure 6.
Heterotopic pancreas complication as acute pancreatitis in a 28-year-old woman with complaint of abdominal pain and nausea (elevated serum lipase level of 1300 U/L). Axial contrast-enhanced CT images show the orthotopic pancreas with a normal appearance (white arrow in A, B). A lobulated mass is seen expanding from the gastric antrum with a similar appearance to the orthotopic pancreas (arrowhead in C–F), with surrounding fat stranding and inflammation. There is also a lumen structure centrally (black arrow in C, D) [19].

Intussusception following HP is an extremely rare phenomenon and occurs more in pediatrics, in the jejumum and ileum and often needs to surgical resection [59, 60].

7. Heterotopic pancreas adenocarcinoma

There are few literature around adenocarcinoma arising from HP, so adequate diagnosis and treatment is important. The estimated incidence of malignancy arising from HP ranges from 0/7 to 1/8%. Guillou et al. suggested the following criteria for diagnosis of malignant transformation of HP: 1-the tumor must be within or near the HP tissue, 2-a direct transition between the pancreas structure and carcinoma must be present, 3-the nonneoplastic HP tissue must consist of fully developed acini and or ductal structures (**Figure** 7) [61, 62].

It is arising from type 1 Heinrich mostly and showed that can be diagnosed by EUS-guided FNA before surgery [63–66]. In the histopathologic examination, the diffuse proliferation of differentiated cells that stain positive for cytokeratin [6].

In pylorus or duodenal HP adenocarcinoma, endoscopy and CT scan both show thickening and stricture of the lumen [6, 21].

Some studies propose early treatment of symptomatic HP more than 1 cm in diameter, particularly if causes obstruction or weight loss. Following patients suggests probably the prognosis of HP-induced adenocarcinoma is better than ordinary pancreas. Adjuvant chemotherapy performed for these patients with FOLFIRINOX and follow-up was uneventful (**Figures** 8 and 9) [65].

8. Treatment

There is a wide range of options in the management of the heterotopic pancreas, from observation to resection of organs. As well as endoscopic mucosal resection (EMR) can be used for the excision of some nodular lesions [40].

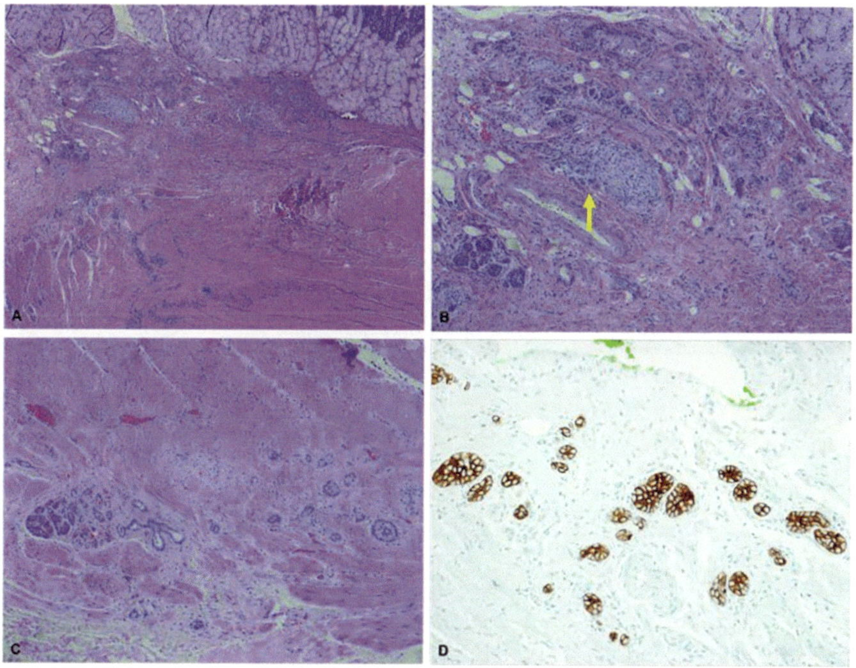

Figure 7.
Histopathological examination. (a) Diffuse proliferation of moderately differentiated adenocarcinoma transmurally (×40). (b) Tumor cells Invasion to nerve bundles (arrow) (×100). (c) heterotopic pancreatic tissue consisting of pancreatic ducts and some acini in the duodenal muscle layer was identified in direct transition to duct-like structures of the adenocarcinoma (×100). (d) stained-positive tumor cells for cytokeratin 7 [6].

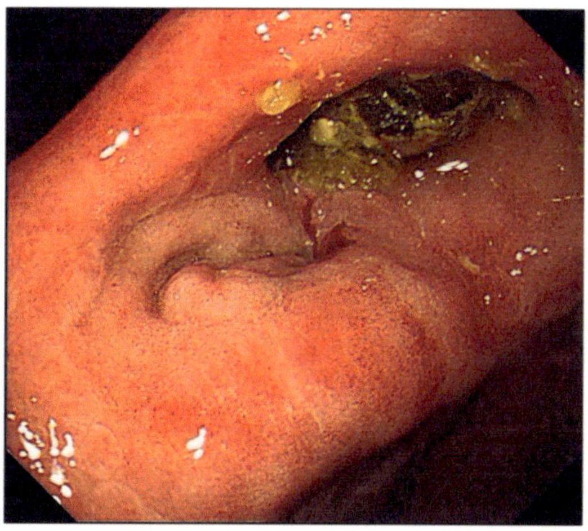

Figure 8.
Malignant heterotopic pancreas in duodenum. Esophagogastroduodenoscopy revealed deformity and stenosis of the duodenal lumen [6].

Endoscopic submucosal dissection is reported to be effective in the resection of complicated HP located in the muscularis propria layer [67].

For asymptomatic cases, observation is acceptable to monitor a patient for a long time, but in symptomatic cases, intervention has better outcomes [68].

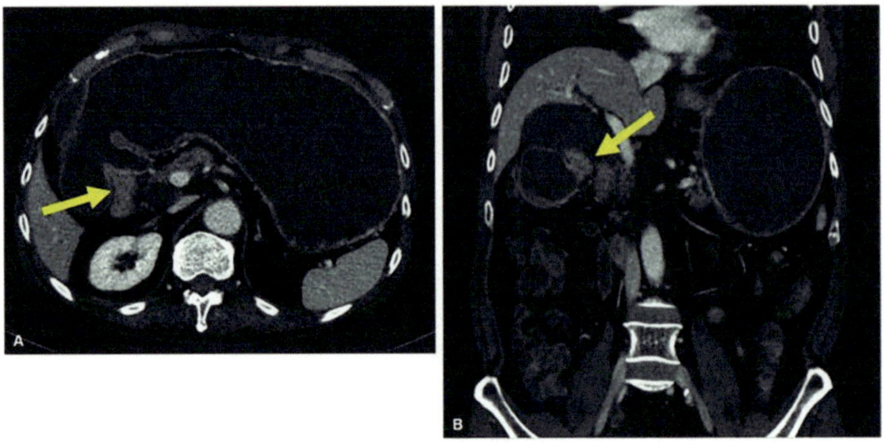

Figure 9.
Abdominal computed tomography showed wall thickness and stenosis of gastroduodenal junction in axial (a) and cronal (b) planes [6].

	n	**Percent (%)**
Distal gastrectomy	84	10.50
Billroth I reconstruction	14	1.70
Billroth II reconstruction	64	8.00
Roux-en-Y reconstruction	6	0.75
Gastric wedge resection	81	10.00
Subtotal gastrectomy	18	2.25
Total gastrectomy	5	0.63
Gastrotomy and local excision	42	5.30
Partial gastrectomy NOS	215	27.00
Pancreaticoduodenectomy	168	21.00
Trans-duodenal excision	19	2.40
Partial duodenectomy	7	0.90
Ampullectomy	2	0.25
Endoscopic submucosal excision	158	19.77
Total procedures	799	100.00

Table 2.
Different surgical and endoscopic procedure and reconstruction were used to resect heterotopic pancreas lesion in 799 patients [25].

It is notable that HP should be considered in patients particularly children with GI symptoms of uncertain origin and resection is advised [69].

In the majority of patients, symptoms dissolve after surgical resection of the lesion in ulcerative or non-ulcerative cases [70, 71]. In asymptomatic patients with pseudocyst formation, observation is a logical way but with recurrent flair up, cyst drainage or surgical resection becomes necessary to avoid further complications such as pancreatic head necrosis and duodenal stricture [51, 52]. In review studies, it is demonstrated that 85% of patients undergoing treatment cured, 9/7% improved and 5.1% not healed [44].

An effective comparison of medical treatment and surgical or endoscopic treatment in the management of HP is needed to reach valuable data for further evaluations (**Table 2**) [32].

Author details

Farajee Soheyla[1,2]

1 General Surgery Department, Madani Hospital, Alborz, Iran

2 Medical Faculty, Alborz University of Medical Science, Alborz, Iran

*Address all correspondence to: sohayla_f7_2012@yahoo.com

References

[1] Gurocak B, Gokturk HS, Kayacetin S, Bakdik S. A rare case of heterotopic pancreas in the stomach which caused closed perforation. The Netherlands Journal of Medicine. 2009;**67**(7):285-287

[2] Bromberg SH, Neto CC, Fernando A, Borger A, Franco MIF, Franca LCM, et al. Pancreatic heterotopias: Clinicopathological analysis of 18 patients. Revista do Colégio Brasileiro de Cirurgiões. 2010;**37**(6):413-419. DOI: 10.1590/S0100-69912010000600007

[3] Martinez NS, Morlock CG, Dockerty MB, Waugh JM, Weber HM. Heterotopic pancreatic tissue involving the stomach. Annals of Surgery. 1958;**147**:1-12

[4] Zhang X, Peng L, Wang Z, Pan F, Ren R, Li Y, et al. Extensive heterotopic pancreas in a rare site: A case report and a review of literature. Medicine (Baltimore). 2023;**102**(9):e32241. DOI: 10.1097/MD.0000000000032241

[5] Pang Y, Liu Y, Liu Q, Hou G. Intraductal papillary mucinous neoplasm arising from heterotopic pancreas in stomach: A case report and review of literature. International Journal of Surgical Pathology. 2023;**31**(5):708-713. DOI: 10.1177/10668969221117990. Epub 2022 Aug 9

[6] Woo CG, Lee J, Son SM. Adenocarcinoma arising from heterotopic pancreas at the first portion of the duodenum: A case report. The Journal of International Medical Research. 2023;**51**(8):3000605231194902. DOI: 10.1177/03000605231194902

[7] Song DE, Kwon Y, Kim KR, Oh ST, Kim JS. Adenocarcinoma arising in gastric heterotopic pancreas: A case report. Journal of Korean Medical Science. 2004;**19**:145-148

[8] Subasinghe D, Sivaganesh S, Perera N, Samarasekera DN. Gastric fundal heterotopic pancreas mimicking a gastrointestinal stromal tumour (GIST): A case report and a brief review. BMC Research Notes. 2016;**22**(9):185. DOI: 10.1186/s13104-016-1995-5

[9] Heinrich H. Ein Beitrag zur Histologie des sogen. Akzessorischen Pankreas. Virchows Archiv A, Pathological Anatomy and Histopathology. 1909;**198**:392-401

[10] Gaspar Fuentes A, Campos Tarrech JM, Fernández Burgui JL, Castells Tejón E, Ruíz Rossello J, Gómez Pérez J, et al. Pancreatic ectopias. Revista Española de las Enfermedades del Aparato Digestivo. 1973;**39**(3):255-268

[11] Khalyfa AA, Aslam R, Spyratos T. Heterotopic pancreas in the esophagus: What do we know?—a review of the literature. Gastro Hep Advances. 2023;**2**(1):144-146

[12] Tanaka K, Tsunoda T, Eto T, Yamada M, Matsuo S, Izawa K. Diagnosis and management of heterotopic pancreas. International Surgery. 1993;**78**:32-35

[13] Okamoto H, Fujishima F, Ishida K, Tsuchida K, Shimizu T, Goto H, et al. Intraductal papillary mucinous neoplasm originating from a jejunal heterotopic pancreas: Report of a case. Surgery Today. 2014;**44**(2):349-353. DOI: 10.1007/s00595-012-0486-0

[14] Kilius A, Samalavicius NE, Danys D, Zaldokas G, Seinin D. Asymptomatic heterotopic pancreas in Meckel's diverticulum: A case report and review

of the literature. Journal of Medical Case Reports. 2015;**9**(9):108. DOI: 10.1186/s13256-015-0576-x

[15] Ulrych J, Fryba V, Skalova H, Krska Z, Krechler T, Zogala D. Premalignant and malignant lesions of the heterotopic pancreas in the esophagus: A case report and review of the literature. Journal of Gastrointestinal and Liver Diseases. 2015;**24**(2):235-239

[16] Shalaby M, Kochman M, L; Lichtenstein, Gary R. Heterotopic pancreas presenting as dysphagia. American Journal of Gastroenterology. 2002;**97**(4):1046-1049. DOI: 10.1111/j.1572-0241.2002.05627.x

[17] Rezvani M, Menias C, Sandrasegaran K, Olpin JD, Elsayes KM, Shaaban AM. Heterotopic pancreas: Histopathologic features, imaging findings, and complications. Radiographics. 2017;**37**(2):484-499

[18] Yi D-F, Yang Q, Zhang P. A case report of adrenal heterotopic pancreas. Asian Journal of Surgery. 2023;**46**(12):5964-5965. DOI: 10.1016/j.asjsur.2023.09.006

[19] Brun-Vergara M, L, Khoshpouri P, Karp J, Sailer A, Pickhardt PJ. Heterotopic pancreatitis. Radio Graphics. 2023;**44**. DOI: 10.1148/rg.230167

[20] Kim DU, Lubner MG, Mellnick VM, Joshi G, Pickhardt PJ. Abdominal Radiology (NY). 2017;**42**(1):216-225

[21] Stock C, Keutgen XM, Pisapia D, Crawford C, Zarnegar R. Heterotopic pancreatic neoplasm presenting as an obstructing mass at the fourth portion of the duodenum. Journal of the Pancreas: JOP. 2011;**12**(3):241-243

[22] Hsia CY, Wu CW, Lui WY. Heterotopic pancreas: A difficult diagnosis. Journal of Clinical Gastroenterology. 1999;**28**:144-147

[23] Christodoulidis G, Zacharoulis D, Barbanis S, Katsogridakis E, Hatzitheofilou K. Heterotopic pancreas in the stomach: A case report and literature review. World Journal of Gastroenterology. 2007;**13**:6098-6100

[24] Samiee-Rad F, Farajee S. Heterotopic pancreas presentation as a fundal submucosal mass, a case report. European Surgery. 2019;**52**:43-47

[25] LeCompte MT, Mason B, Robbins KJ, Yano M, Chatterjee D, Fields RC, et al. Clinical classification of symptomatic heterotopic pancreas of the stomach and duodenum: A case series and systematic literature review. World Journal of Gastroenterology. 2022;**28**(14):1455-1478. DOI: 10.3748/wjg.v28.i14.1455

[26] Trifan A, Târcoveanu E, Danciu M, Huţanaşu C, Cojocariu C, Stanciu C. Gastric heterotopic pancreas: An unusual case and review of the literature. Journal of Gastrointestinal and Liver Diseases. 2012;**21**(2):209-212

[27] Biswas A, Husain EA, Feakins RM, Abraham AT. Heterotopic pancreas mimicking cholangiocarcinoma. Case report and literature review. Journal of the Pancreas: JOP. 2007;**8**:28-34

[28] Armstrong CP, King PM, Dixon JM, Macleod IB. The clinical significance of heterotopic pancreas in the gastrointestinal tract. The British Journal of Surgery. 1981;**68**:384-387. DOI: 10.1002/bjs.1800680606

[29] Lai EC, Tompkins RK. Heterotopic pancreas. Review of a 26 year experience. American Journal of Surgery. 1986;**151**:697-700. DOI: 10.1016/0002-9610(86)90045-

[30] McGarity WC, Perry CW 3rd. Complications of gastric heterotopic pancreas: Two case reports. The American Surgeon. 1971;**37**:77-79

[31] Iijima Y, Iwai S, Yamagata A, et al. Anterior mediastinal ectopic pancreatic cyst incidentally identified by pericarditis: A case report. General Thoracic and Cardiovascular Surgery. 2021;**69**:597-600

[32] Wilde GE, Gakhal M, Sartip KA, Corso MJ, Butt WG. Pancreatitis in initially occult gastric heterotopic pancreas. Clinical Imaging. 2007;**31**:356-359

[33] Sarsenov D, Tırnaksız MB, Doğrul AB, Tanas Ö, Gedikoglu G, Abbasoğlu O. Heterotopic pancreatic pseudocyst radiologically mimicking gastrointestinal stromal tumor. International Surgery. 2015;**100**:486-489

[34] Sandrasegaran K, Maglinte DD, Cummings OW. Heterotopic pancreas: Presentation as jejunal tumor. AJR. American Journal of Roentgenology. 2006;**187**(6):W607-W6095

[35] Eisenberger CF, Gocht A, Knoefel WT, Busch CB, Peiper M, Kutup A, et al. Heterotopic pancreas—clinical presentation and pathology with review of the literature. Hepato-Gastroenterology. 2004;**51**(57):854-858

[36] Karpińska MS, Nienartowicz M, Markowska-Woyciechowska A, Budrewicz-Czapska K. Heterotopic pancreas in the stomach (type II according to Heinrich) - literature review and case report. Polski Przeglad Chirurgiczny. 2011;**83**(3):171-174

[37] Yan HL, Wang SD, Yang JL, Wang Z. Gastrointestinal: Gastric heterotopic pancreas has potential of malignancy requiring appropriate resection. Journal of Gastroenterology and Hepatology. 2022;**37**(12):2205. DOI: 10.1111/jgh.15842. Epub 2022 Apr 20

[38] Sasaki Y, Niwa Y, Hirooka Y, et al. The use of endoscopic ultrasound-guided fine-needle aspiration for investigation of submucosal and extrinsic masses of the colon and rectum. Endoscopy. 2005;**37**:154-160. DOI: 10.1055/s-2004-826152

[39] Sepe PS, Moparty B, Pitman MB, et al. EUS-guided FNA for the diagnosis of GI stromal cell tumors: Sensitivity and cytologic yield. Gastrointestinal Endoscopy. 2009;**70**:254-261. DOI: 10.1016/j.gie.2008.11.038

[40] Lee TH, Wang HP, Huang SF, Wang TH, Lin JT. Endoscopic mucosal resection for treatment of heterotopic pancreas in the stomach. Journal of the Formosan Medical Association. 1999;**98**(9):643-645

[41] Kida M, Kawaguchi Y, Miyata E, et al. Endoscopic ultrasonography diagnosis of subepithelial lesions. Digestive Endoscopy. 2017;**29**:431-443

[42] Park JY, Lee ES, Hwang HW, Park HJ, Kim BJ, Choi CH. Heterotopic pancreas: The added value of endoscopic ultrasound with computed tomography for diagnosis. Medical Ultrasonography. 2021;**23**(1):22-28. DOI: 10.11152/mu-2704. Epub 2020 Nov 10

[43] Chatzipantelis P, Salla C, Karoumpalis I, et al. Endoscopic ultrasound-guided fine needle aspiration biopsy in the diagnosis of gastrointestinal stromal tumors of the stomach. A study of 17 cases. Journal of Gastrointestinal and Liver Diseases. 2008;**17**:15-20

[44] Watson RR, Binmoeller KF, Hamerski CM, et al. Yield and performance characteristics of

endoscopic ultrasound-guided fine needle aspiration for diagnosing upper GI tract stromal tumors. Digestive Diseases and Sciences. 2011;**56**:1757-1762. DOI: 10.1007/s10620-011-1646-6

[45] Elwir S, Glessing B, Amin K, Jensen E, Mallery S. Pancreatitis of ectopic pancreatic tissue: A rare cause of gastric outlet obstruction. Gastroenterology Report (Oxf). 2017;**5**:237-240

[46] Raman SP, Salaria SN, Hruban RH, Fishman EK. Groove pancreatitis: Spectrum of imaging findings and radiology-pathology correlation. AJR. American Journal of Roentgenology. 2013;**201**:W29-W39

[47] Mandal S, Mandal AK. Heterotopic pancreas presenting as a tumour nodule along with perforation and peritonitis is rare: Report of two cases. ANZ Journal of Surgery. 2008;**78**:725

[48] O'Malley RB, Maturen KE, Al-Hawary MM, Mathur AK. Case of the season: Ectopic pancreas. Seminars in Roentgenology. 2013;**48**:188-191

[49] Castell-Monsalve FJ, Sousa-Martin JM, Carranza-Carranza A. Groove pan-creatitis: MRI and pathologic findings. Abdominal Imaging. 2008;**33**(3):342-348

[50] de Ponthaud C, Daire E, Pioche M, Napoléon B, Fillon M, Sauvanet A, et al. Cystic dystrophy in heterotopic pancreas. Journal of Visceral Surgery. 2023;**160**(2):108-117. DOI: 10.1016/j.jviscsurg.2023.03.001. Epub 2023 Mar 23

[51] Jennings RE, Berry AA, Strutt JP, Gerrard DT, Hanley NA. Human pancreas development. Development. 2015;**142**:3126-3137

[52] Bryan DS, Waxman I, Matthews JB. Gastric obstruction due to intramural pseudocyst associated with heterotopic pancreas. Journal of Gastrointestinal Surgery. 2014;**18**:1225-1226

[53] Jain AS, Patel AM, Jain SR, Thakkar A. Accessory pancreatic lobe with gastric duplication cyst: Diagnostic challenges of a rare congenital anomaly. BML Case Reports. 2015;**2015**:bcr2014207751

[54] Sharma DK, Agarwal S, Saran RK, Agarwal AK. Pseudocyst of ectopic pancreas of the duodenal wall masquerading as malignant cystic tumor of pancreas. Saudi Journal of Gastroenterology. 2009;**15**(4):271-273. DOI: 10.4103/1319-3767.56101

[55] Barbu ST, Valeanu D, Muresan A, Munteanu D, Casoinic F. Cystic dystrophy of the duodenal wall in heterotopic pancreas with groove pancreatitis: A diagnostic and therapeutic challenge. Chirurgia. 2018;**113**:418-423

[56] Matsubara K, Ishida M, Morito T, et al. A rare case of enlarged gastric heterotopic pancreas with retention cysts: A case report and literature review. International Journal of Surgery Case Reports. 2020;**74**:284-288

[57] Kawaguchi S, Murakami A, Nishida M. Duodenal heterotopic pancreas with a large retention cyst: A case report and literature review. Internal Medicine. 2023;**62**(5):723-727. DOI: 10.2169/internalmedicine.0227-22. Epub 2022 Jul 22

[58] Gananadha S, Hunt DR. A unique case of pancreatitis and retention cyst in esophageal heterotopic pancreas. Surgical Laparoscopy, Endoscopy & Percutaneous Techniques. 2005;**15**:345-347

[59] Deng KH, Wei DH, Liu W. Ileo-Ileal intussusception by heterotopic pancreas. Clinics and Research in Hepatology and

Gastroenterology. 2023;**47**(7):102179. DOI: 10.1016/j.clinre.2023.102179. Epub 2023 Jul 18

[60] Kechiche N, Makhlouf D, Laamiri R, Zouaoui A, Mani S, Ksiaa A, et al. Intussusception caused by heterotopic pancreas: A Tunisian case series of 5 pediatric patients. Archives of Iranian Medicine. 2022;**25**(12):844-846

[61] Guillou L, Nordback P, Gerber C, Schneider RP. Ductal adenocarcinoma arising in a heterotopic pancreas situated in a hiatal hernia. Archives of Pathology & Laboratory Medicine. 1994;**118**(5):568-571

[62] Makhlouf HR, Almeida JL, Sobin LH. Carcinoma in jejunal pancreatic heterotopia. Archives of Pathology & Laboratory Medicine. 1999;**123**(8):707-711. DOI: 10.5858/1999-123-0707-CIJPH

[63] Yasuda K et al. The diagnosis of submucosal tumors of the stomach by endoscopic ultrasonography. Gastrointestinal Endoscopy. 1989;**35**(1):10-15

[64] Bini R, Voghera P, Tapparo A, Nunziata R, Demarchi A, Capocefalo M, et al. Malignant transformation of ectopic pancreatic cells in the duodenal wall. World Journal of Gastroenterology. 2010;**16**(10):1293-1295. DOI: 10.3748/wjg.v16.i10.1293

[65] Endo S, Saito R, Ochi D, Yamada T, Hirose M, Hiroshima Y, et al. Effectiveness of an endoscopic biopsy procedure using EUS-FNA and EMR-C for diagnosing adenocarcinoma arising from ectopic pancreas: Two case reports and a literature review. Internal Medicine. 2014;**53**(10):1055-1062. DOI: 10.2169/internalmedicine.53.1420

[66] Salah W, Faigel DO. When to puncture, when not to puncture: Submucosal tumors. Endoscopic Ultrasound. 2014;**3**(2):98-108. DOI: 10.4103/2303-9027.131038

[67] Noh JH, Kim DH, Kim S-W, Park YS, Na HK, Ahn JY, et al. Endoscopic submucosal dissection as alternative to surgery for complicated gastric heterotopic pancreas. World Journal of Clinical Cases. 2020;**8**(20):4708-4718. DOI: 10.12998/wjcc.v8.i20.4708

[68] Lee NJ, Hruban RH, Fishman EK. Gastric heterotopic pancreas: Computed tomography with clinicopathologic correlation. Journal of Computer Assisted Tomography. 2017;**41**(5):675-678. DOI: 10.1097/RCT.0000000000000606

[69] Persano G, Cantone N, Pani E, Ciardini E, Noccioli B. Heterotopic pancreas in the gastrointestinal tract in children: A single-center experience and a review of the literature. Italian Journal of Pediatrics. 2019;**45**(1):142. DOI: 10.1186/s13052-019-0738-3

[70] Ormarsson OT, Gudmundsdottir I, Mårvik R. Diagnosis and treatment of gastric heterotopic pancreas. World Journal of Surgery. 2006;**30**:1682-1689

[71] De Castro Barbosa JJ, Dockerty MB, Waugh JM. Pancreatic heterotopia; review of the literature and report of 41 authenticated surgical cases, of which 25 were clinically significant. Surgery, Gynecology & Obstetrics. 1946;**82**:527-542

Chapter 15

Medical Treatment of Acute Pancreatitis

Gulcin Ercan

Abstract

This chapter comprehensively examines the current approaches to managing acute pancreatitis (AP), a complex and potentially life-threatening inflammatory condition. It encompasses the fundamental principles of initial clinical assessment, fluid resuscitation, and pain management while emphasizing evidence-based strategies for nutritional support and pharmacological interventions. Additionally, the chapter explores the judicious use of antibiotics, considerations for minimally invasive and surgical interventions, and the management of systemic and local complications such as infected pancreatic necrosis and vascular complications. Special focus is placed on tailoring treatments based on the etiology of AP, including hypertriglyceridemia-induced AP, and addressing emerging therapeutic modalities such as low-molecular-weight heparins and enteral nutrition techniques. By integrating the latest evidence and expert consensus, this chapter aims to enhance understanding and optimize clinical outcomes for patients with both mild and severe forms of AP.

Keywords: acute pancreatitis, medical management, inflammatory response, pancreatic enzymes, fluid resuscitation

1. Introduction

Acute pancreatitis (AP) is an acute inflammatory process of the pancreas, with mortality rates ranging from 3 to 17%, depending on the severity of the disease and associated complications [1, 2]. Although there are regional and local variations, gallstones and alcohol remain the most common causes of AP [3, 4]. Gallstone-related cases account for 40–60% of AP occurrences, alcohol accounts for 10–20%, and hypertriglyceridemia accounts for 5–10% [3]. While alcohol-induced AP is generally associated with daily alcohol consumption exceeding 50 grams, it is worth noting that less than 5% of chronic alcoholics may develop AP for unexplained reasons [5, 6].

In cases where there is no history of gallstones or significant alcohol use, a serum triglyceride level exceeding 1000 mg/dL suggests hypertriglyceridemia-related AP. Although pancreatitis has been reported due to various agents and medications, the most commonly implicated agents include 6-mercaptopurine, azathioprine, isoniazid, loop diuretics, and didanosine [7, 8].

Recent epidemiological data have indicated that the incidence of AP is increasing globally, with rates ranging from 5 to 80 cases per 100,000 individuals [9]. This rise is attributed to factors such as obesity, metabolic syndrome, and increased alcohol consumption. Notably, AP is among the most common gastrointestinal causes of hospitalizations in the United States, with an annual incidence estimated at 13 to 49 per 100,000 persons. The risk of AP is similar among men and women and increases with age [10].

Understanding the pathophysiology of AP is crucial for effective management. The disease is initiated by prematurely activating digestive enzymes within the pancreas, leading to autodigestion and inflammation. This process can result in systemic inflammatory response syndrome (SIRS) and, in severe cases, multiorgan dysfunction. Early recognition and intervention are vital to prevent progression and reduce mortality [10].

This chapter provides a comprehensive overview of the current strategies for managing acute pancreatitis, a severe inflammatory condition of the pancreas. The chapter covers key aspects such as initial clinical assessment, fluid resuscitation, pain management, nutritional support, and pharmacological agents. It also explores the role of antibiotics, the management of complications such as infected pancreatic necrosis, and the criteria for surgical intervention. Emphasizing evidence-based practices, this chapter aims to outline the most effective treatment approaches, addressing both mild and severe forms of acute pancreatitis, to optimize patient outcomes.

2. Treatment of acute pancreatitis

The primary therapeutic interventions for patients diagnosed with AP include fluid resuscitation, pain management, and nutritional support.

2.1 Fluid resuscitation

Aggressive fluid resuscitation is essential to counteract hypovolemia resulting from third-space fluid losses and decreased intravascular volume [11]. In the absence of contraindications such as cardiovascular, renal, or other significant comorbid conditions, it is recommended to administer isotonic crystalloid solutions—either normal saline or Ringer's lactate—at a rate of 5–10 mL/kg per hour. For patients presenting with hypotension and tachycardia, a more aggressive approach may be warranted, such as an initial bolus of 20 mL/kg over 30 minutes. However, in cases of hypercalcemia, Ringer's lactate is contraindicated due to its calcium content [12].

The choice between normal saline and Ringer's lactate for fluid resuscitation in AP remains a subject of ongoing research. While some studies suggest that Ringer's lactate may reduce systemic inflammation compared to normal saline, the American Gastroenterological Association's 2018 guidelines indicate no definitive superiority of one crystalloid solution over the other [13]. Therefore, the selection should be individualized based on patient-specific factors and clinical judgment [14].

Regarding the use of hydroxyethyl starch (HES) in AP, evidence indicates that it does not confer a mortality benefit and may, in fact, increase the risk of multi-organ failure. Consequently, the administration of HES is generally not recommended in the management of AP [15].

Fluid requirements should be reassessed frequently during the first 6 hours after presentation and subsequently over the next 24–48 hours [16]. Targeted therapy can be adjusted based on parameters such as heart rate, mean arterial pressure, central venous pressure (CVP), urine output, blood urea nitrogen (BUN), and hematocrit levels. Adequate fluid resuscitation is particularly important when initial vital signs are abnormal. The goals include achieving a heart rate below 120 beats per minute, maintaining the mean arterial pressure between 65 and 85 mmHg, ensuring urine output exceeds 0.5–1 mL/kg/hour, keeping hematocrit levels between 35% and 44%, and normalizing BUN levels. Changes in BUN, especially at admission and within the first 24 hours of hospitalization, are effective predictors of mortality [17]. Patients with stable or increasing BUN levels may require additional fluid resuscitation. However, it is important to recognize that low urine output may reflect acute tubular necrosis rather than persistent volume depletion. In such cases, aggressive fluid administration may lead to peripheral and pulmonary edema without improving urine output [17].

Inadequate fluid resuscitation can result in hypotension and acute tubular necrosis [18]. Hemoconcentration persisting beyond 24 hours has been associated with the development of necrotizing pancreatitis, which leads to vascular leak syndrome, third-space fluid loss, and impaired pancreatic perfusion. Therefore, it is crucial to limit aggressive fluid resuscitation to the first 24–48 hours after disease onset. Excessive fluid administration beyond 48 hours is not recommended, as it increases the risk of intubation and abdominal compartment syndrome [19].

In summary, the cornerstone of AP management involves prompt and adequate fluid resuscitation tailored to the patient's clinical status, alongside appropriate pain control and nutritional support. Ongoing assessment and adjustment of therapy are crucial to optimize outcomes and minimize complications.

2.2 Pain control

In patients with AP, abdominal pain is one of the main symptoms, and managing pain is crucial for maintaining hemodynamic stability. Considering the pathophysiology of the disease, the ischemic process caused by vascular leakage and hemoconcentration may lead to pain and, subsequently, lactic acidosis. From this perspective, early fluid replacement is essential not only for hemodynamic stability but also for pain palliation [19].

Several small randomized controlled trials (RCTs) comparing different opioid and non-opioid analgesics in AP patients have not demonstrated any significant superiority of one analgesic over another in terms of efficacy or safety [20–22]. Additionally, a study comparing non-opioid analgesics (intravenous paracetamol, dexketoprofen) with tramadol in AP found them to be similarly effective for pain control [22]. Another study highlighted that, in AP patients, epidural anesthesia was effective not only for pain management but also for improving pancreatic arterial perfusion [23].

Opioids are considered safe and effective agents for pain control in AP patients [20]. Hydromorphone or fentanyl (intravenous) can be used for pain palliation in AP. Fentanyl, in particular, is increasingly preferred due to its better safety profile in patients with renal insufficiency. However, it is important to note that fentanyl, like other opioids, may cause respiratory depression. Fentanyl can be administered in both bolus doses and continuous infusion, and patients should be closely monitored for potential side effects [19].

In recent years, the use of meperidine in AP has increased, as studies suggest that it does not cause an increase in the sphincter of Oddi pressure, unlike morphine [23].

Nevertheless, there is no clinical evidence to suggest that morphine can cause or exacerbate pancreatitis or cholecystitis. Meperidine has a short half-life, and repeated doses may lead to neuromuscular side effects as well as the accumulation of its metabolite, normeperidine, which, though rare, can cause seizures. This risk should be kept in mind when using meperidine [19].

2.3 Nutrition

In patients diagnosed with AP, initiating enteral nutrition as early as possible is crucial due to its protective effects on the intestinal barrier and its role in preventing bacterial translocation. In mild acute pancreatitis (MAP) patients, recovery generally occurs rapidly, and oral feeding is typically feasible within one week, making management with intravenous hydration alone sufficient [24].

In patients with moderately severe acute pancreatitis (MSAP), nutritional support is required if oral intake is unlikely to be sustained within 5–7 days. If the patient does not exhibit ileus, nausea, or vomiting, and if pain severity decreases along with improvements in inflammatory markers, oral feeding can be initiated early (within 24 hours) with a low-fat, soft diet [25, 26].

For some MSAP and severe acute pancreatitis (SAP) patients, oral feeding may not be tolerated due to postprandial pain, nausea, or vomiting caused by luminal compression from fluid collections leading to gastroduodenal inflammation and/or gastric outlet obstruction. If these patients cannot tolerate an oral diet by day 5, enteral nutrition may be necessary. However, once local complications begin to resolve, oral feeding can be resumed as tolerated [19].

2.3.1 Oral nutrition

In a systematic review evaluating randomized studies on patients with (AP), early oral feeding (within ≤48 hours of hospital admission) was found not to increase adverse effects or exacerbate symptoms when compared to delayed oral feeding [27]. In four out of seven studies involving patients with MAP and MSAP, early oral feeding was associated with a reduction in hospital length of stay.

However, conflicting results have been reported in SAP. In a multicenter study comparing early oral feeding (within the first 24 hours) to delayed oral feeding (after 72 hours) in SAP patients, no significant clinical superiority was observed between the groups [28]. In contrast, studies comparing parenteral nutrition and delayed oral feeding (after 48 hours) with early oral feeding (within the first 48 hours) demonstrated the superiority of early oral feeding in terms of reduced rates of infected necrosis, organ failure, hospital length of stay, and mortality [29].

2.3.2 Enteral nutrition

In patients with MSAP and SAP who cannot tolerate oral feeding, enteral nutrition is recommended over parenteral nutrition [4, 30]. In patients with severe or necrotizing pancreatitis who require tube feeding, a feeding tube can be placed either nasogastrically (directly into the stomach) or nasojejunal (beyond the ligament of Treitz) *via* radiological or endoscopic methods. Enteral nutrition is also preferred for patients in intensive care settings, particularly those with organ failure or SIRS, who are unable to tolerate oral intake [19].

Two controlled studies comparing nasogastric and nasojejunal feeding reported no significant differences between the groups in terms of APACHE II scores, CRP levels, pain, or analgesic requirements [31, 32]. However, another small study comparing nasogastric feeding with parenteral nutrition recorded increased pulmonary and total complications in the nasogastric feeding group [33].

Enteral nutrition helps maintain the integrity of the intestinal barrier and prevents bacterial translocation. Compared to parenteral nutrition, enteral feeding has the added advantage of avoiding complications associated with venous access, such as vascular infections. A meta-analysis of eight studies demonstrated that enteral nutrition significantly reduces mortality, multiple organ failure, systemic infections, and the need for surgical interventions compared to parenteral nutrition [34, 35].

Due to reduced pancreatic enzyme secretion in AP, high-protein, low-fat, semi-elemental feeding formulas are preferred as enteral solutions. Enteral feeding should begin at a rate of 20–25 cc per hour and be gradually increased as tolerated to meet daily caloric requirements (25 kcal/kg of ideal body weight). If the patient experiences abdominal pain, vomiting, bloating, or diarrhea, enteral feeding should be discontinued [19].

2.3.3 Parenteral nutrition

Parenteral nutrition should be initiated only in patients who cannot tolerate enteral nutrition or fail to achieve the targeted enteral feeding rate within 48–72 hours, as the addition of parenteral nutrition to enteral feeding may cause adverse effects [36]. Studies conducted on intensive care unit (ICU) patients have reported higher rates of mortality, ICU-associated infections, and the need for renal replacement therapy in those receiving parenteral nutrition compared to enteral nutrition [37].

2.4 Antibiotic therapy

In patients with AP, prophylactic antibiotic use is not recommended regardless of the type (interstitial or necrotizing) or severity (mild, moderate, or severe) of the disease [4]. Even in SAP, studies evaluating the clinical benefits of prophylactic antibiotics have shown no improvement. Furthermore, these studies demonstrated significantly higher mortality and morbidity rates in patients treated with prophylactic antibiotics compared to those who were not [38, 39].

Approximately 20% of AP patients develop extrapancreatic infections, including bloodstream infections, pneumonia, and urinary tract infections [40]. Extrapancreatic infections are associated with increased mortality [17]. When an infection is suspected, antibiotics should be initiated while simultaneously identifying the source of infection. If cultures return negative and no infectious source is identified, antibiotics should be discontinued [19].

2.5 Other treatments

2.5.1 Pentoxifylline

Pentoxifylline, a nonselective phosphodiesterase inhibitor, requires further studies to determine its role in the treatment of AP. In a randomized study with a small sample size involving 28 patients with SAP, pentoxifylline was compared to a placebo when administered within 72 hours of diagnosis or until hospital discharge. The study reported that the number of patients requiring intensive care (0 vs. 4 patients) and those hospitalized for more than 4 days (2 vs. 8 patients) was lower in the pentoxifylline group. However, no significant difference was observed between the two groups in terms of inflammatory marker levels, including circulating tumor necrosis factor-α (TNF-α) [41].

2.5.2 Somatostatin and its analogues

The pathogenesis of AP involves pancreatic autolysis secondary to the activation of digestive enzymes. Somatostatin, a potent inhibitor of pancreatic enzyme secretion, can suppress the activity of the sphincter of Oddi, significantly reduce basal sphincter pressure, stimulate the reticuloendothelial system, protect gastrointestinal mucosal cells and hepatocytes, and decrease interleukin (IL)-6 secretion induced by TNF-α in human pancreatic periacinar myofibroblasts. However, studies have shown that somatostatin does not have a significant effect on complication rates, mortality, pancreatic fistula, or enterocutaneous fistula associated with AP. Additionally, studies investigating its efficacy in preventing post-endoscopic retrograde cholangiopancreatography (ERCP) pancreatitis (PEP) have reported conflicting results. Therefore, based on the current evidence, the routine use of somatostatin in the treatment of AP or the prevention of PEP is not recommended [42, 43].

2.5.3 Antifungals

The use of prophylactic antifungal therapy (e.g., fluconazole) alongside prophylactic or therapeutic antibiotics is not recommended. Fungal infections occur in approximately 9% of cases with necrotizing pancreatitis. However, it remains unclear whether these infections are associated with higher mortality rates [44].

2.5.4 Protease inhibitors

The role of protease inhibitors in the treatment of AP remains uncertain. Meta-analyses have shown that protease inhibitors provide only a marginal reduction in mortality in patients with SAP. Additionally, arterial administration presents another drawback [45]. At present, routine use of protease inhibitors in clinical practice is not recommended [19].

2.5.5 Probiotics

Although the use of probiotics in AP has been increasingly studied in recent years, evidence suggests that their effectiveness is limited. In the largest double-blind RCT conducted by Besselink et al., probiotic prophylaxis was found not to reduce the risk of infectious complications [46]. Moreover, it was associated with a higher incidence of intestinal ischemia and increased mortality. Similarly, a systematic review by Gou et al. reported that probiotics did not reduce the rates of pancreatic infections, hospital length of stay, or mortality [47].

2.5.6 Low molecular weight heparins (LMWH)

In the pancreatic circulation, thrombosis associated with endothelial cell damage, sludge formation, and stasis occurs early in the course of AP, as early as mucous swelling in the acini. The damage starts peripherally and extends toward the center, with fibrin accumulating at the distal end of the thrombus. Factor Xa catalyzes the conversion of prothrombin to thrombin, leading to the formation of fibrin clots. Low molecular weight heparins (LMWH) are molecules that bind to antithrombin III (ATIII) and enhance their activity. By activating ATIII, LMWH strengthens the inhibition of clotting factors Xa and IIa. The heparin-ATIII complex reduces trypsin and chymotrypsin activity and inhibits trypsinogen activation. The anti-inflammatory properties of heparin are distinct from its anticoagulant activity. Heparin reduces leukocyte adhesion to the site of injury and vascular endothelial cells, thereby mitigating inflammatory responses [48].

LMWH has been shown to downregulate endothelin-1 (ET-1), TNF-α, and IL-6, leading to improved microcirculation by reducing microthrombosis formation [49]. Additionally, heparin inhibits pancreatic enzymes and accelerates pancreatic regeneration during the disease course [50]. Experimental and clinical studies have explored the protective effects of heparin in the treatment of AP. Qiu et al. demonstrated the protective effects of LMWH against the development of pancreatic encephalopathy in rats with SAP [51]. Another study showed that LMWH reduces TNF-α and ET-1 levels, positively influencing morphological changes and vascular flow in SAP-induced rats [52]. In a study by Lu et al. involving 256 SAP patients, LMWH significantly reduced the incidence of pancreatic encephalopathy and improved survival rates in SAP [53]. Another study by Lu et al. on SAP patients reported that LMWH reduced mortality rates [54]. In an RCT conducted by Tozlu et al. on patients with MSAP and SAP, while no statistically significant reduction in mortality was observed, LMWH demonstrated significant effects in reducing both local and systemic complications [55].

2.6 Treatments based on etiology

2.6.1 Management of Hypertriglyceridemia

Hypertriglyceridemia is observed in patients with primary or secondary lipid metabolism disorders, including excessive alcohol consumption and poorly controlled diabetes [56]. When triglyceride levels exceed 1000 mg/dL and 2000 mg/dL, the risk of AP is reported to be approximately 5% and 15%, respectively [57]. A recent epidemiological study has found that even a mild increase in triglyceride levels is associated with an elevated risk of AP in susceptible individuals [58]. Another prospective study reported a higher risk of SAP and an increased need for intensive care in patients with hypertriglyceridemia-induced AP [59]. In patients with severe hypertriglyceridemia, maintaining triglyceride levels below 200 mg/dL significantly reduces the risk of recurrent AP episodes [60].

The triglyceride threshold for causing AP is defined as at least 1000 mg/dL by the American Gastroenterological Association (AGA) and the Endocrine Society, and at least 885 mg/dL by the European Society of Cardiology and the European Atherosclerosis Society. Recent systematic reviews have indicated that hypertriglyceridemia-induced AP can be significantly more severe compared to AP caused by other etiologies [61].

As with other causes of AP, the initial treatment of hypertriglyceridemia-induced AP focuses on fluid replacement and pain management. The primary treatment strategies for hypertriglyceridemia include apheresis and insulin therapy. However, no randomized trials have been conducted to directly compare the efficacy of these treatments. The initial therapeutic approach for such patients should be tailored based on the severity of AP and clinical features. If clinical findings include hypocalcemia, lactic acidosis, signs of SIRS, or organ failure, therapeutic plasma exchange (TPE) should be initiated promptly. In patients with MAP or those unable to tolerate TPE, intravenous insulin therapy can be administered to lower triglyceride levels to below 500 mg/dL [62].

2.6.2 Apheresis

Apheresis is a procedure that involves passing blood through a medical device to separate a specific component and returning the remaining components to the body. In patients with hypertriglyceridemia, TPE involves the removal of plasma and its replacement with a colloid solution (albumin or plasma). Currently, no studies directly compare the replacement fluids used in TPE (albumin versus fresh frozen plasma) in hypertriglyceridemic patients. Moreover, the efficacy of TPE in reducing the severity of hypertriglyceridemia-induced AP or other clinically significant endpoints, such as mortality, remains unclear. In a study comparing 20 patients treated with TPE to a control group, no significant differences were found in mortality or systemic complications [63].

2.6.3 Insulin therapy

In SAP associated with hypertriglyceridemia, the goal of insulin therapy is to counteract the stress-induced release of fatty acids from adipocytes, promote intracellular triglyceride formation in adipocytes, and enhance fatty acid metabolism in insulin-sensitive cells. Insulin reduces serum triglyceride levels by increasing the activity of lipoprotein lipase, an enzyme that accelerates the conversion of chylomicrons and very low-density lipoproteins into glycerol and free fatty acids [64]. Additionally, insulin inhibits hormone-sensitive lipase, a key enzyme responsible for breaking down triglycerides in adipocytes and releasing free fatty acids into circulation. Since hypertriglyceridemia is often seen in patients with uncontrolled diabetes, insulin can effectively lower both triglyceride and glucose levels. In this context, a treatment regimen similar to that used in diabetic ketoacidosis can be employed, aiming to maintain blood glucose levels between 150 and 200 mg/dL. This can be achieved by maintaining high plasma insulin levels while preventing hypoglycemia using dextrose-infused solutions as needed. Intravenous insulin is more effective than subcutaneous insulin in cases of severe hypertriglyceridemia, and its titration is easier to manage. Once triglyceride levels fall below 500 mg/dL, insulin therapy can be discontinued [65, 66].

2.6.4 Other treatments

Standard heparin and hemofiltration have also been used in the management of hypertriglyceridemia-induced AP. However, data regarding their use and efficacy remain limited [67].

2.7 Management of Complications

In patients with MSAP or SAP, if signs of sepsis or clinical deterioration are present 72 hours after initial admission, contrast-enhanced abdominal CT imaging is recommended to evaluate for the presence of pancreatic or extrapancreatic necrosis and other local complications [19].

2.7.1 Local complications

The local complications of AP include peripancreatic fluid collection, pancreatic pseudocyst, acute necrotic collection (ANC), and walled-off necrosis (WON). Acute peripancreatic fluid collections and ANCs typically develop within the first 4 weeks after the onset of pancreatitis, while pancreatic pseudocysts and WON generally occur 4 weeks or more after the onset of the disease [30].

2.7.2 Acute Peripancreatic fluid collection

Acute peripancreatic fluid collections typically develop during the early phase of PEP. These collections lack a well-defined wall, are usually asymptomatic, and often resolve spontaneously without the need for drainage. In a study involving patients with interstitial pancreatitis, most acute fluid collections resolved within 7–10 days, and pancreatic pseudocysts developed in only 6.8% of these patients [68].

2.7.3 Pancreatic Pseudocyst

A pancreatic pseudocyst is a well-defined, encapsulated fluid collection with a distinct inflammatory wall, typically located outside the pancreas and containing little to no necrotic material. Pancreatic pseudocysts generally develop more than 4 weeks after the onset of interstitial pancreatic edema. Even when detected *via* ultrasound, it is essential to differentiate pseudocysts from cystic neoplasms, pseudoaneurysms, or duplication cysts using cross-sectional imaging methods such as contrast-enhanced CT or magnetic resonance imaging (MRI). MRI has superior diagnostic accuracy compared to CT for distinguishing WON from simple pseudocysts. However, endoscopic ultrasonography is often sufficient for the diagnostic evaluation of cystic lesions identified on imaging, and additional imaging may not be necessary [69].
On cross-sectional imaging, pancreatic pseudocysts typically exhibit the following characteristics:

- They are generally round or oval in shape and well-demarcated.
- They are typically located outside the pancreas (extraparenchymal).
- The fluid density is homogeneous.
- There are no non-fluid components within the fluid collection.
- A well-defined wall completely encapsulates the fluid.
- No internal septations are present within the cyst cavity [70].

For patients with pancreatic pseudocysts, supportive treatments may include:

- Nasoenteral feeding: Provides pain palliation and nutritional support.

- Proton pump inhibitors (PPIs): Reduce gastric acid secretion and subsequent pancreatic bicarbonate secretion in response.

Drainage is indicated for patients with symptomatic, rapidly enlarging pseudocysts; those with systemic illness due to infected pseudocysts; or those who do not respond to medical therapy. Currently, endoscopic approaches, and less commonly percutaneous drainage, have largely replaced surgical techniques. Criteria for endoscopic drainage are

- The cyst must be mature (with a well-defined wall).
- It must be adjacent to the gastric or duodenal wall.
- The size should be greater than 6 cm.

Endoscopic interventions for pancreatic pseudocysts are

1. Transmural drainage: Accessing the cyst through the gastric or duodenal wall. Balloon dilation followed by the placement of one or more stents.
2. Transpapillary drainage: Draining cysts that are associated with the pancreatic duct. Involves placing a pancreatic stent, with or without pancreatic sphincterotomy [70].

The overall success rate of endoscopic methods for mature pancreatic fluid collections exceeds 90%. Procedure-related outcomes report morbidity rates of 10–15%, resolution rates of 70–80%, and recurrence rates of 10–15% [71, 72]. Endoscopic drainage methods have replaced percutaneous drainage due to lower morbidity, shorter hospital stays, and reduced catheter dwell times. However, percutaneous drainage can still be utilized for accessing retroperitoneal fluid collections, stabilizing septic patients before surgical debridement, or addressing immature collections where endoscopic access is not feasible [73]. In such scenarios, percutaneous catheter drainage serves as a bridging technique for patients too unstable for surgical debridement. In some cases, it may also act as a standalone therapeutic approach [74].

2.7.4 Acute necrotic collections (ANC) and walled-off necrosis (WON)

Necrotizing pancreatitis can present as necrosis involving both pancreatic and peripancreatic tissues. Necrosis can appear as ANC, which contains variable amounts of fluid and necrotic debris but lack a well-defined wall, or as WON, which is characterized by encapsulated pancreatic and/or peripancreatic necrosis with a mature, well-defined wall (**Figure 1**) [19].

Both ANC and WON on imaging share the following features:

- Heterogeneous fluid collections with varying densities of fluid and non-fluid components.
- A well-defined wall completely encapsulating the fluid collection.
- Presence within pancreatic or peripancreatic regions.
- No internal septations in the cyst cavity [19].

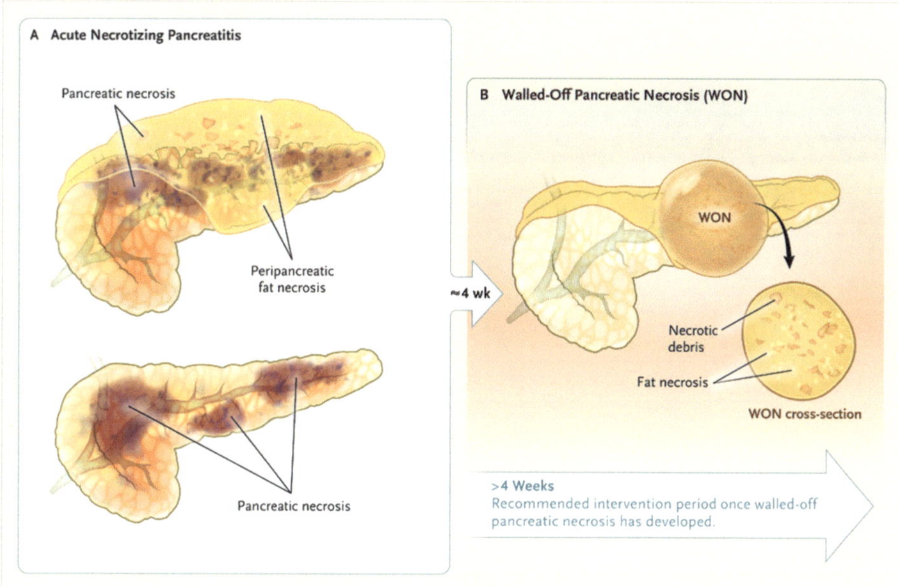

Figure 1.
The progression from acute necrotizing pancreatitis to walled-off pancreatic necrosis (WON). (A) Pancreatic necrosis and peripancreatic fat necrosis are characteristic of acute necrotizing pancreatitis. The necrotic regions seem inflammatory and are limited to the pancreas and surrounding fat tissue. (B) Necrotic pancreatic tissue can develop into walled-off pancreatic necrosis about 4 weeks following acute necrotizing pancreatitis. The picture depicts a well-defined, enclosed area with necrotic debris and fat necrosis. A cross-sectional image reveals the WON's interior structure. Interventions are indicated after ≥4 weeks, when the necrotic tissue has developed a mature wall, making treatments safer [74].

For the treatment of WON, minimally invasive techniques such as percutaneous drainage, endoscopic transmural drainage, and minimally invasive retroperitoneal necrosectomy have been developed. These techniques are as effective as minimally invasive surgery in terms of clinical success for infected and/or symptomatic WON [75]. However, endoscopic approaches have demonstrated lower rates of pancreatic fistulas and reduced hospital stay durations [2]. In a prospective long-term follow-up of 35 patients with SAP, those in the endoscopic approach group exhibited lower rates of diabetes, exocrine insufficiency, and hospital readmissions [76]. The challenges of suboptimal drainage in WON using plastic double-pigtail stents have been recently addressed with the advent of lumen-apposing metal stents (LAMS). LAMS achieves technical success rates exceeding 90%, with numerous studies supporting its clinical efficacy (**Figure 2**) [77, 78].

Complications associated with LAMS include bleeding (1–7%), perforation (1–2%), stent migration (1–6%), and infection (1–11%) [79]. In a randomized controlled trial (RCT) involving 60 patients undergoing endoscopic drainage, no differences in clinical success were observed between the groups treated with LAMS or double-pigtail plastic stents. However, stent-related adverse events were significantly higher with LAMS (32.3%) compared to double-pigtail plastic stents (6.9%) [80].

To minimize adverse events with LAMS, patients should be reassessed within 3–4 weeks, and the stents should be removed if WON has fully or partially resolved. If WON is only partially resolved, replacing the LAMS with double-pigtail plastic stents is recommended, as most of these patients are at risk of developing disconnected duct syndrome [19].

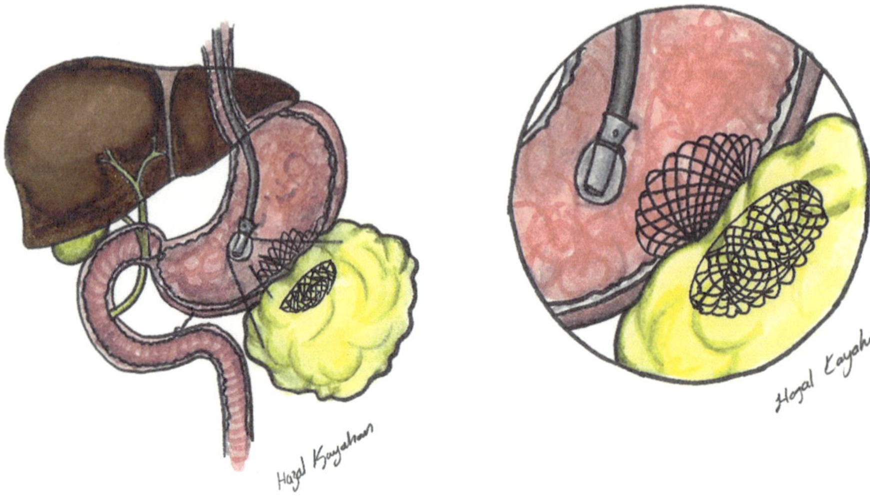

Figure 2.
Creation of a cystgastrostomy with EUS-guided placement of a lumen-apposing metal stent.

2.8 Surgical indications in acute pancreatitis

Conventional absolute indications for surgery in acute pancreatitis include hemorrhage unsuitable for angioembolization, bowel infarction, and perforation. SAP is a risk factor for abdominal compartment syndrome due to visceral and retroperitoneal edema. In cases where nonsurgical treatment fails, surgical abdominal decompression may be required [81].

Other indications for surgical debridement and decompression include infected pancreatic necrosis and symptomatic sterile necrosis characterized by persistent low-grade fever, nausea, lethargy, and anorexia. The goal of pancreatic debridement is to preserve viable pancreatic tissue, control potential pancreatic fistulas, and limit collateral organ damage while removing all necrotic pancreatic and peripancreatic tissue [82]. The surgical indications in acute pancreatitis are summarized:

- Hemorrhages not amenable to angioembolization, bowel infarction, and perforation.

- Infected pancreatic necrosis or symptomatic sterile necrosis characterized by chronic low-grade fever, nausea, lethargy, and anorexia, unresponsive to percutaneous or endoscopic interventions.

- Abdominal compartment syndrome.

- Hemorrhages refractory to endovascular approaches.

- Bowel ischemia or acute necrotizing cholecystitis developing during acute pancreatitis.

- Bowel fistula extending into a peripancreatic collection [19].

2.8.1 Infected necrosis

Pancreatic infection is a leading cause of morbidity and mortality in acute necrotizing pancreatitis. Approximately one-third of patients with pancreatic necrosis develop infected necrosis [83]. There is no correlation between the degree of necrosis and the risk of infection. Although infection can occur early during necrotizing pancreatitis, it is more commonly observed in the late phase (after 10 days) [84]. Most infections (approximately 75%) are monomicrobial and are caused by gut-derived organisms, such as *Escherichia coli*, Pseudomonas, Klebsiella, and Enterococcus. In patients with worsening clinical status (e.g., clinical instability, sepsis physiology, increased white blood cell count, fever) 7–10 days after hospital admission and with evidence of pancreatic or extrapancreatic necrosis, infected necrosis should be suspected [85].

Pancreatic infection should also be considered in the presence of clinical signs of infection and gas-containing necrotic areas on abdominal imaging. In such cases, antimicrobial therapy can be initiated without aspiration for culture sampling [86]. For empirical antibiotic therapy, agents that penetrate pancreatic necrosis should be chosen. Options include monotherapy with a carbapenem or a combination therapy with quinolone, ceftazidime, or cefepime paired with an anaerobic agent such as metronidazole. Some patients with infected necrosis improve clinically without any intervention. However, in certain cases of infected necrosis without WON, temporary percutaneous drainage may be required [87].

2.8.2 Sterile necrosis

If aspirated material is sterile, antibiotics should be discontinued, and conservative management can continue for 4–6 weeks. Antibiotics are not recommended for patients with sterile necrosis to prevent the development of infected necrosis. Sterile necrosis does not require treatment [19].

Intervention (radiological, endoscopic, or surgical) for patients with sterile necrosis without signs of infection (e.g., fever, hypotension, and leukocytosis) is indicated in the following situations:

- 4 to 8 weeks after the onset of AP: Persistent gastric outlet obstruction, bowel obstruction, or biliary obstruction due to mass effect.
- After 8 weeks: Persistent symptoms, including abdominal pain, nausea, vomiting, anorexia, or weight loss.
- After 8 weeks: Symptomatic necrotic collections (pain or obstruction) associated with disconnected duct syndrome (complete transection of the pancreatic duct) [88].

2.9 Peripancreatic vascular complications

2.9.1 Splanchnic venous thrombosis

Splanchnic vein thrombosis (involving the splenic, portal, and/or superior mesenteric veins) is a complication that can occur in 1–24% of patients with AP, depending on the severity of the disease and the imaging modality used [89].

Treatment should focus on the underlying pancreatitis, as thrombosis may resolve spontaneously. Despite the potential risk of bleeding into pancreatic necrosis or fluid collections, anticoagulation should be initiated if the thrombus extends to the portal or superior mesenteric vein or if signs of decompensation due to impaired bowel or liver perfusion are present. In contrast to patients with splanchnic vein thrombosis secondary to chronic pancreatitis, complications such as variceal bleeding are rare in AP patients. Therefore, prophylactic splenectomy is not recommended in AP [90].

2.9.2 Pseudoaneurysms

Pseudoaneurysms are rare but serious complications of AP. They should be suspected in patients with unexplained gastrointestinal bleeding, a sudden drop in hematocrit levels, or a rapid increase in peripancreatic fluid collections [19].

2.9.3 Abdominal compartment syndrome

Abdominal compartment syndrome is defined as a sustained intra-abdominal pressure > 20 mmHg accompanied by new-onset organ failure. Patients with SAP are at high risk of developing intra-abdominal hypertension and abdominal compartment syndrome due to aggressive fluid resuscitation, peripancreatic inflammation, ascites, and ileus-related tissue edema [91]. Patients in the intensive care unit should be monitored for possible abdominal compartment syndrome through serial bladder pressure measurements [92].

2.10 Systemic complications

Patients with AP are at high risk for exacerbations of underlying comorbidities, such as coronary artery disease and chronic lung disease. In addition to treating these exacerbations, management should address other complications, including alcohol withdrawal and hyperglycemia. AP patients also face an increased risk of developing prediabetes and diabetes after the first episode of AP. A meta-analysis of 24 prospective studies involving 1102 patients with a first episode of AP reported that 15% of cases were diagnosed with new-onset diabetes mellitus (DM) within 12 months [93].

3. Conclusions

The management of acute pancreatitis requires a multidisciplinary and evidence-based approach that addresses both the underlying pathology and the systemic complications associated with the disease. This chapter highlights the critical importance of early intervention through adequate fluid resuscitation, pain control, and the timely initiation of enteral nutrition to maintain gut integrity and prevent complications. For severe cases, particularly those involving infected necrosis or SIRS, individualized treatment strategies incorporating antibiotics, minimally invasive procedures, or surgery may be necessary. Advances in understanding the pathophysiology of AP have expanded therapeutic options, such as the targeted use of low-molecular-weight heparins and apheresis for hypertriglyceridemia-induced cases. Ongoing research and refinement of clinical guidelines will continue to shape the management of AP, improving survival rates and reducing the burden of complications. Ultimately, personalized care, informed by patient-specific factors and disease severity, remains pivotal to optimizing outcomes in acute pancreatitis.

Acknowledgements

The author thanks Hazal Kayahan for the figure. The author acknowledges the use of ChatGPT for language polishing of the manuscript.

Conflict of interest

The author declares no conflict of interest.

Appendices and nomenclature

AP	acute pancreatitis
MAP	mild acute pancreatitis
MSAP	moderately severe acute pancreatitis
SAP	severe acute pancreatitis
WON	walled-off necrosis
ANC	acute necrotic collection
SIRS	systemic inflammatory response syndrome
TPD	therapeutic plasma exchange
LAMS	lumen-apposing metal stent
CT	computed tomography
MRI	magnetic resonance imaging
US	ultrasound
ET-1	endothelin-1
TNF-α	tumor necrosis factor-alpha
IL-6	interleukin-6
PPIs	proton pump inhibitors
DM	diabetes mellitus
BISAP	bedside index for severity in acute pancreatitis
CECT	contrast-enhanced computed tomography
ATIII	antithrombin III

Author details

Gulcin Ercan
Department of General Surgery, Sultan 2. Abdulhamid Khan Training and Research Hospital, Istanbul Provincial Directorate of Health, Istanbul, Turkey

*Address all correspondence to: ghepgul@hotmail.com

References

[1] Singh VK, Bollen TL, Wu BU, Repas K, Maurer R, Yu S, et al. An assessment of the severity of interstitial pancreatitis. Clinical Gastroenterology and Hepatology. 2011;**9**(12):1098-1103

[2] van Brunschot S, van Grinsven J, van Santvoort HC, Bakker OJ, Besselink MG, Boermeester MA, et al. Endoscopic or surgical step-up approach for infected necrotising pancreatitis: A multicentre randomised trial. Lancet. 2018;**391**(10115):51-58

[3] Roberts SE, Morrison-Rees S, John A, Williams JG, Brown TH, Samuel DG, et al. The incidence and aetiology of acute pancreatitis across Europe. Pancreatology. 2017;**17**(2):155-165

[4] Tenner S, Baillie J, DeWitt J, Vege SS, American College of Gastroenterology. American College of Gastroenterology guideline: Management of acute pancreatitis. The American Journal of Gastroenterology. 2013;**108**(9):1400-1415;1416. Erratum in: Am J Gastroenterol. 2014;109(2):302

[5] Lankisch PG, Lowenfels AB, Maisonneuve P. What is the risk of alcoholic pancreatitis in heavy drinkers? Pancreas. 2002;**25**(4):411-412

[6] Steinberg W, Tenner S. Acute pancreatitis. The New England Journal of Medicine. 1994;**330**(17):1198-1210

[7] James TW, Crockett SD. Management of acute pancreatitis in the first 72 hours. Current Opinion in Gastroenterology. 2018;**34**(5):330-335

[8] Yadav D, Pitchumoni CS. Issues in hyperlipidemic pancreatitis. Journal of Clinical Gastroenterology. 2003;**36**(1):54-62

[9] Sekimoto M, Takada T, Kawarada Y, et al. JPN guidelines for the management of acute pancreatitis: Epidemiology, etiology, natural history, and outcome predictors in acute pancreatitis. Journal of Hepato-Biliary-Pancreatic Surgery. 2006;**13**:10-24. DOI: 10.1007/s00534-005-1047-3

[10] Mederos MA, Reber HA, Girgis MD. Acute pancreatitis: A review. JAMA. 2021;**325**(4):382-390. DOI: 10.1001/jama.2020.20317

[11] De-Madaria E, Buxbaum JL, Maisonneuve P, et al. Aggressive or moderate fluid resuscitation in acute pancreatitis. The New England Journal of Medicine. 2022;**387**(11):989-1000. DOI: 10.1056/NEJMoa2202884

[12] Guilabert L, Cárdenas-Jaén K, Vaillo-Rocamora A, et al. Normal saline versus lactated Ringer's solution for acute pancreatitis resuscitation, an open-label multicenter randomized controlled trial: The WATERLAND trial study protocol. Trials. 2024;**25**:699. DOI: 10.1186/s13063-024-08539-2

[13] Vege SS, DiMagno MJ, Forsmark CE, Martel M, Barkun AN. Initial medical treatment of acute pancreatitis: American Gastroenterological Association Institute technical review. Gastroenterology. 2018;**154**(4):1103-1139

[14] Gardner TB, Vege SS, Pearson RK, Chari ST. Fluid resuscitation in acute pancreatitis. Clinical Gastroenterology and Hepatology. 2008;**6**(10):1070-1076. DOI: 10.1016/j.cgh.2008.05.005

[15] Tenner S. Initial management of acute pancreatitis: Critical issues during the first 72 hours. The American Journal of Gastroenterology.

2004;**99**(12):2489-2494. DOI: 10.1111/j.1572-0241.2004.40329

[16] Mao EQ, Tang YQ, Fei J, et al. Fluid therapy for severe acute pancreatitis in acute response stage. Chinese Medical Journal. 2009;**122**(2):169-173. DOI: 10.3760/cma.j.issn.0366-6999.2009.02.011

[17] Wu BU, Johannes RS, Sun X, et al. The early prediction of mortality in acute pancreatitis: A large population-based study. Gut. 2008;**57**(12):1698-1703. Available from: https://gut.bmj.com/content/57/12/1698

[18] Whitcomb DC, Muddana V, Langmead CJ, Houghton FD Jr, Guenther A, Eagon PK, et al. Angiopoietin-2, a regulator of vascular permeability in inflammation, is associated with persistent organ failure in patients with acute pancreatitis from the United States and Germany. The American Journal of Gastroenterology. 2010;**105**(10):2287-2292

[19] Binicier ÖB, Patır DÇ. Treatment of acute pancreatitis. Turkiye Klinikleri Journal of Internal Medicine. 2021;**6**:22-38

[20] Basurto, Ona X, Rigau Comas D, Urrútia G. Opioids for acute pancreatitis pain. Cochrane Database of Systematic Reviews. 2013;(7):CD009179. DOI: 10.1002/14651858.CD009179.pub2

[21] Gülen B, Dur A, Serinken M, Karcıoğlu Ö, Sönmez E. Pain treatment in patients with acute pancreatitis: A randomized controlled trial. The Turkish Journal of Gastroenterology. 2016;**27**(2):192-196

[22] Meng W, Yuan J, Zhang C, Bai Z, Zhou W, Yan J, et al. Parenteral analgesics for pain relief in acute pancreatitis: A systematic review. Pancreatology. 2013;**13**(3):201-206

[23] Sadowski SM, Andres A, Morel P, Schiffer E, Frossard JL, Platon A, et al. Epidural anesthesia improves pancreatic perfusion and decreases the severity of acute pancreatitis. World Journal of Gastroenterology. 2015;**21**(43):12448-12456

[24] Lakananurak N, Gramlich L. Nutrition management in acute pancreatitis: Clinical practice consideration. World Journal of Clinical Cases. 2020;**8**(9):1561-1573

[25] Eckerwall GE, Tingstedt BB, Bergenzaun PE, Andersson RG. Immediate oral feeding in patients with mild acute pancreatitis is safe and may accelerate recovery—A randomized clinical study. Clinical Nutrition. 2007;**26**(6):758-763

[26] Moraes JM, Felga GE, Chebli LA, Franco MB, Gomes CA, Gaburri PD, et al. A full solid diet as the initial meal in mild acute pancreatitis is safe and result in a shorter length of hospitalization: Results from a prospective, randomized, controlled, double-blind clinical trial. Journal of Clinical Gastroenterology. 2010;**44**(7):517-522

[27] Vaughn VM, Shuster D, Rogers MAM, Mann J, Conte ML, Saint S, et al. Early versus delayed feeding in patients with acute pancreatitis: A systematic review. Annals of Internal Medicine. 2017;**166**(12):883-892

[28] Bakker OJ, van Brunschot S, van Santvoort HC, Besselink MG, Bollen TL, Boermeester MA. Et al; Dutch pancreatitis study group. Early versus on demand nasoenteric tube feeding in acute pancreatitis. The New England Journal of Medicine. 2014;**371**(21):1983-1993

[29] Li W, Liu J, Zhao S, Li J. Safety and efficacy of total parenteral nutrition

versus total enteral nutrition for patients with severe acute pancreatitis: A meta-analysis. The Journal of International Medical Research. 2018;**46**(9):3948-3958

[30] Banks PA, Bollen TL, Dervenis C, Gooszen HG, Johnson CD, Sarr MG, et al. Classification of acute pancreatitis--2012: Revision of the Atlanta classification and definitions by international consensus. Gut. 2013;**62**(1):102-111

[31] Eatock FC, Chong P, Menezes N, Murray L, McKay CJ, Carter CR, et al. A randomized study of early nasogastric versus nasojejunal feeding in severe acute pancreatitis. The American Journal of Gastroenterology. 2005;**100**(2):432-439

[32] Kumar A, Singh N, Prakash S, Saraya A, Joshi YK. Early enteral nutrition in severe acute pancreatitis: A prospective randomized controlled trial comparing nasojejunal and nasogastric routes. Journal of Clinical Gastroenterology. 2006;**40**(5):431-434

[33] Eckerwall GE, Axelsson JB, Andersson RG. Early nasogastric feeding in predicted severe acute pancreatitis: A clinical, randomized study. Annals of Surgery. 2006;**244**(6):959-965; discussion 965- 7

[34] Marik PE, Zaloga GP. Meta-analysis of parenteral nutrition versus enteral nutrition in patients with acute pancreatitis. BMJ. 2004;**328**(7453):1407

[35] McClave SA, Chang WK, Dhaliwal R, Heyland DK. Nutrition support in acute pancreatitis: A systematic review of the literature. JPEN Journal of Parenteral and Enteral Nutrition. 2006;**30**(2):143-156

[36] Casaer MP, Mesotten D, Hermans G, Wouters PJ, Schetz M, Meyfroidt G, et al. Early versus late parenteral nutrition in critically ill adults. The New England Journal of Medicine. 2011;**365**(6):506-517

[37] Kutsogiannis J, Alberda C, Gramlich L, Cahill NE, Wang M, Day AG, et al. Early use of supplemental parenteral nutrition in critically ill patients: Results of an international multicenter observational study. Critical Care Medicine. 2011;**39**(12):2691-2699

[38] Lee HS, Lee SK, Park DH, Lee SS, Seo DW, Kim MH, et al. Emergence of multidrug resistant infection in patients with severe acute pancreatitis. Pancreatology. 2014;**14**(6):450-453

[39] Mourad MM, Evans R, Kalidindi V, Navaratnam R, Dvorkin L, Bramhall SR, et al. Prophylactic antibiotics in acute pancreatitis: Endless debate. Annals of the Royal College of Surgeons of England. 2017;**99**(2):107-112

[40] Besselink MG, van Santvoort HC, Boermeester MA, Nieuwenhuijs VB, van Goor H, Dejong CH, et al. Dutch acute pancreatitis study group. Timing and impact of infections in acute pancreatitis. The British Journal of Surgery. 2009;**96**(3):267-273

[41] Vege SS, Atwal T, Bi Y, Chari ST, Clemens MA, Enders FT, et al. Pentoxifylline treatment in severe acute pancreatitis: A pilot, double-blind, placebo-controlled, randomized trial. Gastroenterology. 2015;**149**(2):318-20.e3

[42] Bai Y, Ren X, Zhang XF, Lv NH, Guo XG, Wan XJ, et al. Prophylactic somatostatin can reduce incidence of post-ERCP pancreatitis: Multicenter randomized controlled trial. Endoscopy. 2015;**47**(5):415-420

[43] Hu J, Li PL, Zhang T, Chen JP, Hu YJ, Yu Z, et al. Role of somatostatin in preventing post-endoscopic retrograde Cholangiopancreatography (ERCP)

pancreatitis: An update meta-analysis. Frontiers in Pharmacology. 2016;7:489

[44] Trikudanathan G, Navaneethan U, Vege SS. Intra-abdominal fungal infections complicating acute pancreatitis: A review. The American Journal of Gastroenterology. 2011;**106**(7):1188-1192

[45] Seta T, Noguchi Y, Shimada T, Shikata S, Fukui T. Treatment of acute pancreatitis with protease inhibitors: A meta-analysis. European Journal of Gastroenterology & Hepatology. 2004;**16**(12):1287-1293

[46] Besselink MG, van Santvoort HC, Buskens E, Boermeester MA, van Goor H, Timmerman HM, et al. Dutch acute pancreatitis study group. Probiotic prophylaxis in predicted severe acute pancreatitis: A randomised, double-blind, placebo controlled trial. Lancet. 2008;**371**(9613):651-659

[47] Gou S, Yang Z, Liu T, Wu H, Wang C. Use of probiotics in the treatment of severe acute pancreatitis: A systematic review and meta-analysis of randomized controlled trials. Critical Care. 2014;**18**(2):R57. 9

[48] O'Brien T, Dinneen SF, O'Brien PC, Palumbo PJ. Hyperlipidemia in patients with primary and secondary hypothyroidism. Mayo Clinic Proceedings. 1993;**68**(9):860-866

[49] Renzulli P, Jakob SM, Täuber M, Candinas D, Gloor B. Severe acute pancreatitis: Case-oriented discussion of interdisciplinary management. Pancreatology. 2005;**5**(2-3):145-156

[50] Ceranowicz P, Dembinski A, Warzecha Z, Dembinski M, Cieszkowski J, Rembisz K, et al. Protective and therapeutic effect of heparin in acute pancreatitis. Journal of Physiology and Pharmacology. 2008;**59**(Suppl. 4):103-125

[51] Qiu F, Lu XS, Huang YK. Protective effect of low molecular-weight heparin on pancreatic encephalopathy in severe acute pancreatic rats. Inflammation Research. 2012;**61**(11):1203-1209

[52] Qiu F, Lü XS, Huang YK. Effect of low molecular weight heparin on pancreatic micro-circulation in severe acute pancreatitis in a rodent model. Chinese Medical Journal. 2007;**120**(24):2260-2263

[53] Lu XS, Qiu F, Li YX, Li JQ, Fan QQ, Zhou RG, et al. Effect of lower-molecular weight heparin in the prevention of pancreatic encephalopathy in the patient with severe acute pancreatitis. Pancreas. 2010;**39**(4):516-519

[54] Lu XS, Qiu F, Li JQ, Fan QQ, Zhou RG, Ai YH, et al. Low molecular weight heparin in the treatment of severe acute pancreatitis: A multiple Centre prospective clinical study. Asian Journal of Surgery. 2009;**32**(2):89-94

[55] Tozlu M, Kayar Y, İnce AT, Baysal B, Şentürk H. Low molecular weight heparin treatment of acute moderate and severe pancreatitis: A randomized, controlled, open-label study. The Turkish Journal of Gastroenterology. 2019;**30**(1):81-87

[56] de Pretis N, Amodio A, Frulloni L. Hypertriglyceridemic pancreatitis: Epidemiology, pathophysiology and clinical management. United European Gastroenterology Journal. 2018;**6**(5):649-655

[57] Scherer J, Singh VP, Pitchumoni CS, Yadav D. Issues in hypertriglyceridemic pancreatitis: An update. Journal of Clinical Gastroenterology. 2014;**48**(3):195-203

[58] Pedersen SB, Langsted A, Nordestgaard BG. Nonfasting mild-to-moderate hypertriglyceridemia and risk of acute pancreatitis. JAMA. 2016;**176**(12):1834-1842

[59] Nawaz H, Koutroumpakis E, Easler J, Slivka A, Whitcomb DC, Singh VP, et al. Elevated serum triglycerides are independently associated with persistent organ failure in acute pancreatitis. The American Journal of Gastroenterology. 2015;**110**(10):1497-1503

[60] Christian JB, Arondekar B, Buysman EK, Jacobson TA, Snipes RG, Horwitz RI, et al. Determining triglyceride reductions needed for clinical impact in severe hypertriglyceridemia. The American Journal of Medicine. 2014;**127**(1):36-44.e1

[61] Carr RA, Rejowski BJ, Cote GA, Pitt HA, Zyromski NJ. Systematic review of hypertriglyceridemiainduced acute pancreatitis: A more virulent etiology? Pancreatology. 2016;**16**(4):469-476

[62] Ipe TS, Pham HP, Williams LA 3rd. Critical updates in the 7th edition of the American Society for Apheresis guidelines. Journal of Clinical Apheresis. 2018;**33**(1):78-94

[63] Chen JH, Yeh JH, Lai HW, Liao CS. Therapeutic plasma exchange in patients with hyperlipidemic pancreatitis. World Journal of Gastroenterology. 2004;**10**(15):2272-2274

[64] Goldberg IJ. Lipoprotein lipase and lipolysis: Central roles in lipoprotein metabolism and atherogenesis. Journal of Lipid Research. 1996;**37**(4):693-707

[65] Kitabchi AE, Umpierrez GE, Miles JM, Fisher JN. Hyperglycemic crises in adult patients with diabetes. Diabetes Care. 2009;**32**(7):1335-1343

[66] Mikhail N, Trivedi K, Page C, Wali S, Cope D. Treatment of severe hypertriglyceridemia in nondiabetic patients with insulin. The American Journal of Emergency Medicine. 2005;**23**(3):415-417

[67] Alagözlü H, Cindoruk M, Karakan T, Unal S. Heparin and insulin in the treatment of hypertriglyceridemia-induced severe acute pancreatitis. Digestive Diseases and Sciences. 2006;**51**(5):931-933

[68] Lenhart DK, Balthazar EJ. MDCT of acute mild (nonnecrotizing) pancreatitis: Abdominal complications and fate of fluid collections. AJR. American Journal of Roentgenology. 2008;**190**(3):643-649

[69] Dhaka N, Samanta J, Kochhar S, Kalra N, Appasani S, Manrai M, et al. Pancreatic fluid collections: What is the ideal imaging technique? World Journal of Gastroenterology. 2015;**21**(48):13403-13410

[70] ASGE Standards of Practice Committee, Muthusamy VR, Chandrasekhara V, Acosta RD, Bruining DH, Chathadi KV, et al. The role of endoscopy in the diagnosis and treatment of inflammatory pancreatic fluid collections. Gastrointestinal Endoscopy. 2016;**83**(3):481-488

[71] Kahaleh M, Shami VM, Conaway MR, Tokar J, Rockoff T, De La Rue SA, et al. Endoscopic ultrasound drainage of pancreatic pseudocyst: A prospective comparison with conventional endoscopic drainage. Endoscopy. 2006;**38**(4):355-359

[72] Krüger M, Schneider AS, Manns MP, Meier PN. Endoscopic management of pancreatic pseudocysts or abscesses after an EUS-guided 1-step procedure for initial access. Gastrointestinal Endoscopy. 2006;**63**(3):409-416

[73] Ocampo C, Oría A, Zandalazini H, Silva W, Kohan G, Chiapetta L, et al. Treatment of acute pancreatic pseudocysts after severe acute pancreatitis. Journal of Gastrointestinal Surgery. 2007;**11**(3):357-363

[74] Baron TH. Drainage for infected pancreatic necrosis—Is the waiting the hardest part? New England Journal of Medicine. 2021;**385**(15):1433-1435

[75] Yasuda I, Takahashi K. Endoscopic management of walled-off pancreatic necrosis. Digestive Endoscopy. 2021;**33**(3):335-341

[76] Chandrasekaran P, Gupta R, Shenvi S, Kang M, Rana SS, Singh R, et al. Prospective comparison of long term outcomes in patients with severe acute pancreatitis managed by operative and non operative measures. Pancreatology. 2015;**15**(5):478-484

[77] Sharaiha RZ, Tyberg A, Khashab MA, Kumta NA, Karia K, Nieto J, et al. Endoscopic therapy with lumen-apposing metal stents is safe and effective for patients with pancreatic walled-off necrosis. Clinical Gastroenterology and Hepatology. 2016;**14**(12):1797-1803

[78] Law RJ, Chandrasekhara V, Bhatt A, Bucobo JC, Copland AP, Krishnan K, et al. Lumen-apposing metal stents (with videos). Gastrointestinal Endoscopy. 2021;**94**(3):457-470

[79] Nabi Z, Basha J, Reddy DN. Endoscopic management of pancreatic fluid collections-revisited. World Journal of Gastroenterology. 2017;**23**(15):2660-2672

[80] Bang JY, Navaneethan U, Hasan MK, Sutton B, Hawes R, Varadarajulu S, et al. Non-superiority of lumen-apposing metal stents over plastic stents for drainage of walled-off necrosis in a randomized trial. Gut. 2019;**68**(7):1200-1209

[81] Haas B, Nathens AB. Surgical indications in acute pancreatitis. Current Opinion in Critical Care. 2010;**16**(2):153-158

[82] Leppäniemi A, Tolonen M, Tarasconi A, Segovia- Lohse H, Gamberini E, Kirkpatrick AW, et al. 2019 WSES guidelines for the management of severe acute pancreatitis. World Journal of Emergency Surgery : WJES. 2019;**14**:27

[83] Banks PA, Freeman ML. Practice parameters committee of the American college of gastroenterology. Practice guidelines in acute pancreatitis. The American Journal of Gastroenterology. 2006;**101**(10):2379-2400

[84] Bradley EL 3rd, Allen K. A prospective longitudinal study of observation versus surgical intervention in the management of necrotizing pancreatitis. American Journal of Surgery. 1991;**161**(1):19-24; discussion 24-5

[85] Haney CM, Kowalewski KF, Schmidt MW, Koschny R, Felinska EA, Kalkum E, et al. Endoscopic versus surgical treatment for infected necrotizing pancreatitis: A systematic review and meta-analysis of randomized controlled trials. Surgical Endoscopy. 2020;**34**(6):2429-2444

[86] Kylänpää L, Rakonczay Z Jr, O'Reilly DA. The clinical course of acute pancreatitis and the inflammatory mediators that drive it. International Journal of Inflammation. 2012;**2012**:360685

[87] Clancy TE, Ashley SW. Current management of necrotizing pancreatitis. Advances in Surgery. 2002;**36**:103-121

[88] Working Group IAP/APA Acute Pancreatitis Guidelines. IAP/APA evidence-based guidelines for the management of acute pancreatitis. Pancreatology. 2013;**13**(4 Suppl. 2):e1-e15

[89] Nadkarni NA, Khanna S, Vege SS. Splanchnic venous thrombosis and pancreatitis. Pancreas. 2013;**42**(6):924-931

[90] Heider TR, Azeem S, Galanko JA, Behrns KE. The natural history of pancreatitis-induced splenic vein thrombosis. Annals of Surgery. 2004;**239**(6):876-880; discussion 880-2

[91] Radenkovic DV, Bajec D, Ivancevic N, Bumbasirevic V, Milic N, Jeremic V, et al. Decompressive laparotomy with temporary abdominal closure versus percutaneous puncture with placement of abdominal catheter in patients with abdominal compartment syndrome during acute pancreatitis: Background and design of multicenter, randomised, controlled study. BMC Surgery. 2010;**10**:22

[92] De Waele JJ, De Laet I, Kirkpatrick AW, Hoste E. Intra-abdominal hypertension and abdominal compartment syndrome. American Journal of Kidney Diseases. 2011;**57**(1):159-169

[93] Das SL, Singh PP, Phillips AR, Murphy R, Windsor JA, Petrov MS, et al. Newly diagnosed diabetes mellitus after acute pancreatitis: A systematic review and meta-analysis. Gut. 2014;**63**(5):818-831

Chapter 16

Acute Pancreatitis: Nutritional Management

Maria Argente-Pla and Juan Francisco Merino-Torres

Abstract

Acute pancreatitis (AP) is the most common acute gastrointestinal disease requiring hospital admission. AP is characterized by an inflammation of the pancreas, by the intraglandular activation of pancreatic pro-enzymes and concomitant autodigestion of the acini, usually followed by a total structural and functional restoration of the gland. Acute necrotizing pancreatitis is encountered in 20% of patients with AP, being associated with increased morbidity and mortality, and may require artificial nutrition by enteral or parenteral route, as well as additional interventions (endoscopic, radiological, or surgical). Pancreatitis patients should be considered as patients with moderate-to-high nutritional risk due to the catabolic nature of the disease and the impact on the nutritional status during the development of the disease. All patients with mild or moderate AP should undergo validated screening methods; however, patients with severe AP should always be considered at risk of malnutrition. This chapter includes the latest developments in the nutritional management of acute pancreatitis.

Keywords: acute pancreatitis, nutrition, enteral nutrition, nutritional management, pancreas disease

1. Introduction

Acute pancreatitis (AP) is the acute gastrointestinal disease that most frequently requires hospital admission, with favorable evolution in most cases (80%) [1]. AP has an incidence of between 5 and 80/1.000 inhabitants/year. However, there are more severe forms of AP, which represent 15–20% and present with both local (pancreatic necrosis, infection of the necrosis, pancreatic abscess, or pseudocyst) as well as systemic complications (multiple organ failures). Acute necrotizing pancreatitis, with can occur in up to 20% of patients, has a worse prognosis and is associated with rates of early organ failure (38%), need for intervention (38%), and death (15%) [2].

Diagnosis of AP is established by the presence of at least two of the three following criteria [1–3]:

- abdominal pain suggestive of AP: gradual or sudden pain located in the epigastrium that sometimes extends to both hypochondria or to the back. Other symptoms can include fever, nausea and vomiting, tachycardia as well as swollen and tender abdomen.

IntechOpen

- Blood amylase or lipase levels are typically elevated three times the normal level during AP. Amylase values may be normal in patients with alcoholic pancreatitis or hypertriglyceridemia; therefore, the diagnosis should be changed in this population. In addition, intestinal perforation, infarction, obstruction, and abdominal aortic aneurysm can also increase amylase levels. Similarly, lipase can also be elevated in intestinal diseases, cholecystitis, peptic ulcer disease, and biliary obstruction.

- In some cases, when the blood tests are not elevated and the diagnosis is still unclear, abdominal imaging, such as a computed tomography (CT) scan, might be performed.

AP is characterized by an inflammation of the pancreas, by the intraglandular activation of pancreatic pro-enzymes, and concomitant autodigestion of the acini, which is usually followed by a total structural and functional restoration of the gland [1–3].

Several conditions are known to cause acute pancreatitis [4–9]. Of these, gallstones and chronic alcohol use disorder account for approximately two-thirds of cases [4, 5].

Gallstones (including microlithiasis) are the most common cause of acute pancreatitis (40–70% of cases); however, only 3 to 7 percent of patients with gallstones develop pancreatitis. The mechanism by which the passage of gallstones induces pancreatitis is unknown. The reflux of bile into the pancreatic duct due to transient obstruction of the ampulla during the passage of gallstones and an obstruction at the ampulla secondary to stone(s) or edema resulting from the passage of a stone could be the possible initiation event in gallstone pancreatitis [6].

Alcohol is responsible for approximately 25 to 35 percent of cases of acute pancreatitis in the United States. Approximately 10 percent of patients with chronic alcohol use disorder develop attacks of clinically acute pancreatitis that are indistinguishable from other forms of AP. Alcohol may act by increasing the synthesis of enzymes by pancreatic acinar cells to synthesize the digestive and lysosomal enzymes that are thought to be responsible for acute pancreatitis or over-sensitization of acini to cholecystokinin [7].

Other factors that can contribute to the appearance of AP are smoking, certain drugs, and genetic factors. Smoking might increase the risk of acute pancreatitis [8]. There are multiple drugs for which a definite or probable association with acute pancreatitis has been reported [9].

Initial evaluation to determine the etiology of acute pancreatitis includes the patient's history, laboratory evaluation (serum amylase or lipase, triglyceride level, calcium level, and liver biochemistries), and abdominal ultrasound (repeated, if initially negative for gallstones) [4].

Classification. The Atlanta classification has traditionally been used to classify AP. The revised Atlanta classification provides definitions of the clinical and radiological severity of AP [10]. According to the severity, AP is divided into the following:

- Mild acute pancreatitis which is characterized by the absence of organ failure and local or systemic complications. Mild AP does usually not require pancreatic imaging.

- Moderately severe acute pancreatitis which is characterized by one or more transient organ failure(s) (resolves within 48 hours) and/or local or systemic complications without persistent organ failure (>48 hours). Organ failure includes respiratory, cardiovascular, and renal failure.

Systemic complications include exacerbations of pre-existing comorbidities, including congestive heart failure, chronic liver disease, and chronic lung disease. Local complications include interstitial pancreatitis (peripancreatic fluid collections and pancreatic pseudo-cysts), acute necrotic collection, and walled-off necrosis. These patients might require longer hospital stays and have a higher mortality than patients with mild AP.

- Severe acute pancreatitis which is characterized by persistent organ failure that may involve one or multiple organs

Mild to moderately severe pancreatitis is usually self-limiting, and patients can resume oral intake within a few days of AP onset.

However, after acute pancreatitis, especially severe pancreatitis, intestinal barrier dysfunction may occur in up to 60% of patients, leading to bacterial translocation and necrosis infection [1].

2. Acute pancreatitis and malnutrition: Relationship and diagnosis

There are different mechanisms by which a patient with AP can become malnourished. On the one hand, in up to 60% of patients with AP, there may be a dysfunction of the intestinal barrier, which can favor bacterial translocation and infection of necrosis [1]. This may contribute to the increase in catabolism already existing in these patients, especially in severe AP. In addition, alcohol is related to a greater presence of PA and a greater degree of malnutrition [7].

A low or low body mass index (BMI) can also identify patients who are at nutritional risk. However, obesity is a known risk factor for severe AP and is therefore a nutritional risk related to disease severity [11].

For these reasons, all patients with AP should be considered as patients with moderate to high nutritional risk, regardless of the severity of pancreatitis, due its catabolic nature and the impact on the nutritional status as the disease develops during the development of the disease. The *European Society for Clinical Nutrition and Metabolism* (ESPEN) recommends all patients with mild or moderate AP to undergo validated screening methods; however, patients with severe AP should always be considered at risk for malnutrition [12].

There is no specific screening test for malnutrition for patients with AP. However, other validated tools can be used, such as the NRS-2002 malnutrition screening test, which has been validated for hospitalized patients [13].

The use of the GLIM criteria is currently recommended in order to make the diagnosis of malnutrition. To diagnose malnutrition at least one phenotypic criterion and one etiologic criterion should be present. In the case of acute pancreatitis, the etiological criterion would be met by presenting mild-to-moderate inflammation [14], which supports the theory that AP patients are at risk of malnutrition. It would be necessary to investigate the phenotypic criteria in patients with AP to diagnose malnutrition, paying special attention to whether there is weight loss, reduced muscle mass, or low body mass index [14].

3. Nutritional intervention: Indications and requirements

3.1 Indications

Nutritional intervention should be performed in patients with [1]:

- Severe AP: There is systemic inflammatory response syndrome (SIRS) with pancreatic necrosis and multisystemic failure that leads to a hypermetabolic state with catabolic stress and nutrient deficiency. Nutritional treatment is currently considered one of the pillars of treatment for PAG. Recent studies suggest that early enteral nutrition (EN) has more favorable effects on the course of the disease, reducing complications and promoting faster recovery. Parenteral nutrition (PN) would be indicated when it is not possible to cover the necessary caloric requirements with EN or when there is intolerance or contraindication to it (paralytic ileus).

- In those who, presenting mild or moderate BP, have complications, or experience more than 5–7 days without tolerating oral intake.

In patients with moderate AP, prolonged fasting is not recommended and oral feeding should be reintroduced at the earliest opportunity, regardless of serum lipase levels. A soft, low-fat diet is advised as the initial approach for resuming oral intake [1].

3.2 Calculation of nutritional requirements

The caloric and protein requirements of patients with AP can be determined by indirect calorimetry or calculated indirectly using the Harris-Benedict formula or through the calculation of calories and proteins [2]:

- Calories: 25–35 Kcal/Kg/day. The increase in energy expenditure in AP is estimated at 1.49 (1.08–1.78) and could be due to several reasons, including: decreased splanchnic blood flow, acidosis, and bacterial translocation.

- Proteins: 1.2–1.5 gr/Kg/day. It is estimated that nitrogen losses are 20–40 g per day and proteolysis can increase by up to 80%. Patients, who have had decompressive laparotomy performed, present nitrogen losses of around 2 g/L of abdominal fluid lost.

4. Nutrition therapy: Types

The need for nutrition therapy *via* the oral or enteral or parenteral route should be based on the extent of disease and nutrition status of the patient. See **Figure 1.**

4.1 Oral feeding

In cases of mild AP, oral feeding should be initiated as soon as the patient can tolerate it clinically, regardless of serum lipase levels. A low-fat, soft diet is suggested for restarting oral intake in these patients [1].

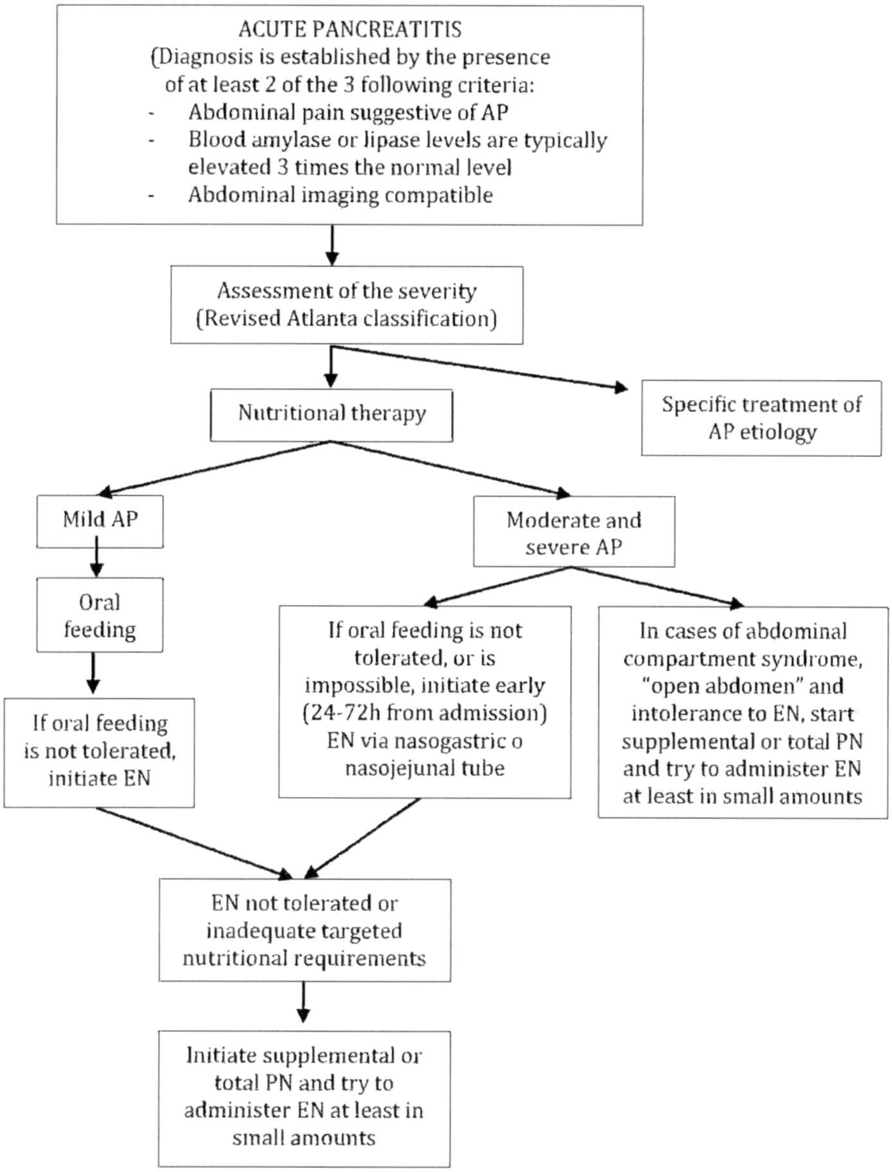

Figure 1.
Algorithm suggesting nutritional management in acute pancreatitis. AP: acute pancreatitis; EN: enteral nutrition; PN: parenteral nutrition. Adapted from Arvanitakis et al. [1].

Hyperlipidemia ranks as the third most frequent cause of AP, accounting for 4–10% of cases, and is associated with a worse prognosis compared to other etiologies. Initial management of hyperlipidemic AP follows standard protocols for the condition. However, subsequent treatment should include tailored measures such as adopting a low-fat diet, promoting weight loss, and administering fibrates. If hypercholesterolemia coexists with hypertriglyceridemia, statins should be added. Effective control of hypertriglyceridemia post-AP reduces the risk of recurrence [3].

Additionally, resuming oral feeding within the first 24 hours after minimally invasive necrosectomy is both feasible and safe, provided the patient's clinical status—hemodynamic stability, septic indicators, and gastric motility—is favorable [6].

When oral intake alone does not meet caloric or protein requirements, oral nutritional supplements should be introduced to ensure adequate nutritional support [1].

4.2 Enteral nutrition

In patients with AP and inability to feed orally, enteral nutrition (EN) is preferred over parenteral nutrition (PN). EN is considered the route of choice in AP and should be tried whenever possible, as it preserves the integrity of the intestinal mucosa, stimulates intestinal motility, prevents bacterial overgrowth, and increases splanchnic blood flow [1]. EN may be used in the presence of pancreatic complications such as ascites, fistulas and pseudocysts [2].

WHEN SHOULD EN BE STARTED?: In case of oral intolerance, EN should be started early in the first 24–72 hours, since if it is feasible, safe and well tolerated, it is associated with benefits with respect to mortality, organ failure, and infectious complications with respect to the later EN.

In several multicenter clinical trials [15–19], no differences were found in terms of infectious complications and deaths between EN started in the first 24 hours after admission and oral diet started within 72 hours after admission, most of the patients included had a mild-to-moderate severe AP. Two studies have concluded that early EN in patients who have undergone a laparotomy causes an increase in the rate of fascial closure, a lower rate of fistula appearance, reduces the appearance of nosocomial infections and reduces hospital costs [11, 20].

EN INFUSION SITE: The administration of EN through a nasogastric tube (NGT) is the choice, reserving administration through a nasojejunal tube (NJT) in cases:

- in those with digestive intolerance due to delayed gastric emptying and/or gastroesophageal reflux, which are experienced by 15% of patients with AP.

- NJT is also preferred in those patients with minimally invasive necrosectomy who are unable to feed orally.

- If there is severe AP and intra-abdominal pressure < 15 mmHg, the nasojejunal route is also preferred, although the nasogastric route could also be used. However, if intra-abdominal pressure is >15 mmHg, EN should be started *via* the nasojejunal route starting at 20 mL/h, increasing the rate as tolerated. Temporary reduction or interruption of EN should be considered when intra-abdominal pressure values increase further with EN. In case of intra-abdominal pressure > 20 mmHg or abdominal compartment syndrome, EN should be temporarily stopped and EN started [1].

Reviewing the literature, no differences have been found between the administration of nutrition through NGT and NJT, but compared to NJT, NGT is easier to place, more convenient and cheaper. Only the guide of the SEMICyUC (*Spanish Society of Intensive, Critical Medicine and Coronary Units*) in its consensus with the SENPE (*Spanish Society of Clinical Nutrition and Metabolism*), indicates that NJT would be indicated in patients with severe acute pancreatitis admitted to the ICU for benefit from 3-lumen NJT (jejunal perfusion while allowing gastric decompression) [21].

The ESPEN European guidelines also recommend the nasogastric route for the administration of EN in patients with AP, reserving the nasojejunal route for cases with digestive intolerance [1].

TYPE OF FORMULA: Regarding the formula of choice for EN, although both standard polymeric formulas and peptide (semi-elemental) formulas are well tolerated, the latest ESPEN clinical guidelines recommend the use of polymeric formulations [1]. However, semi-elemental formulas (small peptide-based medium-chain triglyceride oil formula) could be beneficial in patients with severe AP with malabsorption to improve tolerance.

EN must be able to cover the caloric and protein requirements of each patient. For these reason, hypercaloric and hyperproteic formulas should be considered.

CONTRAINDICATIONS. EN is contraindicated in the presence of digestive intolerance: gastroparesis, prolonged paralytic ileus, severe abdominal pain, intestinal obstruction, intestinal compartment syndrome—intra-abdominal pressure > 20 mmHg—mesenteric ischemia. Approximately 20% of patients with severe AP present this type of complication [1].

Also, EN is not recommended when there is a need for emergency surgery, in which case, parenteral nutrition would be performed.

4.3 Parenteral nutrition

Whenever possible, EN will be used since it is more physiological. However, PN is indicated when the enteral route cannot be used or when it is not sufficient to cover the caloric and protein requirements of the patient.

The indications for PN are [1]:

- Impossibility, failure, or intolerance of EN. In patients with total parenteral nutrition (TPN) due to intolerance to EN, it is recommended to maintain a minimum peptide-type perfusion in the jejunum to maintain the integrity of the intestinal barrier.

- Need to fast due to surgery.

- Worsening of AP symptoms (pain).

- As a complement to EN, when oral or enteral nutrition is not sufficient to cover the nutritional requirements of the patient.

PN requires close monitoring, with monitoring of digital blood glucose levels. In addition, it should not be started before the third day of the hospital stay to reduce metabolic and infectious complications. Switching to EN should be considered when the clinical situation allows doing so. Both peripheral PN and total PN can be administered.

No specific complications of PN are unique to patients with AP and the complications of PN are the same as for other pathologies: mechanical complications (thrombosis, catheter displacement, etc.), infectious, metabolic, and psychological complications.

Regarding PN composition, glucose is the preferred carbohydrate, and intravenous fat emulsions are generally well tolerated and safe as long as triglycerides are below 400 mg/dL [2]. Various clinical guidelines recommend the use of glutamine

(0.2 g/kg/day) in the form of L-glutamine in parenteral nutrition. However, immunonutrition is not important in severe AP, but it is used in a meta-analysis that included 11 clinical trials, and a significant reduction in the appearance of complications was verified. In two meta-analyses (severe AP in one and AP of any severity in the other), a significant decrease in the incidence of infections and mortality was observed. Two other recent meta-analyses showed benefits of glutamine supplementation in raising serum albumin, lowering C-reactive protein levels, and shortening the hospital stay. Nevertheless, all the included studies have a risk of bias due to: small sample sizes, possible heterogeneity in AP severity, and the presence of confounding factors such as interventions that can change the results (drainage, debridement, or surgery).

The oral diet is to be restarted once the symptoms (pain) have disappeared, and the analytical parameters improve. Oral tolerance with a liquid diet is started, simultaneously with PN. While oral intake is progressively increased, PN is reduced until it is completely withdrawn. The diet of choice after the liquid diet is a low-fat diet.

5. Other considerations

Both exocrine and endocrine transient pancreatic insufficiency can occur after AP. Pancreatic function should therefore be monitored, which generally returns to normal again 3 months after abatement of acute pancreatitis. However, routine pancreatic enzyme supplementation is not recommended, only in those patients with documented exocrine pancreatic insufficiency [1].

Endocrine pancreatic function should be checked after about 3 months (by fasting and postprandial blood sugar concentrations, possibly by HbA1c measurement). Severe acute pancreatitis is often followed by diabetes mellitus [4].

Regarding the role of probiotics in AP, they have been found to provide no significant benefit in the pancreatic infection rate, overall infection rate, operation rate, length of hospital stays, and mortality [22]. Furthermore, one of the randomized clinical trials demonstrated higher mortality compared to the placebo group [23]. For this reason, the use of probiotics is not recommended in patients with severe AP [1].

6. Conclusions and recommendations

Management of acute pancreatitis (AP) requires a multidisciplinary team approach, including gastroenterologists, surgeons, endocrinologists, nurses, and nutritionists, due to its complex nature.

Acute necrotizing pancreatitis affects approximately 20% of AP patients, is linked to increased morbidity and mortality, and often necessitates artificial nutrition through enteral or parenteral means, in addition to endoscopic, radiological, or surgical interventions.

Pancreatitis patients are considered at moderate to high nutritional risk due to the disease's catabolic effects and its influence on nutritional status. For this reason, nutritional assessments should be conducted at the time of diagnosis and repeated periodically to prevent and manage malnutrition effectively.

Regarding nutritional intervention, in cases of mild AP, oral feeding should be introduced as soon as clinically appropriate, regardless of serum lipase levels. Enteral nutrition (EN) is recommended over parenteral nutrition (PN) when oral intake is not possible and a standard polymeric diet is the preferred formula. If EN is contraindicated or infeasible, and PN is required, parenteral glutamine supplementation should be administered at 0.20 g/kg per day of L-glutamine.

Probiotics are not recommended for patients with severe AP and pancreatic enzyme replacement should be considered only for patients with confirmed or evident exocrine pancreatic insufficiency and not applied universally.

Conflict of interest

The authors declare no conflict of interest.

Author details

Maria Argente-Pla[1,2]* and Juan Francisco Merino-Torres[1,2,3]

1 Endocrinology and Nutrition Department, La Fe University and Polytechnic Hospital in Valencia, Valencia, Spain

2 Joint Research Unit on Endocrinology, Nutrition and Clinical Dietetics, Health Research Institute La Fe, Valencia, Spain

3 Department of Medicine, Faculty of Medicine, University of Valencia, Valencia, Spain

*Address all correspondence to: mariaargentepla@gmail.com

References

[1] Arvanitakis M, Ockenga J, Bezmarevic M, Gianotti L, Krznarić Ž, Lobo DN, et al. ESPEN guideline on clinical nutrition in acute and chronic pancreatitis. Clinical Nutrition. 2020;**39**:612-631. DOI: 10.1016/j.clnu.2020.01.004

[2] Mirtallo JM, Forbes A, McClave SA, Jensen GL, Waitzberg DL, Davies AR. International consensus guideline committee pancreatitis task force. International consensus guidelines for nutrition therapy in pancreatitis. JPEN Journal of Parenteral and Enteral Nutrition. 2012;**36**:284-291. DOI: 10.1177/0148607112440823

[3] Foster BR, Jensen KK, Bakis G, Shaaban AM, Coakley FV. Revised Atlanta classification for acute pancreatitis: A pictorial essay. Radiographics. 2016;**36**:675-687. DOI: 10.1148/rg.2016150097. Erratum in: Radiographics. 2019;39(3):912

[4] Lankisch PG, Apte M, Banks PA. Acute pancreatitis. Lancet. 2015;**386**(9988):85-96. DOI: 10.1016/S0140-6736(14)60649-8

[5] Forsmark CE, Baillie J. AGA Institute clinical practice and economics committee; AGA Institute governing board. AGA Institute technical review on acute pancreatitis. Gastroenterology. 2007;**132**(5):2022-2044. DOI: 10.1053/j.gastro.2007.03.065

[6] Lerch MM, Saluja AK, Rünzi M, Dawra R, Saluja M, Steer ML. Pancreatic duct obstruction triggers acute necrotizing pancreatitis in the opossum. Gastroenterology. 1993;**104**(3):853-861. DOI: 10.1016/0016-5085(93)91022-a

[7] Yang AL, Vadhavkar S, Singh G, Omary MB. Epidemiology of alcohol-related liver and pancreatic disease in the United States. Archives of Internal Medicine. 2008;**168**(6):649-656. DOI: 10.1001/archinte.168.6.649

[8] Sadr-Azodi O, Andrén-Sandberg Å, Orsini N, Wolk A. Cigarette smoking, smoking cessation and acute pancreatitis: A prospective population-based study. Gut. 2012;**61**(2):262-267. DOI: 10.1136/gutjnl-2011-300566

[9] Nitsche C, Maertin S, Scheiber J, Ritter CA, Lerch MM, Mayerle J. Drug-induced pancreatitis. Current Gastroenterology Reports. 2012;**14**(2):131-138. DOI: 10.1007/s11894-012-0245-9

[10] Banks PA, Bollen TL, Dervenis C, Gooszen HG, Johnson CD, Sarr MG, et al. Acute pancreatitis classification working group. Classification of acute pancreatitis--2012: Revision of the Atlanta classification and definitions by international consensus. Gut. 2013;**62**(1):102-111. DOI: 10.1136/gutjnl-2012-302779

[11] Collier B, Guillamondegui O, Cotton B, Donahue R, Conrad A, Groh K, et al. Feeding the open abdomen. JPEN Journal of Parenteral and Enteral Nutrition. 2007;**31**(5):410-415. DOI: 10.1177/0148607107031005410

[12] Khatua B, El-Kurdi B, Singh VP. Obesity and pancreatitis. Current Opinion in Gastroenterology. 2017;**33**(5):374-382. DOI: 10.1097/MOG.0000000000000386

[13] Bolayir B, Arik G, Yeşil Y, Kuyumcu ME, Varan HD, Kara Ö, et al. Validation of nutritional risk screening-2002 in a hospitalized adult population. Nutrition in

Clinical Practice. 2019;**34**(2):297-303. DOI: 10.1002/ncp.10082

[14] Jensen GL, Cederholm T, Correia MITD, Gonzalez MC, Fukushima R, Higashiguchi T, et al. GLIM criteria for the diagnosis of malnutrition: A consensus report from the global clinical nutrition community. JPEN Journal of Parenteral and Enteral Nutrition. 2019;**43**:32-40. DOI: 10.1002/jpen.1440

[15] Bakker OJ, van Brunschot S, Farre A, Johnson CD, Kalfarentzos F, Louie BE, et al. Timing of enteral nutrition in acute pancreatitis: Meta-analysis of individuals using a single-arm of randomised trials. Pancreatology. 2014;**14**(5):340-346. DOI: 10.1016/j.pan.2014.07.008

[16] Li X, Ma F, Jia K. Early enteral nutrition within 24 hours or between 24 and 72 hours for acute pancreatitis: Evidence based on 12 RCTs. Medical Science Monitor. 2014;**17**:2327-2335. DOI: 10.12659/MSM.892770

[17] Song J, Zhong Y, Lu X, Kang X, Wang Y, Guo W, et al. Enteral nutrition provided within 48 hours after admission in severe acute pancreatitis: A systematic review and meta-analysis. Medicine (Baltimore). 2018;**97**(34):e11871. DOI: 10.1097/MD.0000000000011871

[18] Petrov MS, Pylypchuk RD, Uchugina AF. A systematic review on the timing of artificial nutrition in acute pancreatitis. The British Journal of Nutrition. 2009;**101**(6):787-793. DOI: 10.1017/S0007114508123443

[19] Feng P, He C, Liao G, Chen Y. Early enteral nutrition versus delayed enteral nutrition in acute pancreatitis: A PRISMA-compliant systematic review and meta-analysis. Medicine (Baltimore). 2017;**96**(46):e8648. DOI: 10.1097/MD.0000000000008648

[20] Dissanaike S, Pham T, Shalhub S, Warner K, Hennessy L, Moore EE, et al. Effect of immediate enteral feeding on trauma patients with an open abdomen: Protection from nosocomial infections. Journal of the American College of Surgeons. 2008;**207**(5):690-697. DOI: 10.1016/j.jamcollsurg.2008.06.332

[21] Bordejé L, Lorencio C, Acosta J. Spanish Society of Intensive Care Medicine and Coronary Units-Spanish Society of parenteral and enteral nutrition (SEMICYUC-SENPE). Guidelines for specialized nutritional and metabolic support in the critically ill-patient. In: Update. Consensus of the Spanish Society of Intensive Care Medicine and Coronary Units-Spanish Society of Parenteral and Enteral Nutrition (SEMICYUC-SENPE): Severe Acute Pancreatitis. Med Intensiva. Vol. 35. Spanish; 2011. pp. 33-37. DOI: 10.1016/S0210-5691(11)70007-9

[22] Gou S, Yang Z, Liu T, Wu H, Wang C. Use of probiotics in the treatment of severe acute pancreatitis: A systematic review and meta-analysis of randomized controlled trials. Critical Care. 2014;**18**(2):R57. DOI: 10.1186/cc13809

[23] Besselink MG, van Santvoort HC, van der Heijden GJ, Buskens E, Gooszen HG. Dutch acute pancreatitis study G. New randomized trial of probiotics in pancreatitis needed? Caution advised. Langenbeck's Archives of Surgery. 2009;**394**:191-192. DOI: 10.1007/s00423-008-0419-y

Chapter 17

Integrin αvβ3-Targeted Therapeutic Strategies in Pancreatic Cancers

Zi-Lin Li, Ya-Jung Shih, Chung-Che Tsai, Chih-Yang Wang, Wen-Long Wang, Kuan Wang, Jaqueline Whang-Peng, Ju-Ku Mo and Hung-Yun Lin

Abstract

Pancreatic cancer is a significant health concern, primarily due to challenges in early diagnosis and limited treatment options. The increasing incidence of pancreatic cancers and the lack of effective chemotherapy underscore the need for early detection and efficient therapy. The cell surface integrin αvβ3 overexpresses in most cancers and newly growing endothelial cells crucial in cancer growth and metastasis. Novel nanotechnologies have been developed to target integrin αvβ3 and its functions for detective and therapeutic purposes. This chapter details the importance of the cell target, integrin αvβ3, in pancreatic cancer's development, proliferation, and metastasis. Theranostics, a new therapeutic strategy combined with diagnostics and therapeutics, can help in early cancer detection and monitoring of treatment response. These cutting-edge technologies enable simultaneous diagnosis through imaging and targeted delivery of therapeutics to cancer cells. Nanocarriers, such as liposomes and PLGA, can be used for theranostics to provide a comprehensive approach to potentially revolutionizing the treatment of pancreatic cancer. The potential of nano-drugs, either as standalone treatments or combined with theranostics, will be explored. Combined with currently available anticancer drugs, a target-specific nano-delivery system can provide a personalized treatment approach, where the drug's dosage and the treatment duration can be adjusted based on the patient's response. The elucidation of the targeting and anti-vascular therapeutic effects of the nano-delivery system of target-specific medicine will introduce a new strategic therapy for pancreatic cancers.

Keywords: pancreatic cancer, targeted therapy, integrin αvβ3, nanotechnology, theranostics

1. Introduction

Pancreatic cancers are specified by extremely high mortality and poor prognosis (**Figure 1**). They are primarily ascribed to difficulties in early diagnosis and limited therapeutics. An increasing incidence of this epidemiologically significant cancer and the lack of effective chemotherapy highlight the urgent need for early detection and effective therapy [1]. Integrin αvβ3 (**Figure 1**) is a plasma membrane structural protein essential for extracellular matrix protein-cell interactions. It has been reported in studies related to cancer pathogenesis. Integrin αvβ3 enhances pancreatic tumor progression and metastasis [2–4]. FAK is a downstream signal molecule of integrin

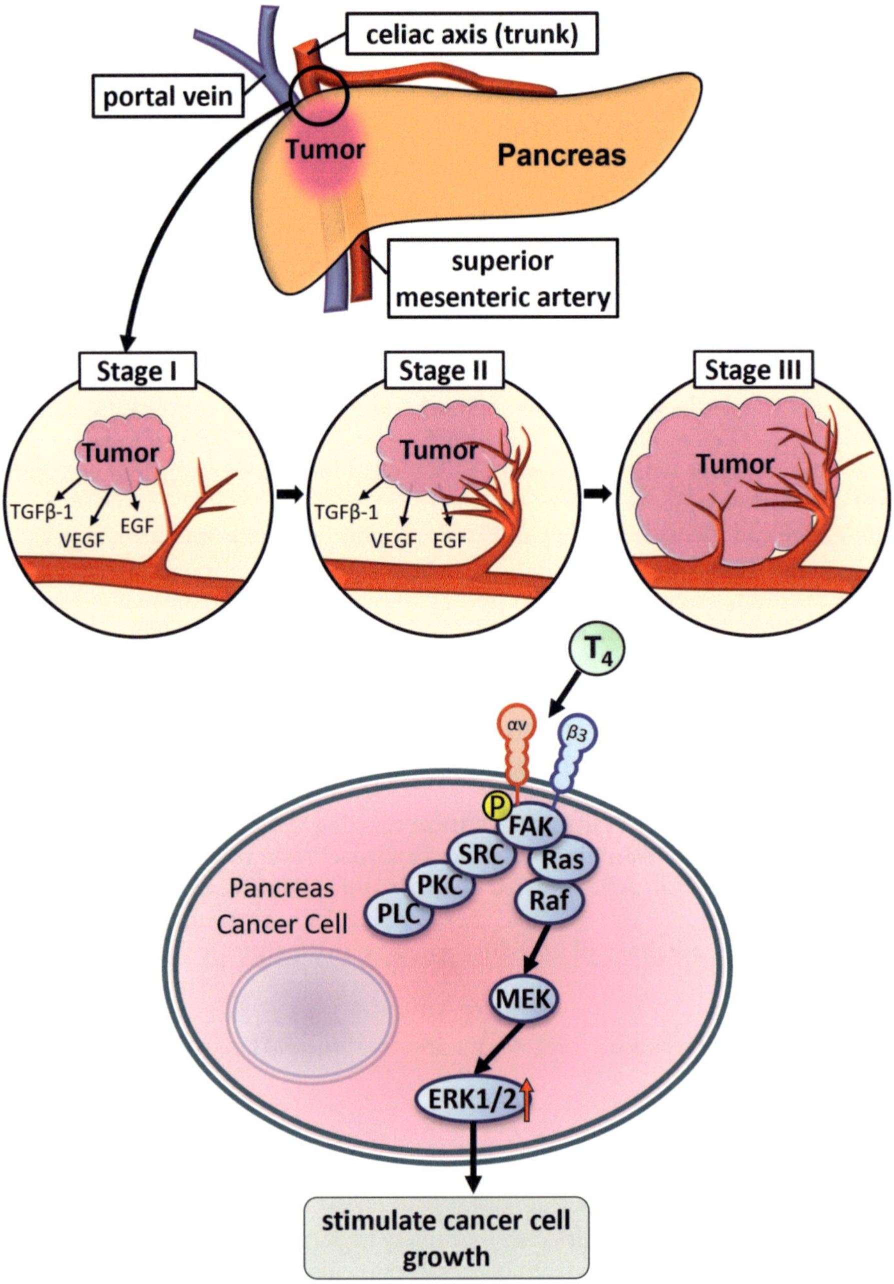

Figure 1.
Stage progressions and integrin αvβ3-dependent signal transduction in pancreatic cancer.

αvβ3. Using membrane-impermeable nanoparticles such as NDAT containing T_4-like ligands provides an attractive handle to modulate integrin αvβ3-dependent signal transduction, cell proliferation, and metastasis extracellular matrix protein-cell interactions from outside the cell surface. We anticipate and explore that integrin αvβ3 will be a new target for the anti-vascular treatment of pancreatic cancer [5]. In the current review, we provide a narrative review of findings in nanoparticle-directed targeting treatment for pancreatic cancers, focusing on biomarker-targeted delivery.

2. Pancreatic cancer

Pancreatic cancer is a leading worldwide cancer death leading cause. The burden caused by pancreatic cancer globally has more than doubled over the past 25 years [6]. Although much of this increase is due to aging populations worldwide, additionally, alcohol intake, obesity, diabetes, and cigarette smoking are risk factors for pancreatic cancer incidence [6]. These risk factors are increasing in many regions of the world prevalently, resulting in an increased age-adjusted incidence of pancreatic cancer. Although not directly modifiable, genetic factors are critical to pancreatic cancer risk and have been identified in hereditary cancer genes associated with hereditary pancreatitis and pathogenic variants in genome-wide association studies. There is currently no practical screening test for pancreatic cancer [7]. Additionally, most patients have locally advanced disease (30 to 35%) or metastatic disease (50 to 55%) at diagnosis. Adjuvant chemotherapy with FOLFIRINOX (fluorouracil, irinotecan, leucovorin, oxaliplatin) after surgery is the standard of care, with an estimated median overall survival of 54.4 months, compared with 35 months for gemcitabine monotherapy (by death score). The hazard ratio for the strata is 0.64 ([95% CI, 0.48-0.86]; $P = 0.003$). Neoadjuvant systemic therapy, with or without radiation therapy and subsequent surgical evaluation, is an accepted treatment approach for resectable and borderline disease. Patients with locally advanced disease unresectable due to extensive vascular involvement, systemic therapy to ensure control of locoregional disease, followed by radiation therapy, may be an option. On the other hand, patients with locally advanced and metastatic pancreatic cancer, multiagent chemotherapy regimens including FOLFIRINOX, gemcitabine/nab-paclitaxel, and irinotecan/nanosomal fluorouracil have 2 to 6 months survival benefit. In the 5 to 7% of patients with pathogenic germline mutations in the (breast cancer gene) BRCA gene and metastatic pancreatic cancer, olaparib, a polyadenosine diphosphate (ADB)-ribose polymerase inhibitor, may prevent progression by improving survival after initial platinum therapy with primary and maintenance treatment options. Pancreatic cancers present several biomarkers during progression [8]. Specific targeted therapies have been developing against cell surface biomarkers [9]. Integrin αvβ3 has been shown to be a good candidate for target therapy. Although increasing therapeutic and imaging technologies dramatically improve survival chances for cancer patients, pancreatic cancer still has a rising incidence and a difficult prognosis. Practically distinguishing this type of malignancy makes it challenging to treat, with no approved early detection method, extended asymptomatic state, restricted therapeutic options, limited treatment options, poor response to chemotherapy, and dense tumor stroma impeding drug delivery. By reducing drug toxicity, increasing tumor accumulation, the ability to modulate the tumor microenvironment, and even improving imaging contrast, it seems that nanotechnology may 1 day give hope for better outcomes in pancreatic cancer. Further conjugating nanoparticles with overexpressed biomarkers amplifies the benefits mentioned, with a potential increase in survival and treatment response [10].

3. Integrin αvβ3 is a specific target for pancreatic cancer

Thyroid hormones, triiodothyronine (T_3) and thyroxine (T_4), have been shown as pro-angiogenic hormones for cancer management. Endogenous circulating hormone levels may promote cancer progression and downregulate the effectiveness of anticancer therapy [11]. Non-canonically, thyroid hormone-modulated angiogenesis is initiated at the cell surface receptor integrin αvβ3 (**Figure 1**), [11]. This integrin αvβ3 is predominantly expressed in tumor cells, proliferating endothelial cells, and tumor stroma-associated cells, emphasizing its potential relevance in angiogenesis and tumor biology. Thyroid hormone-integrin αvβ3 signaling activates intracellular signal transduction pathways commonly associated with angiogenesis. The signal transduction pathways are regulated *via* pro-angiogenic molecules such as vascular endothelial growth factor. Integrin αvβ3 has been interested as a theranostics target for its overexpression in most cancer cells and newly forming blood vessels involved in cancer metastasis. Although thyroid hormone, T_4, plays a vital role in regulating critical metabolisms *via* nuclear hormone receptors, it has been shown recently to stimulate cancer proliferation *via* its specific binding to integrin αvβ3 on the cell surface to activate signal transduction pathways [12, 13]. Thyroid hormone analogs, particularly L-thyroxine (T_4), are relevant to the functions of various cancers. Thyroid hormones, T_4, and, to a lesser extent, T_3, *via* integrin αvβ3 activate the ERK1/2 signal pathway to stimulate cancer cell proliferation. T_4 induces the expression of PCNA, cyclin D1, and c-Myc in both K-ras wild-type HT-29 and mutant HCT-116 cells [14]. On the other hand, thyroid hormone analogues can also crosstalk with the EGFR-Ras signal transduction pathway. The EGFR signal activation and sequential downstream Ras/Raf signal transduction pathway are essential for cancer cell progression. Mutant Ras oncogenes play a critical role in colorectal carcinoma chemoresistance. In addition, chemoresistance may depend partially on the ERK1/2 activation. Although suppressed integrin αvβ3 activation inactivates cancer proliferation, mechanisms involved in thyroid hormone-induced proliferation and the crosstalk between integrin αvβ3 and growth factor receptors in pancreatic cancer are not fully understood.

Tumor immune escape is an essential strategy for tumor survival. Many mechanisms of tumor immune escape exist, including immunosuppression, which has recently become a research hotspot. Programmed cell death protein 1 (PD-1) suppresses immune responses. The transmembrane protein programmed death-ligand 1 (PD-L1) is a co-inhibitory factor of the immune response. PD-L1 promotes self-tolerance by moderating T cells' activation, such as activating apoptosis in antigen-specific T cells or inhibiting apoptosis in regulatory T cells. As an immunosuppressive molecule receptor, PD-1 can inhibit the activation of T lymphocytes and play an essential role in immune escape. PD-1 belongs to the CD28/CTLA-4 family of molecules and negatively regulates PD-1 signaling. PD-L1 can interact with PD-1 to reduce the proliferation of PD-1-positive cells, inhibit their cytokine secretion, and induce apoptosis. In addition to cancer cells, multiple types of host cells in the tumor microenvironment (TME) and lymph nodes, including dendritic cells, macrophages, fibroblasts, and T cells, also express PD-L1 to reduce antitumor immunity [15–17]. Integrin αvβ3 is uniquely sensitive to thyroid hormone T_4 and overexpressed in the cancer cell surface.

4. Nanotechnologies in medicine

Chemotherapy is the standard treatment for local and systemic cancer treatment. Various routes of administration administer anticancer drugs. Some anticancer drugs, such as paclitaxel and docetaxel, have low solubility. Other small-molecule anticancer drugs, cabozantinib and nintedanib, vascular endothelial growth factor receptor (VEGFR) inhibitors and compounds such as curcumin have similar concerns exist with [18–20].

Nanomaterial carriers have recently been developed to avoid biodegradation of therapeutic agents and improve their stability *in vivo*. Many nanoscale delivery systems for cancer treatment, including some nanoparticle formulations that make poorly water-soluble drugs more effective and more accessible to administer orally, are undergoing clinical trials and are increasingly used in clinical practice. This increasing use underscores the practical application of these systems. A key drug-developing challenge is to create new multifunctional nanomaterials with properties that allow specific drugs to cross different biological barriers and target various types of cells, tissues, and organs. Effective nano-delivery systems have ideal loading and release capabilities for therapeutic reagents, high efficacy, long shelf life, and minimal or no side effects [21, 22].

Some nano-delivery systems are both solid (nanocrystals, lipids, polymer nanoparticles) and liquids (including nanoliposomes, nanoemulsions, and nanopolymer vesicles) [23, 24]. The size, hydrophobicity, and charge of nanoparticles determine their physical and chemical properties, including metabolism, absorption, distribution, and excretion. The nanoparticles' sizes are an essential parameter to determine their pharmacokinetics. In addition, the size is also in charge of nanoparticle's interaction with the immune system and their entrance to cells [25]. Surface charge is crucial in determining their cellular uptake and cytotoxicity [26]. The surface properties of nanoparticles determine their hydrophilicity or hydrophobicity, cellular uptake, particle clearance, interaction with plasma proteins, and immune responses [27]. In addition to the release site of a nanoparticle, its biological fate also depends on its chemical and physical properties. Interestingly, nanomaterials with specific surface chemistries can be used to determine the location of bioactive release, allowing therapeutic agents to be released to particular tissues and organs in the body [24].

Another aspect of targeted therapy is to develop nanomaterial carriers. The general size of nanomaterials is about 1 to 100 nanometers, and the usual size of nanomaterial carriers is <200 nm. On the other hand, the endothelial pores on the blood vessel are approximately 10–1000 nm in diameter, allowing nanoparticles to excess within the tumor space due to the increased permeability of blood vessels [25]. Nanoparticles can be accumulated passively with lower lymphatic drainage [25]. To improve the potency and broaden the anticancer properties, the naturally occurring T_4 analogue, tetraiodothyroacetic acid (tetrac), has been covalently bonded *via* a linker with a 200-nm biodegradable nanoparticle to prohibit cell entry of tetrac, named NDAT. In addition, this nanoparticle restricts the action of its hormone receptor on the extracellular domain of plasma membrane integrin αvβ3 (**Figure 2**). This reformulation shows a higher potency than unmodified tetrac at the integrin αvβ3. NDAT affects a broader range of cancer-relevant genes than tetrac.

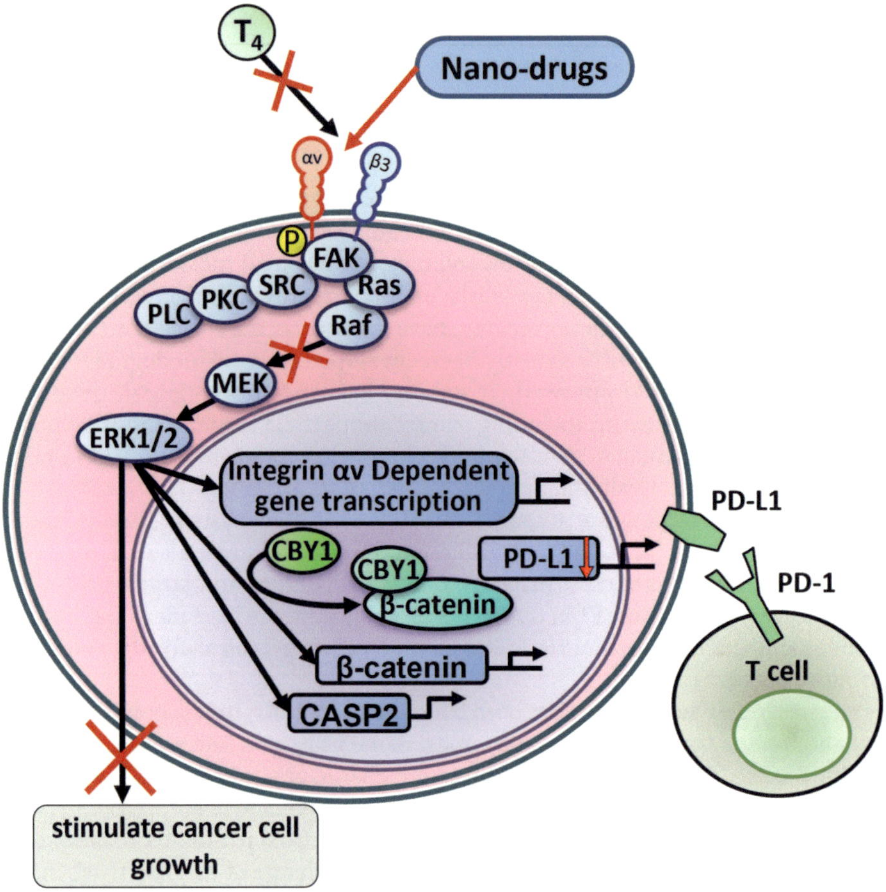

Figure 2.
Interference with integrin αvβ3 signal pathways blocks pancreatic cancer growth.

5. Working mechanisms of tetrac derivatives

Integrin αvβ3 is overexpressed by cancer cells and rapidly dividing endothelial cells. Extracellular matrix proteins are the principal ligands of the integrin αvβ3, but it is also a cell surface small molecule receptor that binds specifically thyroid hormone and thyroid hormone analogs. Thyroid hormones (T_4 and T_3) regulate the expression of specific genes by a mechanism initiated non-genomically [28]. Tetrac, the deaminated analogue of T_4, has anticancer functions effectively against different types of cancer cells, including pancreatic cancer cells (**Figure 2**). Although K-RAS wild-type colorectal cancer HT-29 cells contain far less integrin αvβ3 than K-RAS mutant HCT-116 cells, HT-29 was more sensitive to tetrac derivatives, both tetrac and NDAT [29]. K-RAS status appears to play an essential role in drug resistance [29]. Tetrac derivatives block the transcriptional activities induced by thyroid hormones. On the other hand, tetrac derivates regulate the transcription of cancer cell genes independent of thyroid hormones. These genes are essential to cell survival pathways, controlling the cell cycle, repairing double-strand DNA breaks (DSBs), angiogenesis, apoptosis, and cell export of chemotherapeutic agents [30]. Both tetrac and NDAT bind to tumor cell surface integrin αvβ3, and the agents may have different mechanisms of antiproliferation in colorectal cancer cells [29]. Tetrac modulates the thyroid hormone-induced pro-angiogenic actions at the integrin receptor and agonist-independent anti-angiogenic effects. Additionally, tetrac suppresses endothelial cell growth, migration, and tube formation *via* diminishing the transcription of vascular growth factors/growth factor receptors, hypoxia-inducible factor-1α, pro-angiogenic cytokines, and several other pro-angiogenic genes. Meanwhile, tetrac stimulates the expression of endogenous angiogenesis inhibitors. Tetrac derivatives disturb tumor-associated angiogenesis *via* multiple mechanisms. The anticancer actions of unmodified tetrac and NDAT initiate exclusively at plasma membrane integrin αvβ3. Many effects of the agents are performed by integrin αvβ3 downstream in specific gene expression or altered activities of nuclear corepressor and co-activator protein (**Figure 2**) [31]. Together with its low toxicity and high tissue selectivity, tetrac derivatives are promising candidates for clinical application [11].

In RAS-mutant colorectal cancer cells, tetrac derivatives may overcome chemoresistance to other drugs *via* actions initiated at integrin αvβ3 and involving downstream the EGFR-Ras signaling pathways [12]. *In vitro*, NDAT downregulates αv and β3 monomer expression. *In vivo* in tumor xenografts, similarly, NDAT suppresses the expression of integrin αv and β3. A distinct reduction in tumor weight and viability was observed in xenografts treated with NDAT [32]. Furthermore, NDAT is safe and tolerable in mice treated with high doses [32]. These studies suggest that NDAT is an effective and safe antagonist of integrin αvβ3 expressed in various types of cancer cells, indicating the importance of the targetability and suppression of αvβ3-associated tumor functions. In addition, NDAT suppresses PD-L1 accumulation in mouse xenografts.

Meanwhile, tetrac stimulates the expression of endogenous angiogenesis inhibitors [11]. Tetrac derivatives disturb tumor-associated angiogenesis *via* multiple mechanisms. The anticancer actions of unmodified tetrac and NDAT initiate exclusively at plasma membrane integrin αvβ3. Many effects of the agents are performed by integrin αvβ3 downstream in specific gene expression or altered activities of nuclear corepressor and co-activator protein (**Figure 2**) [31]. Together with its low toxicity and high tissue selectivity, tetrac derivatives are promising candidates for clinical application [11].

6. Current integrin αvβ3-targeted nanoparticles in use

Integrins are a family of plasma membrane heterodimeric glycoproteins that regulate tumor growth, angiogenesis, migration, and metastasis. Thyroid hormones T_4 and, to a lesser extent, T_3 bind cell surface integrin αvβ3 to activate the signal transduction pathways, mainly the ERK1/2 pathway, and stimulate cancer cell growth. Thyroid hormone analogues also engage in crosstalk with the EGFR-Ras pathway. EGFR signal generation and downstream Ras/Raf pathway transduction contribute significantly to tumor cell progression. Mutated RAS oncogenes contribute to chemoresistance in pancreatic cancer cells; chemoresistance may depend in part on the activity of the ERK1/2 pathway.

NDAT has been shown to enhance the first-line chemotherapic agent-induced antiproliferative effects in various types of cancer. Cancer resistance to chemotherapeutic agents is a significant issue in the management of cancer patients. In RAS-mutant CRC cells, tetrac derivatives may overcome chemoresistance to other drugs *via* actions initiated at integrin αvβ3 and involving crosstalk with the EGFR-Ras signaling pathways [12]. The ribonucleotide reductase regulatory subunit M2 (RRM2) overexpression is linked with aggressive cancer behavior and chemoresistance. A stilbenoid phytoalexin resveratrol binds to the cell surface integrin αvβ3 specific site, triggering an inhibitory effect in cancer cells *via* nuclear translocation of cyclooxygenase-2 (COX-2). However, resveratrol paradoxically activates RRM2 gene expression and protein translation in colon cancer cells. NDAT downregulates RRM2 gene expression in cancer cells. RRM2 downregulation, whether achieved by RNA interference or treatment with NDAT, enhanced resveratrol-induced COX-2 gene expression and nuclear uptake, essential to integrin αvβ3-mediated-resveratrol-induced antiproliferation in cancer cells [33].

Combining tetrac and cetuximab inhibits cell proliferation in colorectal cancers with different K-RAS status [14]. The combination of NDAT and cetuximab suppressed more than cetuximab alone on T_4-induced expression of mRNA of proliferative genes such as PCNA, cyclin D1, c-Myc, and RRM2 significantly in HCT-116 cells [14]. The combination of NDAT and cetuximab elevates significantly more T_4-suppressed mRNA expressions of pro-apoptotic genes p53 and ribonucleoside-diphosphate reductase subunit M2 B (RRM2B) than cetuximab alone [14]. Tetrac/NDAT combined with cetuximab significantly reduced cell proliferation in the K-RAS mutant HCT-116 cells compared to cetuximab alone. However, the therapeutic strategy does not show privilege in the K-RAS wild-type cancer cells [14]. Overexpressed PD-L1 promotes cancer cell proliferation and metastasis. Thus, the PD-L1 pathway may stimulate cancer cells to perform an adaptive resistance mechanism *in vivo*. The property of drug resistance attenuates clinical treatment efficacy in cancer patients, such as chemoresistance to gefitinib in colon cancers. Gefitinib (10 mg/kg) suppresses PD-L1 accumulation, while NDAT (1 mg/kg) enhances the inhibitory effect of gefitinib (10 mg/kg) [34].

PD-L1 is a critical regulator that defends tumor cells against immune surveillance. The change in PD-L1 expression correlates with tumorigenic characteristics. The highly expressed PD-L1 is observed in gefitinib-resistant primary CRC cells, Colo_160224, rather than in K-Ras mutant HCT-116 cells. Gefitinib (1 μM and 10 μM) decreased PD-L1 expression in two gefitinib sensitive cancer cell lines. Gefitinib suppressed PD-L1 expression but did not inhibit proliferation through phosphatidylinositol 3-kinase (PI3K) in gefitinib-resistant primary CRC cells. Gefitinib does not inhibit PI3K activation in gefitinib-resistant Colo_160224 cells. About 10 μM gefitinib promoted PD-L1 expression in gefitinib-resistant primary CRC Colo_160224 cells [34]. Inactivated PI3K inactivated PD-L1 expression and CRC Colo_160224 cell growth. However, in Colo_160224 cells, NDAT inhibited PI3K activation and PD-L1 accumulation in gefitinib-resistant. Furthermore, NDAT combined with gefitinib inhibited the phosphorylation of PI3K, the expression of PD-L1, and cell proliferation. NDAT *via* inactivating ERK1/2 downregulates inducible PD-L1 expression and protein accumulation [14] and PI3K [34]. PD-L1 knockdown can also inhibit the proliferation of oral cancer cells [35].

Furthermore, NDAT significantly reduced PD-L1 expression and tumor growth in the HCT-116 (K-RAS mutant) xenograft experiment. By down-regulating PD-L1 expression by blocking PI3K activation, NDAT effectively inhibited cell proliferation in gefitinib-resistant colorectal cancer cells. NDAT's potential to inhibit PI3K-mediated PD-L1 upregulation and reduce proliferation in gefitinib-resistant colorectal cancer cells [34] is a fascinating area of research. Tetrac and NDAT have been shown to inhibit PD-L1 mRNA abundance and PD-L1 protein content in oral cancer cells [35], colorectal cancer cells [14, 34], and breast cancer cells [14]. The potential of NDAT to inhibit PD-L1 expression could be a critical mechanism for its antiproliferative effects on cancer cells, sparking further interest and engagement in this field.

NDAT also enhances anticancer drug delivery and target specificity by payload. NDAT payloaded chemotherapy increases drug delivery to cancers and increases drug efficacy [36]. NDAT can efficiently deliver paclitaxel and doxorubicin to pancreatic or breast cancer orthotopic nude mouse xenografts. NDAT payloaded with anticancer drugs can increase intra-tumoral drug concentrations about 5-fold (paclitaxel; $P < 0.001$) or 2.3-fold (doxorubicin; $P < 0.01$) higher than with conventional systemic drug administration [36]. Reducing tumor volume reflects enhanced xenograft drug uptake and an increased paclitaxel effect with drug delivery by NDAT.

Recently, chemically modified bis-triazole-tetrac conjugated with polyethylene glycol (P-bi-TAT) has shown a higher binding affinity to αvβ3 receptors than tetrac [37]. Noncytotoxic P-bi-TAT induces antiproliferation in pancreatic cancer cells (SUIT2). Microarray experiments assessed the mechanisms of the anticancer activity of P-bi-TAT on SUIT2 cells, and genome-wide profiling identified significant alterations of 1348 genes' expression. Both down-regulated and up-regulated transcripts suggest that a molecular interference at the signaling pathway-associated gene expression is the prevalent mode of P-bi-TAT anticancer activity.

In addition, P-bi-TAT can be used as a radio-sensitizer and chemo-sensitizer that acts on the extracellular domain of the cell surface αvβ3 receptor [37] in a mouse model of pancreatic cancer. P-bi-TAT treatment increased tumor-targeted radiation-induced cell death and decreased tumor size. P-bi-TAT acted as a chemo-sensitizer and enhanced the 5-fluorouracil (5FU) effect in reducing pancreatic tumor weight compared to 5FU monotherapy [37]. P-bi-TAT treatment increased tumor-targeted radiation-induced cell death and decreased tumor size. P-bi-TAT acted as a chemo-sensitizer and enhanced the 5FU effect in decreasing pancreatic tumor weight compared to 5FU monotherapy [37, 38].

Inhibiting immune checkpoints with PD-1/PD-L1 blockade is a promising area of anticancer therapy. Although clinical data have revealed the success of PD-1/PD-L1 blockade as monotherapy or combined with cytotoxic T-lymphocyte-associated protein 4 (CTLA-4) or chemotherapy, the combination with radiotherapy could further boost antitumor immunity. The combined treatment enhances clinical outcomes because of the immunostimulatory effects of radiation. On the other hand, the synergistic PD-1/PD-L1 blockade combined with radiotherapy can be challenged by the complex nature of the TME, including tumor hypoxia.

Immune checkpoint inhibitors against PD-1/PD-L1 have shown good efficacies against solid tumors but have not shown encouraging therapeutic results in pancreatic cancer [39]. Anti-checking point therapies have the potential to be efficacious in pancreatic cancer treatment, and further relevant studies are needed. The reason for the ineffectiveness of anti-PD-1/PD-L1 alone in pancreatic cancer treatment is that pancreatic cancer has an immunosuppressive tumor microenvironment and develops drug resistance during therapy. Anti-PD-1/PD-L1-based combination therapeutic regimens change the immunosuppressive tumor microenvironment to reduce the development of drug resistance in pancreatic cancer [39].

In vitro, a genome-wide gene expression profiling analysis of human glioblastoma (GBM) and acute myelocytic leukemia (AML) cell lines treated with noncytotoxic doses of tetrac derivative (NDAT) conducted by Gennadi V Glinsky et al. has demonstrated a decreased expression of genes related to the radioresistance of cancer cells.

The study found that following the NDAT treatment in AML cells, gene expression of poly ADP-ribose polymerase 9 (PARP9), poly ADP-ribose polymerase 15 (PARP15), as well as signal transducer and activator of transcription 3 (STAT3) are significantly reduced. On the other hand, the expressions of protein kinase, DNA-activated catalytic subunit (PRKDC), EGFR, and CCNDI are reduced in GBM cells significantly [40]. A broader spectrum of genes implicated in cancer cells' radioresistance is observed in NDAT-treated primary patient-derived GBM cells. The potential of tetrac derivatives in improving the therapeutic effects of radiation is significant, and further detailed experimental and clinical studies, including analysis of tumor genomics of individual patients and different tumor types, are needed to understand and utilize this potential fully.

Recently, we have shown that integrin αvβ3 on cancer cells is activated during tumor irradiation *in vitro*. Tetrac blocks this critical change in the physical state of integrin αvβ3. The nuclear corepressor, the silencing mediator for retinoid and thyroid hormone receptor (SMRT), appears to be important in repairing radiation-induced DSBs [41], may implicate thyroid hormone promoting of this mechanism of radioresistance and the vital role of integrin αvβ3 in radioresistance/radiosensitivity [42, 43].

Tetrac radiosensitizes murine glioma GL261 cells [44] and human glioblastoma U87MG cells [45]. Tetrac restores radiosensitivity to resistant human basal cell carcinoma (TE.354.T) cells [46]. NDAT enhances radiosensitivity and inhibits cancer cell growth *in vitro* after X-ray irradiation. NDAT decreases the repair of DSBs induced by radiation [45]. Additionally, tetrac may cause DSBs itself. Tetrac derivatives bind with integrin αvβ3 exclusively to interfere with the binding of T_4 with the RGD binding domain, preventing thyroid hormone-induced cancer cell growth and anti-apoptotic actions on small-cell lung carcinoma xenografts in athymic mice for tumor-targeted radiation. Exposure of U87MG cells of tetrac for 1 hour *in vitro* before radiation causes more than 70% reduction in the repair of X-irradiation-induced DSBs. However, the molecular basis of this action of tetrac on DNA repair has yet to be established [31].

Endogenous T_4 in the intact organism—preclinically in animal models or the clinical setting—is a support mechanism in tumor cells for AKT (protein kinase B)-dependent DSB repair. In cancer cells, the PI3K/AKT/mammalian target of the rapamycin (mTOR) signal transduction pathway is usually disordered, and its excessive activity contributes to tumor cell proliferation [47] and radioresistance, which enhances repair that is induced by radiation DSBs [47, 48]. Although it is unclear how AKT may be stimulated in cancer cells in the radiation setting to generate radioresistance [49], thyroid hormone at physiological levels can activate the AKT pathway through the cell surface integrin αvβ3 [50, 51]. Thyroxine may activate signal STAT3-dependent mechanisms to contribute to tumor radioresistance. STAT3 has been shown to promote radioresistance in various tumors, including gliomas and lung cancer [52]. Nongenomically, thyroxine induces specific tyrosine phosphorylation of STAT3 and activates the protein, subsequently nuclear translocation [53]. Physiological free concentration of T_4 also nongenomically potentiates EGF-induced c-Fos expression that subsequently promotes glioma cell radioresistance [54].

NDAT (1 mg/kg body weight) combined with 5 Gy tumor-targeted irradiation in mice with H1299 xenografts indicates better anticancer efficacy than irradiation alone [54]. In pancreatic cancer and non-small-cell lung cancer, irradiation combined with NDAT treatment demonstrated anticancer efficacy [55].

7. Conclusions

Nanotechnology offers potential improvements in drug delivery and tumor targeting. Due to their size and surface properties, Nanoparticles enhance anticancer drug stability, efficacy, and delivery while minimizing side effects. Thyroid hormones, particularly T_4, interact with integrin αvβ3, influencing cancer cell proliferation. Tetrac, a T_4 analogue, and its nanoparticle derivative NDAT, inhibit this interaction, showing promise in reducing tumor growth and overcoming chemoresistance, especially in K-RAS-mutant cancers. Integrin αvβ3-targeted nanoparticles like NDAT have demonstrated effectiveness in enhancing the antiproliferative effects of chemotherapy, improving drug delivery, and inhibiting PD-L1 expression, a critical factor in immune escape. Its payload with doxorubicin shows promising effectiveness in antiproliferation and inhibiting cell viability, demonstrating NDAT is an effective and safe inhibitor of integrin αvβ3 expression in various cancer types and further indicating its impact on the targetability and suppression of αvβ3-associated tumor functions. New compounds like P-bi-TAT demonstrate higher binding affinity and potent anticancer activity, particularly in pancreatic cancer models. Overall, integrin αvβ3-targeted therapies, combined with advancements in nanotechnology, hold promise for improving outcomes in pancreatic cancer, offering potential new avenues for treatment by enhancing drug delivery, targeting specific cancer pathways, and reducing immune escape mechanisms.

Acknowledgements

The authors express their profound appreciation for the excellent studies conducted by Miss Tin Yi Chu, Miss Yi-Chen Chen, and Dr. Yee-Shin Lee, who graduated from our lab. Dr. Lin deeply appreciates the pivotal role of Dr. Li-Feng Liu, Academic Sinic, in encouraging his science career. The authors respectfully dedicate this article in memory of our best friends and colleagues at Taipei Medical University, Ms. Chao-Nan Hsiung, who sadly passed away in 2024 after battling pancreatic cancer.

Authors' contributions

ZL Li, YJ Shih, C-C Tsai, K Wang, J Whang-Peng, and L-Y Lin conceptualized the study; C-Y Wang, WL Wang, K Wang, J-K Mo, and H-Y Lin contributed to PubMed searching; CC Tsai, ZL Li, K Wang, and H-Y Lin contributed to writing—original draft preparation; C-C Tsai and H-Y Lin contributed to writing—review and editing; H-Y Lin, K Wang, and J Whang-Peng supervised the study.

Funding

This work was supported in part by the Chair Professor Research Fund to Dr. J. Whang-Peng and Dr. K. Wang, by a grant from the Ministry of Science and Technology, Taiwan (MOST 111-2314-B-038-123 to H.-Y. Lin, NSTC112-2320-B-038-021 to K. Wang, and NSTC112-2314-B-038-098 to J. Whang-Peng), and by an integrated grant from the Ministry of Science and Technology, Taiwan (NSTC 112-2314-B-038-003 to J. Whang-Peng, NSTC 112-2314-B-038-004 to H.-Y. Lin, and NSTC 112-2314-B-038-005 to K. Wang).

Conflict of interest

The authors declare no conflict of interest.

Author details

Zi-Lin Li[1†], Ya-Jung Shih[1†], Chung-Che Tsai[1†], Chih-Yang Wang[1], Wen-Long Wang[2], Kuan Wang[3*], Jaqueline Whang-Peng[1,4*], Ju-Ku Mo[1] and Hung-Yun Lin[1]

1 Graduate Institute of Cancer Molecular Biology and Drug Discovery, College of Medical Science and Technology, Taipei Medical University, Taipei, Taiwan

2 Department of Life Science, Fu Jen Catholic University, New Taipei City, Taiwan

3 Graduate Institute of Nanomedicine and Medical Engineering, College of Medical Engineering, Taipei Medical University, Taipei, Taiwan

4 Cancer Center, Wan Fang Hospital, Taipei Medical University, Taipei, Taiwan

*Address all correspondence to: wangk007@gmail.com and jqwpeng@nhri.edu.tw

† These authors contributed equally to this article.

References

[1] Zhang X, Shi S, Zhang B, Ni Q, Yu X, Xu J. Circulating biomarkers for early diagnosis of pancreatic cancer: Facts and hopes. American Journal of Cancer Research. 2018;**8**(3):332-353

[2] Leone F, Cavalloni G, Pignochino Y, Sarotto I, Ferraris R, Piacibello W, et al. Somatic mutations of epidermal growth factor receptor in bile duct and gallbladder carcinoma. Clinical Cancer Research. 2006;**12**(6):1680-1685

[3] Utispan K, Sonongbua J, Thuwajit P, Chau-In S, Pairojkul C, Wongkham S, et al. Periostin activates integrin α5β1 through a PI3K/AKT-dependent pathway in invasion of cholangiocarcinoma. International Journal of Oncology. 2012;**41**(3):1110-1118

[4] Patsenker E, Wilkens L, Banz V, Osterreicher CH, Weimann R, Eisele S, et al. The alphavbeta6 integrin is a highly specific immunohistochemical marker for cholangiocarcinoma. Journal of Hepatology. 2010;**52**(3):362-369

[5] Yin F, Yang C, Wang Q, Zeng S, Hu R, Lin G, et al. A light-driven therapy of pancreatic adenocarcinoma using gold nanorods-based nanocarriers for co-delivery of doxorubicin and siRNA. Theranostics. 2015;**5**(8):818-833

[6] Klein AP. Pancreatic cancer epidemiology: Understanding the role of lifestyle and inherited risk factors. Nature Reviews. Gastroenterology & Hepatology. 2021;**18**(7):493-502

[7] Yang Z, Mitra A, Liu W, Berlowitz D, Yu H. TransformEHR: Transformer-based encoder-decoder generative model to enhance prediction of disease outcomes using electronic health records. Nature Communications. 2023;**14**(1):7857

[8] Yang H, Li W, Ren L, Yang Y, Zhang Y, Ge B, et al. Progress on diagnostic and prognostic markers of pancreatic cancer. Oncology Research. 2023;**31**(2):83-99

[9] Karandish F, Mallik S. Biomarkers and targeted therapy in pancreatic cancer. Biomark Cancer. 2016;**8**(Suppl. 1):27-35

[10] Grapa CM, Mocan L, Crisan D, Florea M, Mocan T. Biomarkers in pancreatic cancer as analytic targets for nanomediated imaging and therapy. Materials (Basel). 2021;**14**(11):3083

[11] Schmohl KA, Nelson PJ, Spitzweg C. Tetrac as an anti-angiogenic agent in cancer. Endocrine-Related Cancer. 2019;**26**(6):R287-r304

[12] Yang YSH, Ko PJ, Pan YS, Lin HY, Whang-Peng J, Davis PJ, et al. Role of thyroid hormone-integrin αvβ3-signal and therapeutic strategies in colorectal cancers. Journal of Biomedical Science. 2021;**28**(1):24

[13] Davis PJ, Mousa SA, Lin HY. Nongenomic actions of thyroid hormone: The integrin component. Physiological Reviews. 2021;**101**(1):319-352

[14] Lee YS, Chin YT, Yang YSH, Wei PL, Wu HC, Shih A, et al. The combination of tetraiodothyroacetic acid and cetuximab inhibits cell proliferation in colorectal cancers with different K-ras status. Steroids. 2016;**111**:63-70

[15] Peng Q, Qiu X, Zhang Z, Zhang S, Zhang Y, Liang Y, et al. PD-L1 on dendritic cells attenuates T cell activation and regulates response to immune checkpoint blockade. Nature Communications. 2020;**11**(1):4835

[16] Cha JH, Chan LC, Li CW, Hsu JL, Hung MC. Mechanisms controlling

PD-L1 expression in cancer. Molecular Cell. 2019;**76**(3):359-370

[17] Guo S, Yuan J, Meng X, Feng X, Ma D, Han Y, et al. Cancer-associated fibroblasts: Just on the opposite side of antitumour immunity? International Immunopharmacology. 2023;**122**:110601

[18] Narvekar M, Xue HY, Eoh JY, Wong HL. Nanocarrier for poorly water-soluble anticancer drugs–barriers of translation and solutions. AAPS PharmSciTech. 2014;**15**(4):822-833

[19] Loftsson T, Brewster ME. Pharmaceutical applications of cyclodextrins: Basic science and product development. The Journal of Pharmacy and Pharmacology. 2010;**62**(11):1607-1621

[20] Ismael GF, Rosa DD, Mano MS, Awada A. Novel cytotoxic drugs: Old challenges, new solutions. Cancer Treatment Reviews. 2008;**34**(1):81-91

[21] Bilia AR, Piazzini V, Guccione C, Risaliti L, Asprea M, Capecchi G, et al. Improving on nature: The role of nanomedicine in the development of clinical natural drugs. Planta Medica. 2017;**83**(5):366-381

[22] Kloss FR, Offermanns V, Kloss-Brandstätter A. Comparison of allogeneic and autogenous bone grafts for augmentation of alveolar ridge defects-A 12-month retrospective radiographic evaluation. Clinical Oral Implants Research. 2018;**29**(11):1163-1175

[23] Borel T, Sabliov CM. Nanodelivery of bioactive components for food applications: Types of delivery systems, properties, and their effect on ADME profiles and toxicity of nanoparticles. Annual Review of Food Science and Technology. 2014;**5**:197-213

[24] Ganesan P, Karthivashan G, Park SY, Kim J, Choi DK. Microfluidization trends in the development of nanodelivery systems and applications in chronic disease treatments. International Journal of Nanomedicine. 2018;**13**:6109-6121

[25] Hoshyar N, Gray S, Han H, Bao G. The effect of nanoparticle size on in vivo pharmacokinetics and cellular interaction. Nanomedicine (London, England). 2016;**11**(6):673-692

[26] Fröhlich E, Roblegg E. Models for oral uptake of nanoparticles in consumer products. Toxicology. 2012;**291**(1-3):10-17

[27] Ajdary M, Moosavi MA, Rahmati M, Falahati M, Mahboubi M, Mandegary A, et al. Health concerns of various nanoparticles: A review of their in vitro and in vivo toxicity. Nanomaterials (Basel). 2018;**8**(9):634

[28] Mousa SA, Hercbergs A, Lin HY, Keating KA, Davis PJ. Actions of thyroid hormones on thyroid cancers. Frontiers in Endocrinology (Lausanne). 2021;**12**:691736

[29] Chin YT, He ZR, Chen CL, Chu HC, Ho Y, Su PY, et al. Tetrac and NDAT induce antiproliferation via integrin αvβ3 in colorectal cancers with different K-RAS status. Frontiers in Endocrinology (Lausanne). 2019;**10**:130

[30] Davis PJ, Glinsky GV, Lin HY, Leith JT, Hercbergs A, Tang HY, et al. Cancer cell gene expression modulated from plasma membrane integrin αvβ3 by thyroid hormone and nanoparticulate tetrac. Frontiers in Endocrinology (Lausanne). 2014;**5**:240

[31] Davis PJ, Sudha T, Lin HY, Mousa SA. Thyroid hormone, hormone analogs, and angiogenesis. Comprehensive Physiology. 2015;**6**(1):353-362

[32] Chang TC, Chin YT, Nana AW, Wang SH, Liao YM, Chen YR, et al. Enhancement by nano-diamino-tetrac of antiproliferative action of gefitinib on colorectal cancer cells: Mediation by EGFR sialylation and PI3K activation. Hormones and Cancer. 2018;**9**(6):420-432

[33] Nana AW, Wu SY, Yang YS, Chin YT, Cheng TM, Ho Y, et al. Nano-diamino-tetrac (NDAT) enhances resveratrol-induced antiproliferation by action on the RRM2 pathway in colorectal cancers. Hormones and Cancer. 2018;**9**(5):349-360

[34] Huang TY, Chang TC, Chin YT, Pan YS, Chang WJ, Liu FC, et al. NDAT targets PI3K-mediated PD-L1 upregulation to reduce proliferation in gefitinib-resistant colorectal cancer. Cells. 2020;**9**(8):1830

[35] Lin SJ, Chin YT, Ho Y, Chou SY, Sh Yang YC, Nana AW, et al. Nano-diamino-tetrac (NDAT) inhibits PD-L1 expression which is essential for proliferation in oral cancer cells. Food and Chemical Toxicology. 2018;**120**:1-11

[36] Sudha T, Bharali DJ, Yalcin M, Darwish NH, Debreli Coskun M, Keating KA, et al. Targeted delivery of paclitaxel and doxorubicin to cancer xenografts via the nanoparticle of nano-diamino-tetrac. International Journal of Nanomedicine. 2017;**12**:1305-1315

[37] Sudha T, Godugu K, Glinsky GV, Mousa SA. Triazole modified tetraiodothyroacetic acid conjugated to polyethylene glycol, a thyrointegrin α(v)β(3) antagonist as a radio- and chemo-sensitizer in pancreatic cancer. Biomedicine. 2022;**10**(4):795

[38] Liu L, Huang X, Shi F, Song J, Guo C, Yang J, et al. Combination therapy for pancreatic cancer: Anti-PD-(L)1-based strategy. Journal of Experimental & Clinical Cancer Research. 2022;**41**(1):56

[39] Zhang H, Duan XR, Xing LY, Jia YX, Zhou JY, Ma JJ. Exploring novel systemic therapies for pancreatic cancer: A review of emerging anti-PD-1/PD-L1 combination therapy. Neoplasma. 2022;**69**(5):995-1007

[40] Glinsky GV, Hercbergs A, Mousa SA, Lin HY, Davis PJ. Additional considerations in cancer cell radioresistance, integrin αvβ3 and thyroid hormones. Endocrine Research. Aug-Nov 2024;**49**(4):251-254

[41] Yu J, Palmer C, Alenghat T, Li Y, Kao G, Lazar MA. The corepressor silencing mediator for retinoid and thyroid hormone receptor facilitates cellular recovery from DNA double-strand breaks. Cancer Research. 2006;**66**(18):9316-9322

[42] Monferran S, Skuli N, Delmas C, Favre G, Bonnet J, Cohen-Jonathan-Moyal E, et al. Alphavbeta3 and alphavbeta5 integrins control glioma cell response to ionising radiation through ILK and RhoB. International Journal of Cancer. 2008;**123**(2):357-364

[43] Ou J, Luan W, Deng J, Sa R, Liang H. αV integrin induces multicellular radioresistance in human nasopharyngeal carcinoma via activating SAPK/JNK pathway. PLoS One. 2012;**7**(6):e38737

[44] Hercbergs A, Davis PJ, Davis FB, Ciesielski MJ, Leith JT. Radiosensitization of GL261 glioma cells by tetraio-dothyroacetic acid (tetrac). Cell Cycle. 2009;**8**(16):2586-2591

[45] Hercbergs AH, Lin HY, Davis FB, Davis PJ, Leith JT. Radiosensitization and production of DNA double-strand breaks in U87MG brain tumor cells induced by

tetraiodothyroacetic acid (tetrac). Cell Cycle. 2011;**10**(2):352-357

[46] Leith JT, Davis PJ, Mousa SA, Hercbergs AA. In vitro effects of tetraiodothyroacetic acid combined with X-irradiation on basal cell carcinoma cells. Cell Cycle. 2017;**16**(4):367-373

[47] Mehta M, Khan A, Danish S, Haffty BG, Sabaawy HE. Radiosensitization of primary human glioblastoma stem-like cells with low-dose AKT inhibition. Molecular Cancer Therapeutics. 2015;**14**(5):1171-1180

[48] Golding SE, Morgan RN, Adams BR, Hawkins AJ, Povirk LF, Valerie K. Pro-survival AKT and ERK signaling from EGFR and mutant EGFRvIII enhances DNA double-strand break repair in human glioma cells. Cancer Biology & Therapy. 2009;**8**(8):730-738

[49] Han X, Xue X, Zhou H, Zhang G. A molecular view of the radioresistance of gliomas. Oncotarget. 2017;**8**(59):100931-100941

[50] Cheng SY, Leonard JL, Davis PJ. Molecular aspects of thyroid hormone actions. Endocrine Reviews. 2010;**31**(2):139-170

[51] Davis PJ, Goglia F, Leonard JL. Nongenomic actions of thyroid hormone. Nature Reviews. Endocrinology. 2016;**12**(2):111-121

[52] Luwor RB, Stylli SS, Kaye AH. The role of Stat3 in glioblastoma multiforme. Journal of Clinical Neuroscience. 2013;**20**(7):907-911

[53] Lin HY, Shih A, Davis FB, Davis PJ. Thyroid hormone promotes the phosphorylation of STAT3 and potentiates the action of epidermal growth factor in cultured cells. The Biochemical Journal. 1999;**338**(Pt. 2):427-432

[54] Liu ZG, Jiang G, Tang J, Wang H, Feng G, Chen F, et al. c-Fos over-expression promotes radioresistance and predicts poor prognosis in malignant glioma. Oncotarget. 2016;**7**(40):65946-65956

[55] Sudha T, Rehman MU, Darwish NHE, Coskun MD, Satti JA, Davis PJ, et al. Nano-targeting of thyrointegrin $\alpha v\beta 3$ receptor in solid tumors and impact on radiosensitization. Radiation Research. 2021;**196**(4):375-385